Patient-Specific Implants in Musculoskeletal (Orthopedic) Surgery

Patient-Specific Implants in Musculoskeletal (Orthopedic) Surgery

Editor

Maximilian Rudert

MDPI • Basel • Beijing • Wuhan • Barcelona • Belgrade • Manchester • Tokyo • Cluj • Tianjin

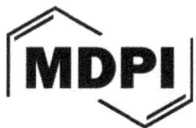

Editor
Maximilian Rudert
Department of Orthopedics
University of Wuerzburg
Wuerzburg
Germany

Editorial Office
MDPI
St. Alban-Anlage 66
4052 Basel, Switzerland

This is a reprint of articles from the Special Issue published online in the open access journal *Journal of Personalized Medicine* (ISSN 2075-4426) (available at: www.mdpi.com/journal/jpm/special_issues/patientspecific_implants).

For citation purposes, cite each article independently as indicated on the article page online and as indicated below:

LastName, A.A.; LastName, B.B.; LastName, C.C. Article Title. *Journal Name* **Year**, *Volume Number*, Page Range.

ISBN 978-3-0365-4248-5 (Hbk)
ISBN 978-3-0365-4247-8 (PDF)

© 2022 by the authors. Articles in this book are Open Access and distributed under the Creative Commons Attribution (CC BY) license, which allows users to download, copy and build upon published articles, as long as the author and publisher are properly credited, which ensures maximum dissemination and a wider impact of our publications.
The book as a whole is distributed by MDPI under the terms and conditions of the Creative Commons license CC BY-NC-ND.

Contents

About the Editor vii

Maximilian Rudert
Taking the Next Step in Personalised Orthopaedic Implantation
Reprinted from: *J. Pers. Med.* **2022**, *12*, 365, doi:10.3390/jpm12030365 1

Andre F. Steinert, Lennart Schröder, Lukas Sefrin, Björn Janßen, Jörg Arnholdt and Maximilian Rudert
The Impact of Total Knee Replacement with a Customized Cruciate-Retaining Implant Design on Patient-Reported and Functional Outcomes
Reprinted from: *J. Pers. Med.* **2022**, *12*, 194, doi:10.3390/jpm12020194 5

Juliana Habor, Maximilian C. M. Fischer, Kunihiko Tokunaga, Masashi Okamoto and Klaus Radermacher
The Patient-Specific Combined Target Zone for Morpho-Functional Planning of Total Hip Arthroplasty
Reprinted from: *J. Pers. Med.* **2021**, *11*, 817, doi:10.3390/jpm11080817 17

Klaus Schlueter-Brust, Johann Henckel, Faidon Katinakis, Christoph Buken, Jörg Opt-Eynde and Thorsten Pofahl et al.
Augmented-Reality-Assisted K-Wire Placement for Glenoid Component Positioning in Reversed Shoulder Arthroplasty: A Proof-of-Concept Study
Reprinted from: *J. Pers. Med.* **2021**, *11*, 777, doi:10.3390/jpm11080777 35

Carlos González-Bravo, Miguel A. Ortega, Julia Buján, Basilio de la Torre and Loreto Barrios
Wear Risk Prevention and Reduction in Total Hip Arthroplasty. A Personalized Study Comparing Cement and Cementless Fixation Techniques Employing Finite Element Analysis
Reprinted from: *J. Pers. Med.* **2021**, *11*, 780, doi:10.3390/jpm11080780 43

Cyrus Anthony Pumilia, Lennart Schroeder, Nana O. Sarpong and Gregory Martin
Patient Satisfaction, Functional Outcomes, and Implant Survivorship in Patients Undergoing Customized Unicompartmental Knee Arthroplasty
Reprinted from: *J. Pers. Med.* **2021**, *11*, 753, doi:10.3390/jpm11080753 59

Kevin Döring, Kevin Staats, Stephan Puchner and Reinhard Windhager
Patient-Specific Implants for Pelvic Tumor Resections
Reprinted from: *J. Pers. Med.* **2021**, *11*, 683, doi:10.3390/jpm11080683 69

Kim Huber, Bernhard Christen, Sarah Calliess and Tilman Calliess
True Kinematic Alignment Is Applicable in 44% of Patients Applying Restrictive Indication Criteria—A Retrospective Analysis of 111 TKA Using Robotic Assistance
Reprinted from: *J. Pers. Med.* **2021**, *11*, 662, doi:10.3390/jpm11070662 83

Sonja A. G. A. Grothues and Klaus Radermacher
Variation of the Three-Dimensional Femoral J-Curve in the Native Knee
Reprinted from: *J. Pers. Med.* **2021**, *11*, 592, doi:10.3390/jpm11070592 95

Céline Saphena Moret, Benjamin Luca Schelker and Michael Tobias Hirschmann
Clinical and Radiological Outcomes after Knee Arthroplasty with Patient-Specific versus Off-the-Shelf Knee Implants: A Systematic Review
Reprinted from: *J. Pers. Med.* **2021**, *11*, 590, doi:10.3390/jpm11070590 105

Peter Savov, Lars-Rene Tuecking, Henning Windhagen and Max Ettinger
Individual Revision Knee Arthroplasty Is a Safe Limb Salvage Procedure
Reprinted from: *J. Pers. Med.* **2021**, *11*, 572, doi:10.3390/jpm11060572 119

Felix Wunderlich, Maheen Azad, Ruben Westphal, Thomas Klonschinski, Patrick Belikan and Philipp Drees et al.
Comparison of Postoperative Coronal Leg Alignment in Customized Individually Made and Conventional Total Knee Arthroplasty
Reprinted from: *J. Pers. Med.* **2021**, *11*, 549, doi:10.3390/jpm11060549 131

Feng-Yu Liu, Chih-Chi Chen, Chi-Tung Cheng, Cheng-Ta Wu, Chih-Po Hsu and Chih-Yuan Fu et al.
Automatic Hip Detection in Anteroposterior Pelvic Radiographs—A Labelless Practical Framework
Reprinted from: *J. Pers. Med.* **2021**, *11*, 522, doi:10.3390/jpm11060522 139

Alexander J. Nedopil, Connor Delman, Stephen M. Howell and Maury L. Hull
Restoring the Patient's Pre-Arthritic Posterior Slope Is the Correct Target for Maximizing Internal Tibial Rotation When Implanting a PCL Retaining TKA with Calipered Kinematic Alignment
Reprinted from: *J. Pers. Med.* **2021**, *11*, 516, doi:10.3390/jpm11060516 147

Martin Schulze, Georg Gosheger, Sebastian Bockholt, Marieke De Vaal, Tymo Budny and Max Tönnemann et al.
Complex Bone Tumors of the Trunk—The Role of 3D Printing and Navigation in Tumor Orthopedics: A Case Series and Review of the Literature
Reprinted from: *J. Pers. Med.* **2021**, *11*, 517, doi:10.3390/jpm11060517 159

Tajrian Amin, William C.H. Parr and Ralph J. Mobbs
Opinion Piece: Patient-Specific Implants May Be the Next Big Thing in Spinal Surgery
Reprinted from: *J. Pers. Med.* **2021**, *11*, 498, doi:10.3390/jpm11060498 179

Haseeb Sultan, Muhammad Owais, Chanhum Park, Tahir Mahmood, Adnan Haider and Kang Ryoung Park
Artificial Intelligence-Based Recognition of Different Types of Shoulder Implants in X-ray Scans Based on Dense Residual Ensemble-Network for Personalized Medicine
Reprinted from: *J. Pers. Med.* **2021**, *11*, 482, doi:10.3390/jpm11060482 191

Andrea Angelini, Michele Piazza, Elisa Pagliarini, Giulia Trovarelli, Andrea Spertino and Pietro Ruggieri
The Orthopedic-Vascular Multidisciplinary Approach Improves Patient Safety in Surgery for Musculoskeletal Tumors: A Large-Volume Center Experience
Reprinted from: *J. Pers. Med.* **2021**, *11*, 462, doi:10.3390/jpm11060462 219

Wiebke K. Guder, Jendrik Hardes, Markus Nottrott, Lars E. Podleska and Arne Streitbürger
Highly Cancellous Titanium Alloy (TiAl$_6$V$_4$) Surfaces on Three-Dimensionally Printed, Custom-Made Intercalary Tibia Prostheses: Promising Short- to Intermediate-Term Results
Reprinted from: *J. Pers. Med.* **2021**, *11*, 351, doi:10.3390/jpm11050351 235

Sebastian Philipp von Hertzberg-Boelch, Mike Wagenbrenner, Jörg Arnholdt, Stephan Frenzel, Boris Michael Holzapfel and Maximilian Rudert
Custom Made Monoflange Acetabular Components for the Treatment of Paprosky Type III Defects
Reprinted from: *J. Pers. Med.* **2021**, *11*, 283, doi:10.3390/jpm11040283 245

About the Editor

Maximilian Rudert

Maximilian Rudert currently works at the Department of Orthopaedics König-Ludwig-Haus, University of Wuerzburg. Maximilian does research in Orthopedic Surgery, Surgery and Oncology. Their current project is 'Patient-specific knee arthroplasty', 'minimally invasive hip arthroplasty through the direct anterior approach', and 'revision arthroplasty of the hip and knee'.

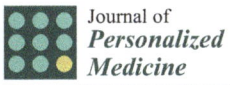

Editorial

Taking the Next Step in Personalised Orthopaedic Implantation

Maximilian Rudert

Orthopaedic Department, König-Ludwig-Haus, University of Wuerzburg, D-97074 Wuerzburg, Germany; m-rudert.klh@uni-wuerzburg.de

Citation: Rudert, M. Taking the Next Step in Personalised Orthopaedic Implantation. *J. Pers. Med.* **2022**, *12*, 365. https://doi.org/10.3390/jpm12030365

Received: 9 February 2022
Accepted: 25 February 2022
Published: 27 February 2022

Publisher's Note: MDPI stays neutral with regard to jurisdictional claims in published maps and institutional affiliations.

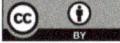

Copyright: © 2022 by the author. Licensee MDPI, Basel, Switzerland. This article is an open access article distributed under the terms and conditions of the Creative Commons Attribution (CC BY) license (https://creativecommons.org/licenses/by/4.0/).

Most of the treatments in medicine are patient specific, are they not?

We examine patients, make individual diagnoses and adapt our therapy to the specific case. The more precisely we are in our efforts to record all parameters that could influence our therapy, the more individual our treatment will become for the patient. Machine Learning, Neural Networks, and Big Data management will help us to overcome the endless story of biomedical statistical approaches concerning outcome data in orthopaedics [1]. Hopefully we can find out in the long term who exactly is suitable for which therapy. One problem in orthopaedics is that new treatment approaches, such as patient-specific instruments, are applied equally to all patients without it being possible to demonstrate differences in the treatment result.

Why should we bother with individualization of our implants and techniques, if we adapt our therapy to patients anyway? The more we try to pigeonhole the patient, which is often forced to us by treatment guidelines and classifications we use, the more likely we are not to achieve individual treatment. Looking at the neighbouring field of oncologic treatment, nobody would question that individualization of tumour therapy with personalized instruments like antibodies has led to thriving of this field in terms of success in patient survival and positive responses to alternatives for conventional treatments. The same seems to happen to the field of orthopaedic surgery although not strikingly obvious because outcome does not equal survival in most of our cases.

Nonetheless, tumour surgery is a good way of looking at things in orthopaedic personalization, but from a different angle. The defects that arise from tumours and their surgical removal are so different that only in rare cases do they not require any adjustment to the standard [2]. This has been the case for decades, but the techniques that are available to us are becoming more and more sophisticated and allow better restorations [3–6]. The same is actually true for defects in revision arthroplasty and spinal surgery [7–9]. Since more and more revisions are re-revisions, the defects and collateral damage become bigger with every episode of loosening and consecutive operation. 3D printing technologies allow for visualization of the defects on templates that can be used to understand our treatment approach. Still, in order to simplify the treatment, we classify the defects, which, firstly, is not easy and, secondly, does not always make sense [10,11]. Again we come into the dilemma of small numbers, very individual anatomical requirements and a multitude of confounders, which make a statistical analysis practically impossible [1]. Furthermore, three-dimensional defects can change during the operative procedure. A lot of experience is therefore necessary in order to anticipate this and either fit bones using resection guides or tolerate inaccuracies where possible.

Modern alignment techniques in primary knee arthroplasty have also adopted the concepts of individualization of the implant position and soft tissue tension to approximate the preoperative situation. In this way, the individual anatomical requirements of the patient are taken into account and the joint is not put into a predicament in which it has never been before. This is intended to increase the outcome and satisfaction [12–14]. The use of patient-specific implants in primary endoprosthetics follows a comparable principle. Due to the optimal alignment and size as well as the shape of the implants, the physiological load transfer should be maintained in the entire movement of the joints [15–18].

Artificial intelligence-based recognition of different types of implants and detection of the region of interest in standard x-rays will help to improve treatment by gathering big data [19,20]. With these large amounts of data, it will be easier to optimize standard situations for the individual patient and his or her specific anatomical requirements [21,22]. Ultimately, however, this information only helps us if we can put it into practice on the patient. Augmented reality and robotic systems will help us to translate the planning [23]. Personally, I strongly believe that these new technologies will bring us further in successful and, above all, adapted therapy for our patients.

Funding: This research received no external funding.

Institutional Review Board Statement: This Editorial did not require ethical approval.

Informed Consent Statement: Not applicable.

Data Availability Statement: See References to the Editorial.

Conflicts of Interest: The authors declare no conflict of interest.

References

1. Hewett, T.E.; Webster, K.E. EDITORIAL: The Use of Big Data to Improve Human Health—How Experience from Other Industries Will Shape the Future. *Int. J. Sports Phys. Ther.* **2021**, *16*, 29856. [CrossRef] [PubMed]
2. Rudert, M.; Holzapfel, B.M.; Pilge, H.; Rechl, H.; Gradinger, R. Partial pelvic resection (internal hemipelvectomy) and endoprosthetic replacement in periacetabular tumors. *Oper. Orthop. Traumatol.* **2012**, *24*, 196–214. [CrossRef] [PubMed]
3. Angelini, A.; Piazza, M.; Pagliarini, E.; Trovarelli, G.; Spertino, A.; Ruggieri, P. The Orthopedic-Vascular Multidisciplinary Approach Improves Patient Safety in Surgery for Musculoskeletal Tumors: A Large-Volume Center Experience. *J. Pers. Med.* **2021**, *11*, 462. [CrossRef]
4. Döring, K.; Staats, K.; Puchner, S.; Windhager, R. Patient-Specific Implants for Pelvic Tumor Resections. *J. Pers. Med.* **2021**, *11*, 683. [CrossRef] [PubMed]
5. Guder, W.K.; Hardes, J.; Nottrott, M.; Podleska, L.E.; Streitbürger, A. Highly Cancellous Titanium Alloy (TiAl6V4) Surfaces on Three-Dimensionally Printed, Custom-Made Intercalary Tibia Prostheses: Promising Short- to Intermediate-Term Results. *J. Pers. Med.* **2021**, *11*, 351. [CrossRef]
6. Schulze, M.; Gosheger, G.; Bockholt, S.; De Vaal, M.; Budny, T.; Tönnemann, M.; Pützler, J.; Bövingloh, A.S.; Rischen, R.; Hofbauer, V.; et al. Complex Bone Tumors of the Trunk—The Role of 3D Printing and Navigation in Tumor Orthopedics: A Case Series and Review of the Literature. *J. Pers. Med.* **2021**, *11*, 517. [CrossRef] [PubMed]
7. Amin, T.; Parr, W.C.H.; Mobbs, R.J. Opinion Piece: Patient-Specific Implants May Be the Next Big Thing in Spinal Surgery. *J. Pers. Med.* **2021**, *11*, 498. [CrossRef]
8. Savov, P.; Tuecking, L.R.; Windhagen, H.; Ettinger, M. Individual Revision Knee Arthroplasty Is a Safe Limb Salvage Procedure. *J. Pers. Med.* **2021**, *11*, 572. [CrossRef]
9. von Hertzberg-Boelch, S.P.; Wagenbrenner, M.; Arnholdt, J.; Frenzel, S.; Holzapfel, B.M.; Rudert, M. Custom Made Monoflange Acetabular Components for the Treatment of Paprosky Type III Defects. *J. Pers. Med.* **2021**, *11*, 283. [CrossRef]
10. Horas, K.; Arnholdt, J.; Steinert, A.F.; Hoberg, M.; Rudert, M.; Holzapfel, B.M. Acetabular defect classification in times of 3D imaging and patient-specific treatment protocols. *Orthopade* **2017**, *46*, 168–178. [CrossRef]
11. Schierjott, R.A.; Hettich, G.; Graichen, H.; Jansson, V.; Rudert, M.; Traina, F.; Weber, P.; Grupp, T.M. Quantitative assessment of acetabular bone defects: A study of 50 computed tomography data sets. *PLoS ONE* **2019**, *14*, e0222511. [CrossRef] [PubMed]
12. Huber, K.; Christen, B.; Calliess, S.; Calliess, T. True Kinematic Alignment Is Applicable in 44% of Patients Applying Restrictive Indication Criteria—A Retrospective Analysis of 111 TKA Using Robotic Assistance. *J. Pers. Med.* **2021**, *11*, 662. [CrossRef] [PubMed]
13. Nedopil, A.J.; Delman, C.; Howell, S.M.; Hull, M.L. Restoring the Patient's Pre-Arthritic Posterior Slope Is the Correct Target for Maximizing Internal Tibial Rotation When Implanting a PCL Retaining TKA with Calipered Kinematic Alignment. *J. Pers. Med.* **2021**, *11*, 516. [CrossRef] [PubMed]
14. Pumilia, C.A.; Schroeder, L.; Sarpong, N.O.; Martin, G. Patient Satisfaction, Functional Outcomes, and Implant Survivorship in Patients Undergoing Customized Unicompartmental Knee Arthroplasty. *J. Pers. Med.* **2021**, *11*, 753. [CrossRef] [PubMed]
15. Grothues, S.A.G.A.; Radermacher, K. Variation of the Three-Dimensional Femoral J-Curve in the Native Knee. *J. Pers. Med.* **2021**, *11*, 592. [CrossRef]
16. Moret, C.S.; Schelker, B.L.; Hirschmann, M.T. Clinical and Radiological Outcomes after Knee Arthroplasty with Patient-Specific versus Off-the-Shelf Knee Implants: A Systematic Review. *J. Pers. Med.* **2021**, *11*, 590. [CrossRef]
17. Wunderlich, F.; Azad, M.; Westphal, R.; Klonschinski, T.; Belikan, P.; Drees, P.; Eckhard, L. Comparison of Postoperative Coronal Leg Alignment in Customized Individually Made and Conventional Total Knee Arthroplasty. *J. Pers. Med.* **2021**, *11*, 549. [CrossRef]

18. Steinert, A.F.; Schroder, L.; Sefrin, L.; Janssen, B.; Arnholdt, J.; Rudert, M. The Impact of Total Knee Replacement with a Customized Cruciate-Retaining Implant Design on Patient-Reported and Functional Outcomes. *J. Pers. Med.* **2022**, *12*, 194. [CrossRef]
19. Liu, F.Y.; Chen, C.C.; Cheng, C.T.; Wu, C.T.; Hsu, C.P.; Fu, C.Y.; Chen, S.C.; Liao, C.H.; Lee, M.S. Automatic Hip Detection in Anteroposterior Pelvic Radiographs—A Labelless Practical Framework. *J. Pers. Med.* **2021**, *11*, 522. [CrossRef]
20. Sultan, H.; Owais, M.; Park, C.; Mahmood, T.; Haider, A.; Park, K.R. Artificial Intelligence-Based Recognition of Different Types of Shoulder Implants in X-ray Scans Based on Dense Residual Ensemble-Network for Personalized Medicine. *J. Pers. Med.* **2021**, *11*, 482. [CrossRef]
21. González-Bravo, C.; Ortega, M.A.; Buján, J.; Torre, B.D.; Barrios, L. Wear Risk Prevention and Reduction in Total Hip Arthroplasty. A Personalized Study Comparing Cement and Cementless Fixation Techniques Employing Finite Element Analysis. *J. Pers. Med.* **2021**, *11*, 780. [CrossRef] [PubMed]
22. Habor, J.; Fischer, M.; Tokunaga, K.; Okamoto, M.; Radermacher, K. The Patient-Specific Combined Target Zone for Morpho-Functional Planning of Total Hip Arthroplasty. *J. Pers. Med.* **2021**, *11*, 817. [CrossRef] [PubMed]
23. Schlueter-Brust, K.; Henckel, J.; Katinakis, F.; Buken, C.; Opt-Eynde, J.; Pofahl, T.; Rodriguez y Baena, F.; Tatti, F. Augmented-Reality-Assisted K-Wire Placement for Glenoid Component Positioning in Reversed Shoulder Arthroplasty: A Proof-of-Concept Study. *J. Pers. Med.* **2021**, *11*, 777. [CrossRef] [PubMed]

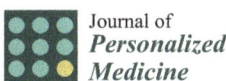

Article

The Impact of Total Knee Replacement with a Customized Cruciate-Retaining Implant Design on Patient-Reported and Functional Outcomes

Andre F. Steinert [1,2], Lennart Schröder [1,3], Lukas Sefrin [1], Björn Janßen [1], Jörg Arnholdt [1,3] and Maximilian Rudert [1,*]

1. Department of Orthopaedic Surgery, König-Ludwig-Haus, Julius-Maximilians-University Würzburg, Brettreichstraße 11, D-97074 Würzburg, Germany; andre.steinert@campus-nes.de (A.F.S.); Lennart.Schroeder@med.uni-muenchen.de (L.S.); lsef@gmail.de (L.S.); bjoern_janssen@web.de (B.J.); Joerg.Arnholdt@med.uni-muenchen.de (J.A.)
2. Rhön Klinikum, Campus Bad Neustadt, EndoRhön Center for Joint Replacement, Teaching Hospital of the Phillipps University Marburg, Von Guttenberg Str. 11, D-97616 Bad Neustadt, Germany
3. Department of Orthopaedics and Trauma Surgery, Musculoskeletal University Center Munich (MUM), University Hospital, Ludwigs-Maximilians-University Munich, Marchionistr. 15, D-81377 Munich, Germany
* Correspondence: m-rudert.klh@uni-wuerzburg.de; Tel.: +49-931-803-1101; Fax: +49-931-803-1109

Abstract: Purpose: To treat patients with tricompartmental knee osteoarthritis (OA), a customized cruciate-retaining total knee arthroplasty (CCR-TKA) system can be used, including both individualized instrumentation and implants. The objective of this monocentric cohort study was to analyze patient-reported and functional outcomes in a series of patients implanted with the second generation of this customized implant. Methods: At our arthroplasty center, we prospectively recruited a cohort of patients with tricompartmental gonarthrosis to be treated with total knee replacement (TKA) using a customized cruciate-retaining (CCR) implant design. Inclusion criteria for patients comprised the presence of intact posterior cruciate and collateral ligaments and a knee deformity that was restricted to <15° varus, valgus, or flexion contracture. Patients were assessed for their range of motion (ROM), Knee Society Score (KSS), Western Ontario and McMaster University osteoarthritis index (WOMAC), and short form (SF)-12 physical and mental scores, preoperatively, at 3 and 6 months, as well as at 1, 2, 3, and 5 years of follow-up (FU) postoperatively. Results: The average age of the patient population was 64 years (range: 40–81), the average BMI was 31 (range: 23–42), and in total, 28 female and 45 male patients were included. Implant survivorship was 97.5% (one septic loosening) at an average follow-up of 2.5 years. The KSS knee and function scores improved significantly ($p < 0.001$) from, respectively, 41 and 53 at the pre-operative visit, to 92 and 86, respectively, at the 5-year post-operative time point. The SF-12 Physical and Mental scores significantly ($p < 0.001$) improved from the pre-operative values of 28 and 50, to 50 and 53 at the 5-year FU, respectively. Patients experienced significant improvements in their overall knee range of motion, from 106° at the preoperative visit to 122°, on average, 5 years postoperatively. The total WOMAC score significantly ($p < 0.001$) improved from 49.1 preoperatively to 11.4 postoperatively at 5-year FU. Conclusions: Although there was no comparison to other implants within this study, patients reported high overall satisfaction and improvement in functional outcomes within the first year from surgery, which continued over the following years. These mid-term results are excellent compared with those reported in the current literature. Comparative long-term studies with this device are needed. Level of evidence 3b (individual case–control study).

Keywords: patient-specific; custom-made implant; total knee arthroplasty; TKA; knee replacement; tricompartmental knee osteoarthritis; iTotal

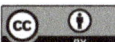

1. Introduction

Advanced knee osteoarthritis (OA) is a disabling disease frequently requiring knee replacement surgery. Despite overall improvements over the past few decades in total knee arthroplasty (TKA), surgical procedures, and implant design, recent studies have shown that approximately 19% of patients treated with TKA continue to experience discomfort in their treated joint [1–3]. Inappropriate size, fit, and positioning of the implant components including rotational and coronal alignment have emerged among the key factors that lead to a higher risk of implant failure, poor outcomes, and high revision rates over time [4].

To overcome these limitations, several novel surgical techniques in TKA surgery have been explored in recent years [5]. Patient-specific knee prostheses have been introduced to provide an ideal coverage of the bony surfaces of the tibia and the femur and are shaped to address the patient-specific J-curve anatomy of the bones [6,7]. The second generation (G2) of a patient-specific cruciate-retaining TKA system iTotal™ (CCR-TKA) comprises custom-made implants as well as instrumentation and represents a new approach for the treatment of patients with tricompartmental knee OA. Based on computed tomography (CT) scans of the affected limb and computer-aided design and manufacturing (CAD/CAM) protocols, this system aims to achieve an optimal fit of implant components and instruments [8,9]. Using this implant technology, encouraging initial clinical and radiographic results have been reported for unicompartmental (UKA) [10,11] and bicompartmental (BKA) knee arthroplasty [12–14].

Therefore, the aim of this prospective longitudinal clinical study was to analyze the clinical outcome of the treatment of tricompartmental knee OA with CCR-TKA with a follow-up of up to 5 years.

2. Methods

2.1. Patients

In this single-center study at a German university arthroplasty center, a cohort of 73 patients was recruited prospectively from November 2012 until January 2017 to undergo TKA with the iTotal® CR G2 knee replacement (Conformis Inc., Billerica, MA, USA). Patients were diagnosed with end-stage tricompartmental osteoarthritis, and individuals with compromised posterior cruciate or collateral ligaments or having a varus/valgus deformity or fixed extensor lag >15° were excluded. Other exclusion criteria were: active local or systemic infection, immunodeficiency, RA or other forms of inflammatory joint disease, prior arthroplasty of the affected knee, and prior history of failed implant surgery of the joint to be treated, including high tibial osteotomy (HTO). An Ethics Committee approval was obtained from the Institutional Review Board (IRB) of the Julius-Maximilians University Medical Center (approval number 2016101401), and all patients signed an informed consent prior to participation. All surgeries were performed by two high-volume surgeons (first and senior author) using a standard medial parapatellar arthrotomy, under adherence to the standards of Good Clinical Practice (GCP). Patient enrollment and sampling were conducted to include subsequent cases willing to participate and to meet the inclusion criteria after a learning curve with this implant system of 6 months.

2.2. Custom Cruciate-Retaining TKA Implant and Planning

The CCR-TKA implant used has a CE marking and is approved by the United States Food and Drug Administration (FDA). A CT scan of the affected leg was conducted for every patient preoperatively by scanning the knee, the femoral head, and the talus center in accordance with a standard protocol (http://www.conformis.com/healthcare-professionals/imaging-professionals, accessed on 25 January 2022) as previously described [8,9]. The cemented, fixed-bearing, patient-specific implant was designed based on the patient's bone geometry, defining shape and size of the metal implant components, as well as the disposable bone-cutting jigs [8]. A correction of the mechanical axes towards neutral, as well as a preservation of the joint line including the distal and the posterior femoral condylar offset and the tibial slope was implemented in the implant design process [7].

Representative images of the CCR-TKA knee implant are shown in Figure 1A–D. It comprises three components: a femoral shield, a tibial tray, and an optional patellar component, including a separate medial and lateral insert of the tibia with different heights that correspond to the condylar offsets of the femur. The femoral shield and tibial tray were manufactured using a cobalt–chromium–molybdenum alloy, the tibial inserts and the patellar component using ultra-high-molecular-weight polyethylene, while the disposable cutting jigs were made from nylon via 3D printing.

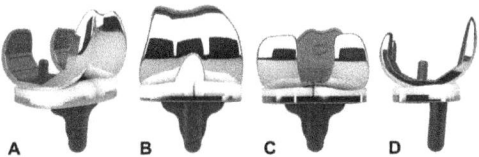

Figure 1. Representative images of the patient-specific, cruciate-retaining iTotal CR G2 total knee replacement. (**A**) Antero-medial, (**B**) anterior, (**C**) posterior, and (**D**) lateral view of the device. Please note that the medial and lateral polyethylene inserts have different heights that correspond to the condylar offset of the femur.

A typical 3D planning protocol (iView®) is shown in Figure 2, comprising representative images of the patient's anatomic and implants' features of the tibia (A) and femur (B), as well as the projected thicknesses of the respective tibial and femoral bone cuts for self-control (Figure 2A,B).

2.3. Surgical Technique

The detailed surgical procedure has been previously described [8]. In brief, following a medial parapatellar arthrotomy, the surgical procedure included 6 different steps, that were facilitated by the use of the provided patient-specific bone resection jigs and iView® protocol, allowing confirmation of all performed bone cuts against the surgical plan for self-control. Specifically, the instrumentation kit comprised 6 different femoral (F1–6) and 5 separate tibial (T1–5) jigs for cutting and drilling. The surgical steps were distal femoral resection (required jigs: F1–3), proximal tibial resection (jig: T1), balancing of extension and flexion gap (jigs: T2, T3), femoral preparation (jigs: F4, F5), trialing (jigs: F6, T4), and final tibial preparation (jig: T5), before the final implantation of the components was performed. Notably, the surgeon had two options for the tibial cuts, with two different T1 instruments facilitating the tibial cut either with a patient-specific slope (shown in red) or with a fixed slope of 5° (shown in black), as shown in the tibial images of the iView® (Figure 2A). Additionally, testing of the trial components could be performed with three individually designed T4 jigs with 1 mm incremental heights. Thereby, the CCR-TKA system allows for kinematic testing using anatomic trial components, where the most appropriate tibial insert heights for the medial (6 mm, 7 mm, or 8 mm) and lateral (A, B, C with custom thicknesses; see iView® bottom row (Figure 2)) knee joint space may be identified before the final components are implanted. Patella resurfacing is performed if necessary, using standard oval dome patellae. Cementing, wound closure, and rehabilitation protocols were in accordance with standard TKA procedures.

2.4. Outcome Parameters

Several clinical outcome scores were assessed pre-operatively and compared to post-operative outcomes at 3 and 6 months, as well as at 1-, 2-, 3- and 5-year post-OP. The Knee Society Scoring System (KSS) by Insall et al. was assessed. It consists of 2 separate subscales: (1) a "Knee" score (100 points total) which considers pain (50 points), stability (25 points), and range of motion (25 points) with deductions for flexion contractures, extension lag, and malalignment, and (2) a "Function" score (100 points total) that utilizes walking distance (50 points) and stair climbing (50 points) with deduction for the use of a walking aid [15,16].

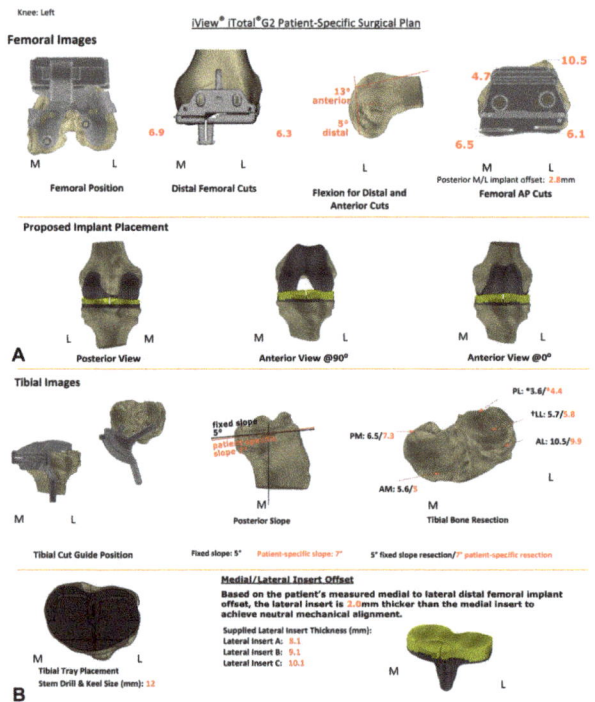

Figure 2. Representative patient-specific surgical plan (iView®). Upper images (**A**) show the positioning of the respective drill guide, cutting jigs, and implant for femoral preparation, and the projected thickness of the cut bone is given in red for self-control. Lower images (**B**) show the positioning of the respective cutting jig and implant for tibial preparation, and the projected thickness of the bone cut is given for self-control. Please note that a fixed cut of 5° slope (black numbers) or a patient-specific slope cut guide (here 7°; red numbers) can be chosen, and asterisks (*) indicate a point 5 mm from edge.

The Western Ontario and McMaster Universities Osteoarthritis Index (WOMAC) was used as a patient-reported outcome measure for knee osteoarthritis, that included the subscales "Pain" (5 items; 50 points), "Stiffness" (2 items; 20 points), and "Function" (17 items; 170 points), with a range from 0 (= no pain/stiffness/problems) to 10 (= extreme pain/stiffness/impossible to do) points for each item [17]. The relative WOMAC scores, i.e., for the total WOMAC score as well as for the subscales, were then calculated from the point values by multiplication × 100 and divided by the maximum score value [17,18].

We also assessed the Short Form (SF) 12 Health Survey, which is a 12-item, patient-reported survey of patient health, that evaluates eight dimensions of health status [19]. Scores in the range of 0–100 are given for each subscale, and higher scores represent better health. Norm-based scoring of each 0–100 scale is then carried out by standardization of each subscale relative to a Z-Score that is 50 on average in the population, with a standard deviation of 10 [19]. Finally, two aggregate summary measures can be derived, a physical (PCS) and a mental (MCS) health subscores, to determine the overall mental and physical well-being [19].

Any device-related adverse event that was observed or reported by the patient was evaluated, and implant survivorship was calculated for patients that had completed a follow-up of a minimum of 2 years post-OP or were revised prior to the 2-year time point.

Radiographic evaluations were also performed prior to surgery and one week post-surgery using a strict antero-posterior (AP) view, a lateral view (including a referencing sphere), as well as a skyline view. The fit of the metal components was assessed, and a deviation of ≥1 mm overhang/underhang was considered as abnormal.

2.5. Statistical Analysis

Demographic information including age, BMI, and gender is presented as descriptive statistics, i.e., averages, proportions, minimum and maximum values. Outcome measures such as ROM, KSS, WOMAC, and SF-12 scores are presented as descriptive statistics using averages, ranges, and standard deviations (SD). To determine the significance of changes in outcome measures between follow-up time points, a two-ailed Student's t-test assuming unequal variances was performed, since the study reports on longitudinal data within the same cohort comparing pre- to respective postoperative data. A p-value of <0.05 was considered to indicate statistical significance. All statistical analyses were conducted using the build-in functions in Microsoft Excel (Microsoft Inc., Redmond, WA, USA).

3. Results

3.1. Study Population and Intraoperative Parameters

Patients' demographics are shown in Table 1. Of the 73 patients included, 41 required right-knee implants, and 32 left implants; the average age of the patient population was 64 years (range: 40–81), the average BMI was 31 (range: 23–42), while 28 female and 45 male patients were recruited (Table 1). In 37 (51%) cases, surgery was performed under general anesthesia, and in 36 cases (49%), spinal anesthesia was administered. The average time of surgery was 93 min (range 66 to 142 min, SD 16.6).

Table 1. Demographic profile of patients enrolled in the study.

Metric		Min	Max
Knees (N)	73	-	-
Patient Gender (% Female)	38%	-	-
Mean Age at Surgery (years)	64	40	81
Mean Body Mass Index (BMI)	31	23	42

3.2. Complications and Survival

By the time of the last follow-up, there had been one revision at 8 months postoperatively due to septic loosening of the implant, resulting in an implant survival rate of 98.6% at the time of the final follow-up. One patient required further surgical intervention due to progression of retro-patellar osteoarthritis, which included revision of the tibial plateau inserts and implantation of a patellar button. There were three manipulations under anesthesia (MUA) for reduced range of motion due to arthrofibrosis at 3, 4, and 9 months after surgery.

3.3. Outcome Parameters

Preoperatively, patients showed an average ROM of 106° (range, 70° to 125°, SD 14.4) for their knee to be treated (Figure 3). At 3 months post-OP, a similar ROM was observed, with an average of 106° (range, 75° to 125°, SD 12.3). From 3 to 6 months, a significant increase in ROM was observed, with an average of 112° (range, 85° to 125°, SD 11; $p = 0.007$) at 6 months post-OP. This significant increase in ROM continued during the following 6 months, with an average of 119° (range, 100° to 125°, SD 6.1; $p = 0.003$) observed 1 year post-OP. The range of motion after CCR-TKA reached a plateau at approximately 2 years, with averages of 122° (range, 105° to 125°, SD 5.7), 122° (range, 100° to 125°, SD 6.1), and 122° (range 115° to 125°, SD 4.7) at 2, 3, and 5 years post-OP, respectively (Figure 3).

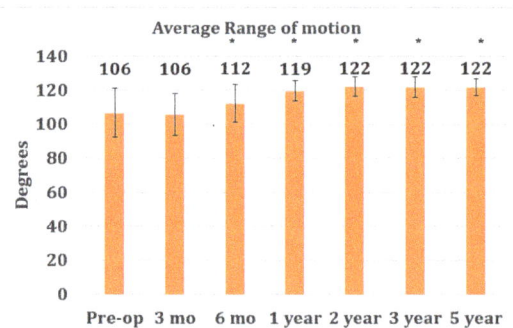

Figure 3. Average range of motion at pre-operative and follow-up time points after CCR-TKA surgery. The graph reports averages +/− SD. Asterisks (*) indicate statistical significance compared with the pre-op control, as determined by Student's *t*-test ($p < 0.05$).

When evaluating the results for the KSS-Function- and KSS-Knee-Score, a statistically significant increase was observed in both scores from pre-OP (Function: 53, Knee: 41) to 3 months (Function 74, Knee: 79; $p < 0.001$) and further to 6 months (Function: 84, Knee: 90; $p < 0.001$) post-OP (Figure 4). The score results reached a plateau 1 year after surgery (Function: 89, Knee: 92; $p < 0.001$) and showed no further significant changes during the follow-up period (Figure 4).

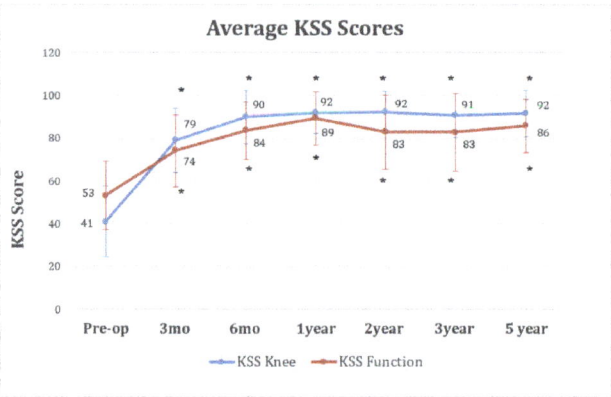

Figure 4. Average Knee Society Scores (KSS) for patients enrolled in the study, including the knee (blue) and function (red) subscores. The graphs reports averages +/− SD. Asterisks (*) indicate statistical significance compared with the pre-op control, as determined by Student's *t*-test ($p < 0.05$).

Similar results were observed in the analysis of the overall WOMAC-Score results. A significant decrease was observed from an average preoperative WOMAC-Score of 49 (range, 100 to 6, SD 20.9) to an average of 21 (range 80 to 0, SD 17; $p < 0.001$) at 3 months and an average of 13 (range, 80 to 0, SD 16; $p = 0.002$) at 6 months post-OP. The WOMAC-Score results at 6 months were not found significantly different from those at up to 5 years postoperatively, with an average of 9 (range, 56 to 0, SD 15.2) at 1 year, an average of 8 (range 36 to 0, SD 10) at 2 years, an average of 20 (range 72 to 0, SD 14) at 3 years, and an average of 17 (range 34 to 0, SD 8) at 5 years post-OP (Figure 5). The respective subscores WOMAC Pain, WOMAC Stiffness, and WOMAC Function followed this pattern, without major differences during the 5-year time course (Figure 5).

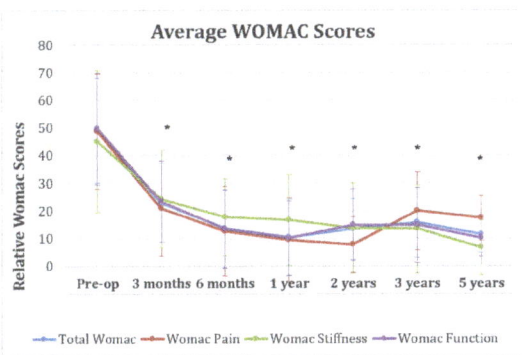

Figure 5. Average Western Ontario and Mc Master Index (WOMAC) for patients enrolled in the study, including the total score (blue), as well as the pain (red), stiffness (green), and function (blue) subscores over time. The graphs reports averages +/− SD. Asterisks (*) indicate statistical significance for all WOMAC scores (total WOMAC, WOMAC pain, WOMAC Stiffness, WOMAC Function) at the respective timepoint compared with the pre-op control scores, as determined by Student's t-test ($p < 0.05$).

Lastly, in both, the SF-12-Physical- and the SF-12-Mental-Score showed an increase from the averages of 28 (range, 14 to 50, SD 7.7) and 49.9 (range, 29 to 69) preoperatively to averages of 39.8 (range, 22 to 54, SD 8.6) and 57.6 (range, 35 to 66, SD 7.1) at 3 months, averages of 45.4 (range 20 to 57, SD 8.6) and 57.9 (range, 29 to 64, SD 6.3) at 6 months, averages of 48.7 (range, 20 to 57, SD 9.5) and 56.5 (range, 43 to 65, SD 4.5) at 1 year, averages of 45.3 (range, 15 to 56, SD 11) and 52.5 (range, 34 to 60, SD 6.5) at 2 years, averages of 44.2 (range, 15 to 57, SD 11) and 53.8 (range, 35 to 61, SD 5.9) at 3 years, and averages of 50 (range, 32 to 57, SD 9.1) and 52.5 (range, 32 to 61, SD 9.5) at 5 years post-OP, respectively (Figure 6). However, only differences in the physical part of the SF-12 were found statistically significant ($p < 0.001$).

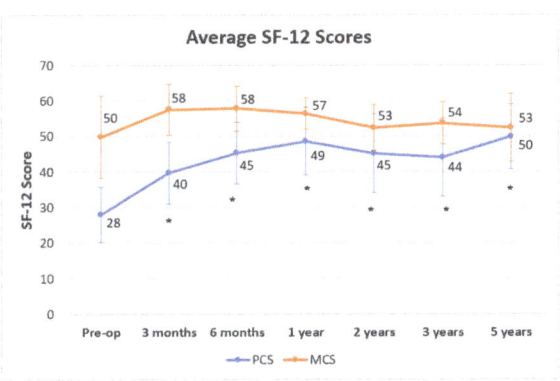

Figure 6. Average Short Form (SF)-12 scores from the pre-operative time point up to the 5-year post-operative time point for patients enrolled in the study, including physical (PCS, blue) and mental (MCS, orange) subscores. The graph reports averages +/− SD. Asterisks (*) indicate statistical significance in comparison with the pre-op control, as determined by Student's t-test ($p < 0.05$).

All knees treated were routinely evaluated radiographically pre- and postoperatively and showed and ideal implant fit without any over- or underhang of the components.

4. Discussion

TKA is performed increasingly more often in relation to the high demands of physical activity and quality of life even in old ages. However, around 20–30% of TKA patients remain unsatisfied with their surgical procedure, and factors such as implant malalignment and component oversizing have shown to be among the most common reasons for postoperative complaints [2,4]. Moreover, the clinical outcomes after TKA surgery in the young patient population are worse than previously thought, with high expectations of the surgical procedure being evident [20,21]. This discrepancy between unsatisfactory results and rising expectations for the TKA procedure is driving implant manufacturers and surgeons alike to improve the surgical techniques as well as the instruments and implants used [5,7]. Recent studies have highlighted the variability of knee joint geometry among individuals [22,23]. The idea of implant customization is thought to address this variability. In this context, the C-TKA used in this study aims to achieve an individual implant fit, to recreate patients' individual joint geometry and kinematics, and therefore to improve the postoperative clinical and functional outcomes [8]. This is facilitated by manufacturing the femoral implant according to the individual J-curve anatomy of the patient derived from preoperative computed-tomography (CT) scans of the knee. The accuracy of the femoral component positioning in this CCR-TKA system can be further confirmed by the agreement of the measured thickness of the posterior femoral condyle resection with the preoperative iView® plan (Figure 2). The tibial component is designed to restore the patient-specific slope and the asymmetric tibial plateau, while the ligament balance may be fine-tuned using different insert heights medially and laterally [8]. According to initial biomechanical studies, this individualized design approach may lead to the restoration of more physiological knee kinematics compared to OTS implants in vitro [24,25] and in vivo [26].

This implant system has been shown to facilitate precise implant positioning and correction of the mechanical axis in radiographic studies [9,27]. The data presented in these studies are consistent with the results of an intraoperative observational study that compared the rotational alignment of the tibial component according to the method of Cobb et al. using this CCR-TKA implant system with that achieved with various OTS-TKA systems and demonstrated improved tibial component rotation with preserved cortical bone coverage for the CCR-TKA [28]. As both implant fit and rotational alignment have been shown to correlate with clinical outcomes and satisfaction [29], these previous radiological findings are in agreement with the results of our analysis that show very good patient-reported outcomes and high satisfaction at mid-term follow-up.

To date, only limited clinical data are available on this CCR-TKA system. In an intra-hospital analysis, reduced blood loss and length of stay (LOS) in the hospital has been observed for CCR-TKA compared with OTS implants at comparable tourniquet and surgical times in a cohort of 621 patients [30]. A different study compared selected hospital outcomes in a consecutive series of patients undergoing TKA using either a customized implant or an OTS implant design. The authors observed significantly lower transfusion rates and fewer adverse events at discharge and after 90 days [24]. Although hospital metrics after CCR-TKA were not assessed in this single-arm study, promising observations regarding perioperative data using CCR-TKA made in these previous studies may have been associated with high patient-reported outcomes that were systematically obtained up to 5 years post-OP in this study cohort.

This study has several limitations, and the results should be interpreted accordingly. First, there was no control group for comparison, and therefore no comparison could be made between outcomes of patients with CCR-TKA and those of patients with OTS-TKA or with TKA implanted utilizing different alignment philosophies such as mechanical or kinematic alignment. Second, there was no blinding at any stage of the procedure, and therefore the high patient-reported outcomes may have been influenced by the patient's awareness of having received a custom-made implant. Third, the OA knees included were not phenotyped according to alignment principles, which are currently under discussion. We believe that varus and valgus deformities of varying severity should be considered distinct entities of the disease, as proposed by the group of Hirschmann et al. [31]. In addition, a larger number of patients and longer study periods are needed to delineate and correlate results with phenotypes and surgical approaches. Lastly, because each implant is unique, general statements about this implant system are difficult to make, although the principles of mechanical axis reconstruction, joint line restoration, and J-curve anatomy are valid and incorporated into each CCR-TKA implant.

However, taking these limitations into account, high clinical outcomes were observed with CCR-TKA that can be compared with those of other OTS-TKA systems at mid-term follow-up. Regarding postoperative ROM, CCR-TKA showed similar or even better results compared to a previous study that assessed ROM for the Attune PS und Press-Fit-Condylar (PFC) Sigma PS TKA systems (DePuy/Synthes, New Brunswick, NJ, USA; 5° vs. 16°) at 2 years of follow-up [32], which are thought to have even higher ROM compared to the respective CR versions. Similarly, patients treated with CCR-TKA showed constantly high ROM (122° at 3–5 years FU; Figure 3), which is in contrast to results observed with the Scorpio CR TKA system, which showed a decrease in ROM 2 years postoperatively [33]. In a different study on the Genesis II TKA system (Fa. Smith & Nephew, London, UK), the authors reported worse ROM at 5 years postoperatively than in this study with the CCR-TKA (114° vs. 122°) [34].

The KSS scoring results observed with the CCR-TKA were somewhat comparable to those with the Attune PS und PFC Sigma PS TKA systems (DePuy Synthes) at 2 and 3 years [32], the Genesis II TKA system [34], and the Attune system using a rotating platform (DePuySynthes) [35] at 5 years postoperatively. Palmer et al. reported almost similar "Knee-subscores" with the Triathlon CR (Stryker Orthopaedics, Kalamazoo, MI, USA), but inferior results compared to the CCR-TKA in the "Function-subscore" (72 vs. 83 points) 2 years postoperatively [36].

In the studies by Harato et al. and Powell et al., WOMAC scores for the PFC Sigma CR or the Genesis II TKA systems at 5 years of follow-up were similar to those in this study [34,35]. In contrast Chaudhary et al. observed worse subscores for "Pain" (14.9 vs. 13.7 points) and "Function" (23.5 vs. 14.9 points) at 2 years postoperatively with the Scorpio CR TKA system compared to the results with the CCR-TKA [33].

Regarding the SF-12 scores, the Genesis II TKA system (Smith & Nephew Inc.) showed worse results in the PCS subscore (42.5 vs. 50.0 points), while the MCS subscore was the same compared to the results observed with the CCR-TKA at the same postoperative timepoint [34]. The PFC Sigma (DePuy Synthes) in comparison showed worse results for both PCS and MCS subscores [35], and the Triathlon CR (Stryker Inc.) showed worse score results for the PCS, while the MCS was at the same level [37] compared with the CCR-TKA at 5 years of follow-up.

However, none of these studies directly compared CCR-TKA with OTS-TKA, and therefore the power of all these comparisons is limited, because different study populations and observers were involved. Furthermore, it may be doubted that differences in postoperative outcomes between TKA knee designs can be elucidated by the use of quality-of-life scores such as the SF-12 or the WOMAC, as they are influenced by a variety of other factors besides knee kinematics and perception of the artificial knee. Perhaps, more refined patient-reported outcome measures such as the "Forgotten Joint Score" may be able to elaborate such differences, especially when they are used in a comparative and blinded fashion over longer periods of time [38]. Further, more refined analytical tools such as regression analysis could be applied in a comparative investigational setup, allowing for more detailed information in which variables matter most in the comparison of different TKA designs and alignment principles and of the extent and level of confidence.

Nonetheless, this study presents promising mid-term clinical outcome data using this patient-specific implant system. Our observations are also supported by the Orthopaedic Data Evaluation Panel in the United Kingdom (ODEP) (http://www.odep.org.uk, accessed on 25 January 2022), who awarded the Conformis iTotal® CR knee replacement system a

"5A" rating, based on strong evidence of implant performance over 5 years, including low revision rates as indicated in the UK's National Joint Registry (NJR).

5. Conclusions

In summary, this study demonstrates that good clinical outcomes may be achieved with this CT-based fixed-bearing CCR-TKA system, which are consistent with existing radiological, preclinical, and early clinical data. Further follow-up studies, including long-term comparative studies of clinical outcomes parameters, are needed to clarify whether this system is a valuable alternative treatment modality for patients with tricompartmental knee OA.

Author Contributions: All authors contributed to the study conception and design. Surgeries were performed by A.F.S. and M.R.; Material preparation and data collection was performed by B.J., L.S. (Lukas Sefrin), J.A. and A.F.S.; Data analysis was performed by B.J., L.S. (Lukas Sefrin), L.S. (Lennart Schroeder), and A.F.S.; The manuscript was written by A.F.S. and M.R. All authors commented on previous versions of the manuscript. All authors have read and agreed to the published version of the manuscript.

Funding: This publication was supported by the Open Access Publication Fund of the University of Wuerzburg.

Institutional Review Board Statement: Approval for this retrospective data analysis was given by the institution's review board (Reference number 2016101401).

Informed Consent Statement: All participants gave informed consent to this data analysis.

Data Availability Statement: The datasets used and/or analyzed during the current study are available from the corresponding author on reasonable request.

Acknowledgments: We are grateful to Sumesh Zingde for his help with data analysis and statistics.

Conflicts of Interest: No benefit in any form have been received or will be received from a commercial party related, directly or indirectly, to the subject of this article. A.F.S. acted as a teaching consultant for ConforMIS Inc., and M.R. received institutional support for training activities from Conformis Inc.

References

1. Noble, P.C.; Conditt, M.A.; Cook, K.F.; Mathis, K.B. The John Insall Award: Patient expectations affect satisfaction with total knee arthroplasty. *Clin. Orthop. Relat. Res.* **2006**, *452*, 35–43. [CrossRef] [PubMed]
2. Bourne, R.B.; Chesworth, B.M.; Davis, A.M.; Mahomed, N.N.; Charron, K.D. Patient satisfaction after total knee arthroplasty: Who is satisfied and who is not? *Clin. Orthop. Relat. Res.* **2010**, *468*, 57–63. [CrossRef] [PubMed]
3. Parvizi, J.; Nunley, R.M.; Berend, K.R.; Lombardi, A.V., Jr.; Ruh, E.L.; Clohisy, J.C.; Hamilton, W.G.; Della Valle, C.J.; Barrack, R.L. High level of residual symptoms in young patients after total knee arthroplasty. *Clin. Orthop. Relat. Res.* **2014**, *472*, 133–137. [CrossRef] [PubMed]
4. Nam, D.; Nunley, R.M.; Barrack, R.L. Patient dissatisfaction following total knee replacement: A growing concern? *Bone Joint J.* **2014**, *96*, 96–100. [CrossRef]
5. Batailler, C.; Swan, J.; Sappey Marinier, E.; Servien, E.; Lustig, S. New Technologies in Knee Arthroplasty: Current Concepts. *J. Clin. Med.* **2020**, *10*, 47. [CrossRef]
6. Steinert, A.F.; Sefrin, L.; Hoberg, M.; Arnholdt, J.; Rudert, M. Individualized total knee arthroplasty. *Orthopade* **2015**, *44*, 294–301. [CrossRef]
7. Steinert, A.F.; Holzapfel, B.M.; Sefrin, L.; Arnholdt, J.; Hoberg, M.; Rudert, M. Total knee arthroplasty. Patient-specific instruments and implants. *Orthopade* **2016**, *45*, 331–340. [CrossRef] [PubMed]
8. Steinert, A.F.; Sefrin, L.; Jansen, B.; Schroder, L.; Holzapfel, B.M.; Arnholdt, J.; Rudert, M. Patient-specific cruciate-retaining total knee replacement with individualized implants and instruments (iTotal CR G2). *Oper. Orthop. Traumatol.* **2021**, *33*, 170–180. [CrossRef]
9. Arnholdt, J.; Kamawal, Y.; Horas, K.; Holzapfel, B.M.; Gilbert, F.; Ripp, A.; Rudert, M.; Steinert, A.F. Accurate implant fit and leg alignment after cruciate-retaining patient-specific total knee arthroplasty. *BMC Musculoskelet Disord* **2020**, *21*, 699. [CrossRef] [PubMed]
10. Arnholdt, J.; Holzapfel, B.M.; Sefrin, L.; Rudert, M.; Beckmann, J.; Steinert, A.F. Individualized unicondylar knee replacement: Use of patient-specific implants and instruments. *Oper. Orthop. Traumatol.* **2017**, *29*, 31–39. [CrossRef] [PubMed]
11. Koeck, F.X.; Beckmann, J.; Luring, C.; Rath, B.; Grifka, J.; Basad, E. Evaluation of implant position and knee alignment after patient-specific unicompartmental knee arthroplasty. *Knee* **2011**, *18*, 294–299. [CrossRef]

12. Arnholdt, J.; Kamawal, Y.; Holzapfel, B.M.; Ripp, A.; Rudert, M.; Steinert, A.F. Evaluation of implant fit and frontal plane alignment after bi-compartmental knee arthroplasty using patient-specific instruments and implants. *Arch. Med. Sci.* **2018**, *14*, 1424–1431. [CrossRef]
13. Beckmann, J.; Steinert, A.F.; Huber, B.; Rudert, M.; Kock, F.X.; Buhs, M.; Rolston, L. Customised bi-compartmental knee arthroplasty shows encouraging 3-year results: Findings of a prospective, multicenter study. *Knee Surg. Sports Traumatol. Arthrosc* **2020**, *28*, 1742–1749. [CrossRef]
14. Steinert, A.F.; Beckmann, J.; Holzapfel, B.M.; Rudert, M.; Arnholdt, J. Bicompartmental individualized knee replacement: Use of patient-specific implants and instruments (iDuo). *Oper. Orthop. Traumatol.* **2017**, *29*, 51–58. [CrossRef]
15. Insall, J.N.; Dorr, L.D.; Scott, R.D.; Scott, W.N. Rationale of the Knee Society clinical rating system. *Clin. Orthop. Relat. Res.* **1989**, *248*, 13–14. [CrossRef]
16. Noble, P.C.; Scuderi, G.R.; Brekke, A.C.; Sikorskii, A.; Benjamin, J.B.; Lonner, J.H.; Chadha, P.; Daylamani, D.A.; Scott, W.N.; Bourne, R.B. Development of a new Knee Society scoring system. *Clin. Orthop. Relat. Res.* **2012**, *470*, 20–32. [CrossRef] [PubMed]
17. Bellamy, N.; Buchanan, W.W.; Goldsmith, C.H.; Campbell, J.; Stitt, L.W. Validation study of WOMAC: A health status instrument for measuring clinically important patient relevant outcomes to antirheumatic drug therapy in patients with osteoarthritis of the hip or knee. *J. Rheumatol.* **1988**, *15*, 1833–1840. [PubMed]
18. Stucki, G.; Meier, D.; Stucki, S.; Michel, B.A.; Tyndall, A.G.; Dick, W.; Theiler, R. Evaluation of a German version of WOMAC (Western Ontario and McMaster Universities) Arthrosis Index. *Z Rheumatol.* **1996**, *55*, 40–49.
19. Ware, J., Jr.; Kosinski, M.; Keller, S.D. A 12-Item Short-Form Health Survey: Construction of scales and preliminary tests of reliability and validity. *Med. Care* **1996**, *34*, 220–233. [CrossRef]
20. Hepinstall, M.S.; Rutledge, J.R.; Bornstein, L.J.; Mazumdar, M.; Westrich, G.H. Factors that impact expectations before total knee arthroplasty. *J. Arthroplast.* **2011**, *26*, 870–876. [CrossRef]
21. Gandhi, R.; Davey, J.R.; Mahomed, N. Patient expectations predict greater pain relief with joint arthroplasty. *J. Arthroplast.* **2009**, *24*, 716–721. [CrossRef]
22. Meier, M.; Zingde, S.; Best, R.; Schroeder, L.; Beckmann, J.; Steinert, A.F. High variability of proximal tibial asymmetry and slope: A CT data analysis of 15,807 osteoarthritic knees before TKA. *Knee Surg. Sports Traumatol. Arthrosc.* **2020**, *28*, 1105–1112. [CrossRef]
23. Meier, M.; Zingde, S.; Steinert, A.; Kurtz, W.; Koeck, F.; Beckmann, J. What Is the Possible Impact of High Variability of Distal Femoral Geometry on TKA? A CT Data Analysis of 24,042 Knees. *Clin. Orthop. Relat. Res.* **2019**, *477*, 561–570. [CrossRef] [PubMed]
24. Culler, S.D.; Martin, G.M.; Swearingen, A. Comparison of adverse events rates and hospital cost between customized individually made implants and standard off-the-shelf implants for total knee arthroplasty. *Arthroplast. Today* **2017**, *3*, 257–263. [CrossRef] [PubMed]
25. Patil, S.; Bunn, A.; Bugbee, W.D.; Colwell, C.W., Jr.; D'Lima, D.D. Patient-specific implants with custom cutting blocks better approximate natural knee kinematics than standard TKA without custom cutting blocks. *Knee* **2015**, *22*, 624–629. [CrossRef] [PubMed]
26. Zeller, I.M.; Sharma, A.; Kurtz, W.B.; Anderle, M.R.; Komistek, R.D. Customized versus Patient-Sized Cruciate-Retaining Total Knee Arthroplasty: An In Vivo Kinematics Study Using Mobile Fluoroscopy. *J. Arthroplast.* **2017**, *32*, 1344–1350. [CrossRef] [PubMed]
27. Ivie, C.B.; Probst, P.J.; Bal, A.K.; Stannard, J.T.; Crist, B.D.; Sonny Bal, B. Improved radiographic outcomes with patient-specific total knee arthroplasty. *J. Arthroplast.* **2014**, *29*, 2100–2103. [CrossRef]
28. Schroeder, L.; Martin, G. In Vivo Tibial Fit and Rotational Analysis of a Customized, Patient-Specific TKA versus Off-the-Shelf TKA. *J. Knee Surg.* **2019**, *32*, 499–505. [CrossRef]
29. Klasan, A.; Twiggs, J.G.; Fritsch, B.A.; Miles, B.P.; Heyse, T.J.; Solomon, M.; Parker, D.A. Correlation of tibial component size and rotation with outcomes after total knee arthroplasty. *Arch. Orthop. Trauma Surg.* **2020**, *140*, 1819–1824. [CrossRef]
30. Schwarzkopf, R.; Brodsky, M.; Garcia, G.A.; Gomoll, A.H. Surgical and Functional Outcomes in Patients Undergoing Total Knee Replacement with Patient-Specific Implants Compared with "Off-the-Shelf" Implants. *Orthop. J. Sports Med.* **2015**, *3*, 2325967115590379. [CrossRef]
31. Hirschmann, M.T.; Moser, L.B.; Amsler, F.; Behrend, H.; Leclerq, V.; Hess, S. Functional knee phenotypes: A novel classification for phenotyping the coronal lower limb alignment based on the native alignment in young non-osteoarthritic patients. *Knee Surg. Sports Traumatol. Arthrosc.* **2019**, *27*, 1394–1402. [CrossRef] [PubMed]
32. Ranawat, C.S.; White, P.B.; West, S.; Ranawat, A.S. Clinical and Radiographic Results of Attune and PFC Sigma Knee Designs at 2-Year Follow-Up: A Prospective Matched-Pair Analysis. *J. Arthroplast.* **2017**, *32*, 431–436. [CrossRef]
33. Chaudhary, R.; Beaupre, L.A.; Johnston, D.W. Knee range of motion during the first two years after use of posterior cruciate-stabilizing or posterior cruciate-retaining total knee prostheses. A randomized clinical trial. *J. Bone Joint Surg. Am.* **2008**, *90*, 2579–2586. [CrossRef]
34. Harato, K.; Bourne, R.B.; Victor, J.; Snyder, M.; Hart, J.; Ries, M.D. Midterm comparison of posterior cruciate-retaining versus -substituting total knee arthroplasty using the Genesis II prosthesis. A multicenter prospective randomized clinical trial. *Knee* **2008**, *15*, 217–221. [CrossRef] [PubMed]

35. Powell, A.J.; Crua, E.; Chong, B.C.; Gordon, R.; McAuslan, A.; Pitto, R.P.; Clatworthy, M.G. A randomized prospective study comparing mobile-bearing against fixed-bearing PFC Sigma cruciate-retaining total knee arthroplasties with ten-year minimum follow-up. *Bone Joint J.* **2018**, *100-B*, 1336–1344. [CrossRef] [PubMed]
36. Palmer, J.; Sloan, K.; Clark, G. Functional outcomes comparing Triathlon versus Duracon total knee arthroplasty: Does the Triathlon outperform its predecessor? *Int. Orthop.* **2014**, *38*, 1375–1378. [CrossRef]
37. Scott, C.E.; Clement, N.D.; MacDonald, D.J.; Hamilton, D.F.; Gaston, P.; Howie, C.R.; Burnett, R. Five-year survivorship and patient-reported outcome of the Triathlon single-radius total knee arthroplasty. *Knee Surg. Sports Traumatol. Arthrosc.* **2015**, *23*, 1676–1683. [CrossRef]
38. Behrend, H.; Giesinger, K.; Giesinger, J.M.; Kuster, M.S. The "forgotten joint" as the ultimate goal in joint arthroplasty: Validation of a new patient-reported outcome measure. *J. Arthroplast.* **2012**, *27*, 430–436.e431. [CrossRef]

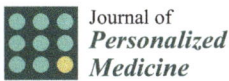

Journal of
Personalized Medicine

Article

The Patient-Specific Combined Target Zone for Morpho-Functional Planning of Total Hip Arthroplasty

Juliana Habor [1,†], Maximilian C. M. Fischer [1,†], Kunihiko Tokunaga [2], Masashi Okamoto [3] and Klaus Radermacher [1,*]

1. Chair of Medical Engineering, Helmholtz-Institute for Biomedical Engineering, RWTH Aachen University, 52074 Aachen, Germany
2. Niigata Hip Joint Center, Kameda Daiichi Hospital, Niigata City 950-0165, Japan
3. Department of Radiology, Kameda Daiichi Hospital, Niigata City 950-0165, Japan
* Correspondence: radermacher@hia.rwth-aachen.de
† These authors contributed equally to this work.

Abstract: Background Relevant criteria for total hip arthroplasty (THA) planning have been introduced in the literature which include the hip range of motion, bony coverage, anterior cup overhang, leg length discrepancy, edge loading risk, and wear. The optimal implant design and alignment depends on the patient's anatomy and patient-specific functional parameters such as the pelvic tilt. The approaches proposed in literature often consider one or more criteria for THA planning. but to the best of our knowledge none of them follow an integrated approach including all criteria for the definition of a patient-specific combined target zone (PSCTZ). **Questions/purposes** (1) How can we calculate suitable THA implant and implantation parameters for a specific patient considering all relevant criteria? (2) Are the resulting target zones in the range of conventional safe zones? (3) Do patients who fulfil these combined criteria have a better outcome score? **Methods** A method is presented that calculates individual target zones based on the morphology, range of motion and load acting on the hip joint and merges them into the PSCTZ. In a retrospective analysis of 198 THA patients, it was calculated whether the patients were inside or outside the Lewinnek safe zone, Dorr combined anteversion range and PSCTZ. The postoperative Harris Hip Scores (HHS) between insiders and outsiders were compared. **Results** 11 patients were inside the PSCTZ. Patients inside and outside the PSCTZ showed no significant difference in the HHS. However, a significant higher HHS was observed for the insiders of two of the three sub-target zones incorporated in the PSCTZ. By combining the sub-target zones in the PSCTZ, all PSCTZ insiders except one had an HHS higher than 90. **Conclusions** The results might suggest that, for a prosthesis implanted in the PSCTZ a low outcome score of the patient is less likely than using the conventional safe zones by Lewinnek and Dorr. For future studies, a larger cohort of patients inside the PSCTZ is needed which can only be achieved if the cases are planned prospectively with the method introduced in this paper. **Clinical Relevance** The method presented in this paper could help the surgeon combining multiple different criteria during THA planning and find the suitable implant design and alignment for a specific patient.

Keywords: total hip arthroplasty; preoperative planning; patient-specific THA; target zone; safe zone; leg length discrepancy; range of motion; edge loading

1. Introduction

Major complications of total hip arthroplasty (THA) and reasons for revisions are infections, dislocations, wear and loosening [1–3]. Different studies found dislocation rates of 0.2% to 10% [4]. When considering 1% and over one million THA surgeries per year worldwide [4], the absolute numbers of dislocations would be over 10,000 cases per year. The number of young and active patients is increasing [5]. The revision rate for patients younger than fifty is higher than in older patients [6]. This indicates that more active lifestyle puts higher demands on the prosthesis [4]. The complications could be addressed by a proper choice of the implant components (size and shape, or implant parameters) and their alignment (position and orientation, or implantation parameters) within the patient's bony structures. Various methods for finding suitable or optimal parameters have been introduced in the literature. Often, the term safe zone describes cup orientations with a low risk for dislocation. In this paper, a more general term, namely target zone, is used to describe a comprehensive set of suitable implant and implantation parameters (and not only the cup orientation).

There are studies using statistical analysis to find a correlation between the clinical outcome and the implant and implantation parameters. Lewinnek suggested aligning the cup with an inclination of $40° \pm 10°$ and anteversion of $15° \pm 10°$ (the so-called Lewinnek safe zone) in order to reduce the dislocation risk [7]. However, studies showed that the majority of dislocated or revised hips had cup orientations within the safe zone [8–10]. Other safe zones [11–20] and rules for combined anteversion of the cup and stem [16,17,21–23] were suggested. Dorr et al., for instance, found a safe range for combined anteversion of $25°$ to $50°$ [23]. However, these safe zones and ranges are not consistent with each other.

Further publications introduced methods for deriving optimal parameters by considering certain criteria, such as the range of motion (ROM) and prosthetic impingement [24–32], bony impingement [33–37], bony cup coverage [38–40], leg length discrepancy, wear rate and edge loading risk [31,32,41–44]. Dislocation is either caused by a levering-out motion due to impingement, or sliding-out motion when the resulting hip force is directed outside of the cup [31]. The hip force affects the wear rate and edge loading which influences the longevity of the implant.

The methods in literature often include one or more criteria but to the best of our knowledge none considers all criteria at once. Consequently, in many cases only a few relevant criteria are evaluated quantitatively whereas others are considered only implicitly or neglected in the daily clinical routine of the patient-specific surgical planning process. Often, a compromise between conflicting objectives has to be found. For instance, positioning the cup for maximal ROM might reduce the bony cup coverage. The cup and stem positioning, the caput–collum–diaphyseal (CCD) angle and the neck length have an influence on the leg length discrepancy but also on the hip force.

The pelvic tilt which has a high variability among different patients and between different postures (supine, standing, sitting) has a direct influence on the functional cup orientation [45–47]. Algorithms for calculating the changed cup orientation due to the pelvic tilt have been introduced [48–52]. Some THA planning methods include the pelvic tilt during calculation of edge loading [41] or during ROM analysis [29].

The aim of this study is to investigate the following questions:

1. How can we calculate suitable THA implant and implantation parameters for a specific patient considering the most relevant criteria?
2. Are the resulting target zones inside conventional safe zones?
3. Do patients with implantations fulfilling these combined criteria have a better outcome score?

2. Material and Methods

2.1. Patient-Specific Target Zone Calculation

We developed a method for calculating the patient-specific combined target zone (PSCTZ) incorporating a more comprehensive set of relevant criteria from (currently) three different target zones addressing different objectives of an optimal implant and implantation planning (Figure 1). Single target zones are calculated based on criteria related to the morphology, ROM, and load situation which are then merged into the PSCTZ. Other criteria can be added in a modular fashion. Hence, the PSCTZ is the overlap of all single target zones.

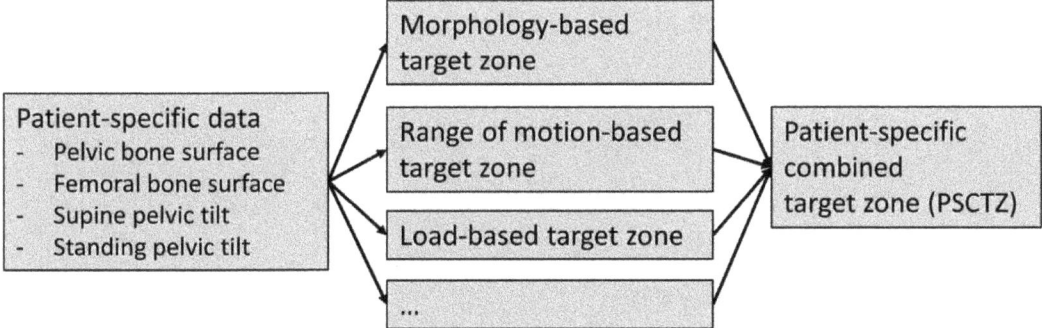

Figure 1. Overview of the concept for patient-specific combined target zone calculation.

Patient-specific morphological and functional data including surface models of the pelvis and femur and the pelvic tilt of functional positions for daily living are needed to calculate each target zone. The surface models can be reconstructed from CT data as in most CT-based planning and navigation systems [53–55]. The pelvic tilt can be derived, for instance, from lateral radiographs [56], EOS imaging combined with CT [57], inclinometers [52] or navigated ultrasound [58,59].

The considered implant parameters are cup size, head/neck ratio, CCD angle and neck length. The considered implantation parameters are cup inclination, cup anteversion, 3D cup position, 3D stem position, stem ante-torsion, stem adduction, and stem flexion. These relate to the pelvic or femoral bone coordinate system. In the current study, the pelvic coordinate system is based on the anterior pelvic plane (APP). The center of rotation is the origin. For the pelvis in standing position, the APP is tilted relative to the frontal plane according to the patient-specific standing tilt, and the line connecting the left and right anterior superior iliac spine is parallel to the horizontal axis. The femoral coordinate system is based on the table top position [60] and the mechanical axis, with the center of rotation being the origin. The femur is in neutral position if the mechanical axis is parallel to the vertical axis and the line connecting the posterior condyles is parallel to the frontal plane.

The implant design and alignment influence the relative alignment of the pelvis and femur. The cup position defines the center of rotation. The femoral alignment depends on the stem position, stem orientation and the CCD angle, since these parameters change the head center position. Hence, a transformation is applied to the femur in order to realign the mechanical axis to the vertical axis.

2.1.1. Morphology-Based Target Zone

The criteria considered in the morphology-based target zones are related to the bony anatomy of the patient. The cup coverage, anterior cup overhang, distance prior to cup penetration, and the leg length discrepancy are calculated (Figure 2).

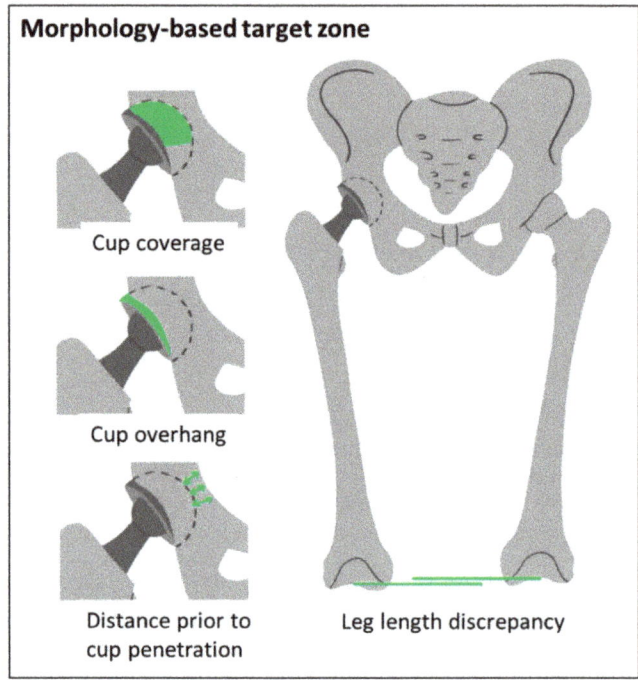

Figure 2. Criteria considered for the morphology-based target zone.

The cup is modelled as hemisphere. The overlapping area between the hemisphere and the acetabulum is determined for calculation of the percentage of coverage, similar to a method proposed by Ueno et al. [39]. The surface of the cup counts as covered if it overlaps by more than 0.5 mm. Then, it is determined which part of the uncovered area of the cup is overhanging and the maximal anterior cup overhang is calculated. Furthermore, the shortest distance from the outer shell of the cup and the medial surface of the pelvic bone is calculated, defining the distance prior to cup penetration. Lastly, the leg length discrepancy is determined by comparing the height of the intercondylar notch on both sides. The bones are neutrally aligned for all calculations.

All implant and implantation parameters that satisfy the following criteria are considered as within the morphology-based target zone:

- A bony coverage of at least 65%.
- An anterior cup overhang of less than 12 mm.
- A distance prior to cup penetration of at least 1 mm,
- A maximal leg length discrepancy of ±8 mm.

A minimum cup coverage of 60% measured in anterior-posterior radiographs [40] or 61.2% measured on the upper portion of a 3D cup model [39] were recommended in recent studies. A more conservative threshold of 65% was chosen here. A study showed that patients with iliopsoas impingement on the acetabular cup which might induce pain had anterior cup overhang of more than 12 mm measured in CT data [61]. The distance prior to penetration was considered in automated planning methods [62,63]. A limit of 1 mm was chosen in order to prevent penetration. A leg length discrepancy of 10 mm was stated as a critical threshold [64]. A more conservative 8 mm was chosen here. These thresholds can be adjusted to the individual patient or other standard values.

2.1.2. ROM-Based Target Zone

The criteria considered in the ROM-based target zones are related to the prosthetic and bony impingement risk while performing a target ROM (Figure 3). The target ROM can be defined based on literature data [27,30,65,66] and might be adapted based on patient-specific characteristics and requirements.

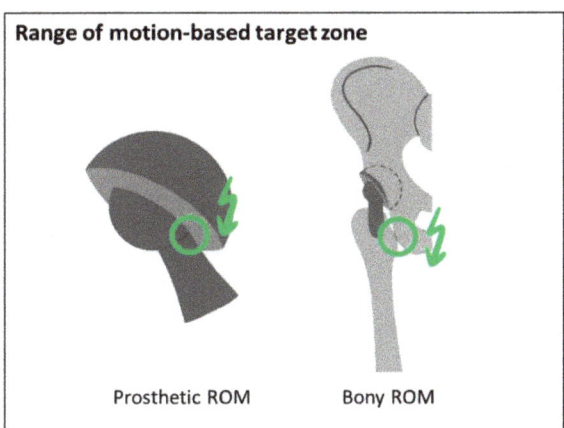

Figure 3. Criteria considered for the ROM-based target zone.

A method introduced by our group is used for calculating the prosthetic ROM-based target zone [29]. Impingement is detected using a 3D to 2D mapping and a 2D distance map function and by evaluating the position of the neck axis relative to the cup limits, including the head/neck ratio. The pelvic tilt angle in standing position is applied to the pelvis before performing the motion of the femur defined by the target ROM relative to the pelvis [29]. In this study, the target ROM proposed by Sugano was selected defined by 120° flexion, 40° extension, 40° abduction and 40° internal rotation at 90° flexion [66]. Additionally, the supine pelvic tilt was considered in the calculation of the ROM-based safe zone, with a modified target ROM with 90° flexion, 5° extension, 30° internal rotation at 90° flexion and 30° external rotation at neutral flexion. For calculating bony impingement, our method was extended to incorporate arbitrary surface shapes. Potential impingement points (PIP) are derived by calculating the intersection of the femoral and pelvic surface with spheres of different radii positioned in the hip joint center. Figure 4A shows the PIP between the femur and the pelvis. Then, the mapping as described by Hsu is performed to calculate the minimal distance to impingement [29]. Figure 4B shows exemplarily the results of the mapping function for a flexion motion. Figure 4C shows the resulting minimal distances for each PIP. Instead of evaluating the absolute distance, the decrease compared to the preoperative situation is calculated for the bony ROM.

All implant and implantation parameters that satisfy the following criteria are considered as within the ROM-based target zone:

- No prosthetic impingement: distance to prosthetic impingement greater than 0°.
- A decrease of the bony ROM of less than 5° compared to the preoperative situation.

These thresholds can be adjusted to the individual patient or other standard values. Due to a slight medialization of the rotation center, most patients had a slight decrease of the bony ROM. Therefore, a small threshold for bony ROM decrease of 5° was chosen arbitrarily.

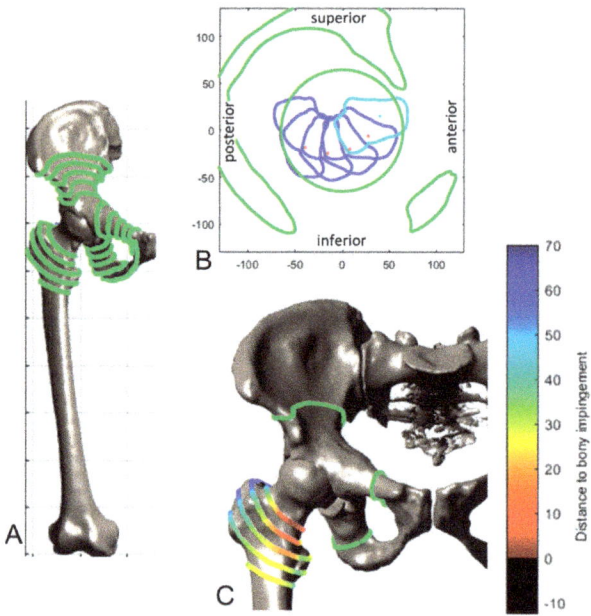

Figure 4. 3D and 2D visualization of possible impinging points (PIP). (**A**): The PIPs are depicted in green on the femur and pelvis. (**B**): 2D mapping containing the cup and pelvic limits (green) for an exemplary flexion motion of the femur (blue). (**C**): The femoral PIP color-coded by the minimal distance to impingement.

2.1.3. Load-Based Target Zone

The amplitude and orientation of the resulting hip force and the resulting minimal distance to edge loading are calculated for the load-based target zone and compared to the preoperative situation (Figure 5).

The resulting hip force in one-leg stance as a surrogate for the peak force phase of level walking is calculated. Firstly, a cadaver template is patient-specifically adapted. The TLEM2.0 cadaver is individually scaled by deforming the femur and pelvis based on bony landmarks of the patient's preoperative data, as well as the bony and prosthetic landmarks of the postoperative data. Then the pelvis of the scaled template is aligned by the patient-specific standing pelvic tilt. The scaled and aligned template serves as input to calculate the hip force using an approach proposed by our group [67]. Then, the contact patch between the femoral head and the cup is calculated using a model described by Imado et al. [68]. The distance to edge loading is defined as the minimal angular distance of the boundary of the contact patch to the rim of the cup. This was calculated using the same method as for calculating the distance to impingement, as described above and in [29].

All implant and implantation parameters that satisfy the following criteria are considered as within the load-based target zone:

- No edge loading: a minimal distance to edge loading greater than $0°$.
- No increase of the resulting hip force: a decrease of the resulting hip force compared to the preoperative situation.

These thresholds can be adjusted to the individual patient or other standard values.

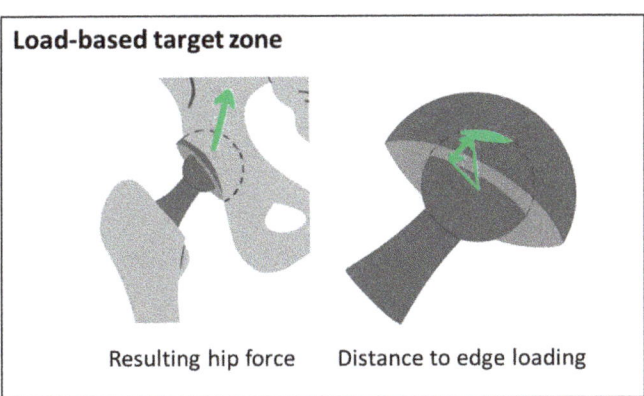

Figure 5. Criteria considered for the load-based target zone.

2.2. Retrospective Analysis

Figure 6 gives an overview of the study design. All patients were operated using conventional preoperative planning and CT-based navigation by one surgeon (KT). For the retrospective analysis, the anatomical and functional data needed for the PSCTZ calculation were extracted from the preoperative data. The actual implant and implantation parameters were extracted from the postoperative data. Whether the patients were inside the PSCTZ, the Lewinnek safe zone and combined anteversion, and whether the patients inside the target zones have a better outcome, were analyzed.

The data of 201 THA patients was retrospectively selected to apply the method described above. There were 171 female and 30 male patients with a mean age of 62.9 years (range 34 to 91 years), a mean height of 1.56 m (range 1.40 to 1.82 m), a mean weight of 57.1 kg (range 35.9 to 103.8 kg), resulting in a mean BMI of 23.4 kg/m^2 (range 16.6 to 34.5 kg/m^2).

The diagnoses before surgery were osteoarthritis (183 patients), idiopathic osteonecrosis of the femoral head (six patients), subchondral insufficient fracture of the femoral head (six patients), femoral acetabular impingement (five patients) and acetabular fracture (one patient). All THA were performed using an anterolateral modified Watson-Jones approach in the lateral position. The CT-based planning and navigation systems used were LEXI ZedHip, Brainlab VectorVision Hip 3.5 or Stryker Hip Navigation. Implanted cups include Zimmer Continuum, Zimmer G7 OsseoTi, Kyocera SQRUM and Stryker Trident. The stems used were CLS, Modulus, Kyocera J-Taper HO, Stryker Accolade and Stryker Accolade II. Pre- and postoperative supine CT images with an isometric pixel spacing of 0.76 mm and a slice thickness and distance of 1 mm of the entire pelvis and both femurs and standing EOS images of the lower extremities including the entire pelvis were acquired from each patient. One patient was eliminated from the study due to missing slices in the postoperative CT images. The postoperative Harris Hip Score (HHS) [69] after one year was available for 199 patients. Therefore, the cohort consisted of 198 patients.

The preoperative CT images were semi-automatically segmented. The thresholds for bone were set to 200 and 2000 Hounsfield units. The surfaces were processed as described in a previous paper of our group [70]. The resulting meshes had a minimum and maximum edge length of 0.5 and 100 mm and a maximum deviation of 0.05 mm compared to the CT segmentation. The surface data served as the input for the PSCTZ calculation. The pelvic landmarks and coordinate system were automatically identified using the ITP method [70]. The landmarks required for the calculation of the femoral coordinate system were detected using the A&A method [71]. The automatically detected landmarks were reviewed and additional landmarks were manually identified by one experienced expert. To measure the preoperative standing pelvic tilt, the segmented surface of the pelvis was registered to the biplanar EOS images using the CT2EOS method [57].

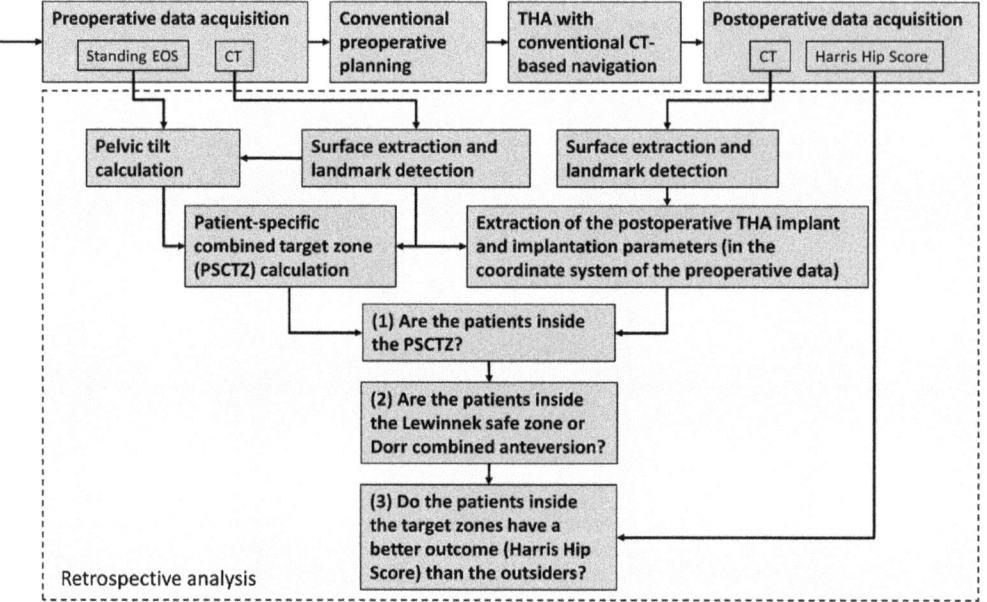

Figure 6. Overview of the retrospective study design.

The bony surfaces of the postoperative CT images were reconstructed similar to the preoperative data. Areas with strong artifacts induced by the implant were omitted. The implants were segmented using a threshold of 2000 Hounsfield units. In case of a ceramic inlay, the cup and the head were manually separated by using a sphere. Spheres and circles were fitted to the reconstructed surfaces of the cup and stem to derive the center of rotation, neck axis, neck, head and outer cup radius and cup orientation. The cup orientation is calculated according to Murray's radiographic definition [72] relative to the pelvic coordinate system. Two landmarks were manually selected on the proximal and distal end of the surface model of the stem to define the stem axis (similar to [73]). The neck and stem axis were used to calculate the stem orientation, stem position, CCD angle and neck length using homogenous matrix operations [74]. The postoperative were registered to the preoperative bone models to describe the implant alignment relatively [57].

Subsequently, it was evaluated which patients were inside the PSCTZ, Lewinnek safe zone and Dorr combined anteversion range. The HHS was used for a comparison of the outcome of the patients inside and outside the target and safe zones. The HHS is not normally distributed. Therefore, two-sided Wilcoxon rank sum test was performed to test the difference. The statistical significance level was set at $\alpha = 0.05$. It was also evaluated whether the age was similar between the insiders and outsiders using the same method.

3. Results

Complications after THA were the followings: two dislocations, one impingement, five psoas syndromes, eight greater trochanter fractures, one acetabular fracture, two peroneal nerve palsies, one sciatic nerve palsy, one stem subsidence and one ectopic ossification. The number of patients inside the morphology-based, ROM-based, load-based and inside all three single target zones and, therefore, inside the PSCTZ are listed in Table 1. The calculated values of each criterion are presented in Table 2.

Table 1. Number of patients inside and outside the conventional and patient-specific target zones and their median HHS and age.

			Inside				Outside		
	n		Median (Min., Max.)	Percentage of Insiders below a HHS of 95 (%)	n		Median (Min., Max.)	Percentage of Insiders below a HHS of 95 (%)	p
Lewinnek safe zone	176	HHS	99 (63, 100)	20	22	HHS	95 (71, 100)	50	0.002
		Age	62 (34, 91)			Age	70 (54, 85)		0.000
Dorr combined anteversion	133	HHS	99 (70, 100)	24	65	HHS	99 (63, 100)	23	0.771
		Age	63 (34, 87)			Age	62 (38, 91)		0.600
Patient-specific target zones									
Morphology-based	70	HHS	100 (74, 100)	14	128	HHS	99 (63, 100)	29	0.022
		Age	62 (38, 87)			Age	63 (34, 91)		0.256
ROM-based	42	HHS	98 (70, 100)	26	156	HHS	99 (63, 100)	23	0.481
		Age	67 (51, 82)			Age	63 (34, 91)		0.110
Load-based	162	HHS	99 (70, 100)	20	36	HHS	97 (63, 100)	39	0.029
		Age	62 (34, 87)			Age	70 (38, 91)		0.008
PSCTZ	11	HHS	100 (87, 100)	18	187	HHS	99 (63, 100)	24	0.466
		Age	62 (52, 82)			Age	63 (34, 91)		0.972

Table 2. Calculated values of each criterion of the PSCTZ.

Criterion	Median (Q1 to Q3, Min. to Max.)	Mean ± SD
Cup coverage (%)	79.6 (72.0 to 86.6, 49.8 to 97.7)	78.7 ± 9.8
Max. Anterior cup overhang (mm)	9.1 (4.4 to 14.8, 0.0 to 38.5)	9.9 ± 7.2
Distance prior to cup penetration (mm)	2.0 (0.4 to 3.7, −4.5 to 9.1)	2.0 ± 2.6
Leg length discrepancy (mm)	0.8 (−3.8 to 5.2, −48.1 to 27.0)	0.8 ± 8.4
Distance to prosthetic impingement (°)	−0.4 (−4.1 to 2.2, −17.1 to 10.6)	−1.1 ± 5.1
Decrease of bony ROM (°)	0.6 (−4.6 to 6.3, −32.7 to 18.3)	−0.2 ± 8.9
Min. distance to edge loading (°)	5.6 (1.6 to 8.7, −14.9 to 21.6)	5.1 ± 6.3
Decrease of the resulting hip force (%BW)	−0.6 (−1.0 to −0.3, −8.7 to 2.4)	−0.7 ± 0.9

Figure 7 shows four exemplary cases which are inside none, one, two or all three patient-specific target zones.

The distribution of the cup orientation and combined anteversion of the patients inside and outside the PSCTZ and the range of the conventional safe zones are shown in Figure 8. Two PSCTZ insiders were outside the Lewinnek safe zone and two outside the Dorr combined anteversion range.

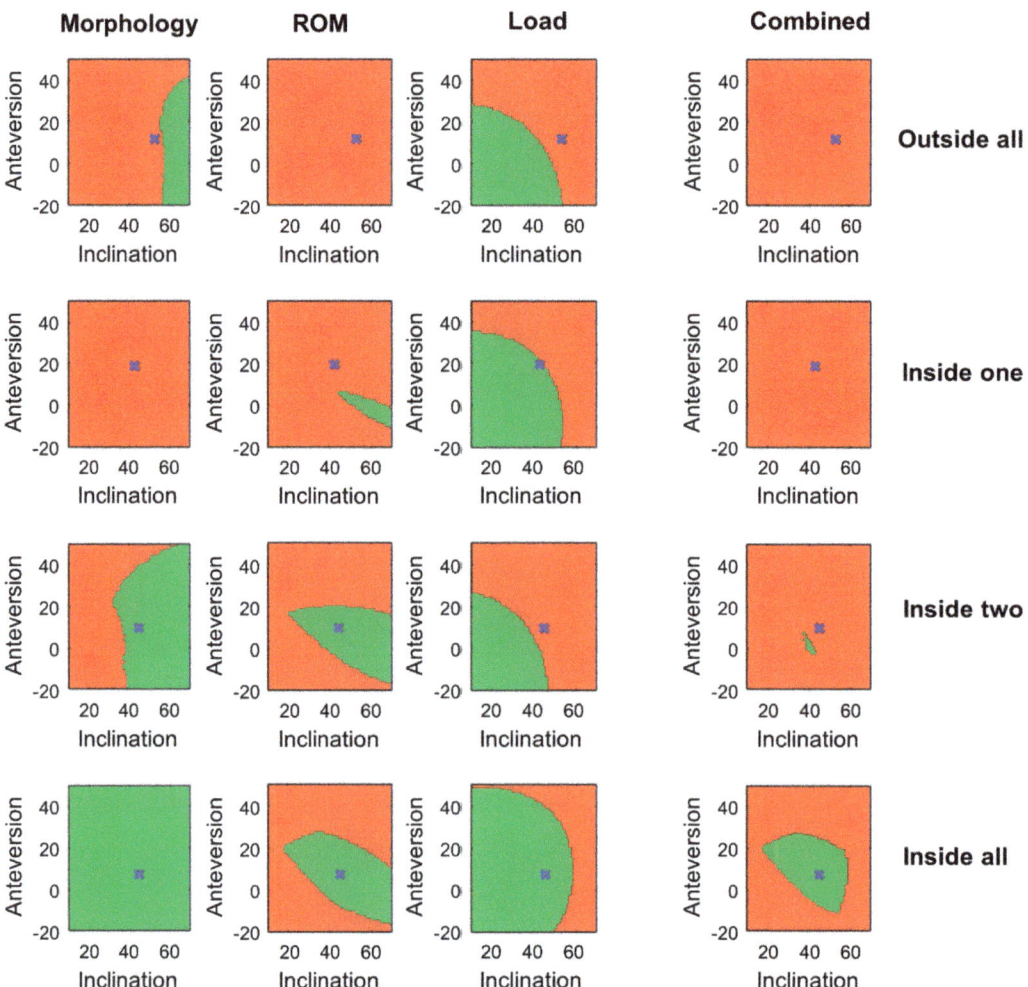

Figure 7. Patient-specific morphology-based, ROM-based, load-based and combined target zone for four exemplary cases. The target zones for the implant and implantation parameters based on the postoperative CT data is shown. The blue x marks the measured postoperative cup orientation.

The HHS of the patients inside and outside the conventional safe zones are shown in Figure 9 and Table 1. Patients inside the Lewinnek safe zone had a significantly higher HHS and are also significantly younger compared to the outsiders. No significant difference existed regarding the HHS and age between insiders and outsiders for the Dorr combined anteversion range.

Figure 10 and Table 1 show the HHS of the patients inside and outside the individual target zones. Insiders of the morphology-based target zone had a significantly higher score than the outsiders. No significant difference in age was found. No significant difference was found between insiders and outsiders of the ROM-based target zone regarding HHS and age. For the load-based target zone, insiders had a significant higher median HHS and a significant younger age compared to the outsiders. No significant difference between the two groups was evident for the PSCTZ. In all single target zones, some insiders have low

HHS. Only if the target zones were combined into the PSCTZ were almost all patients with a low HHS removed.

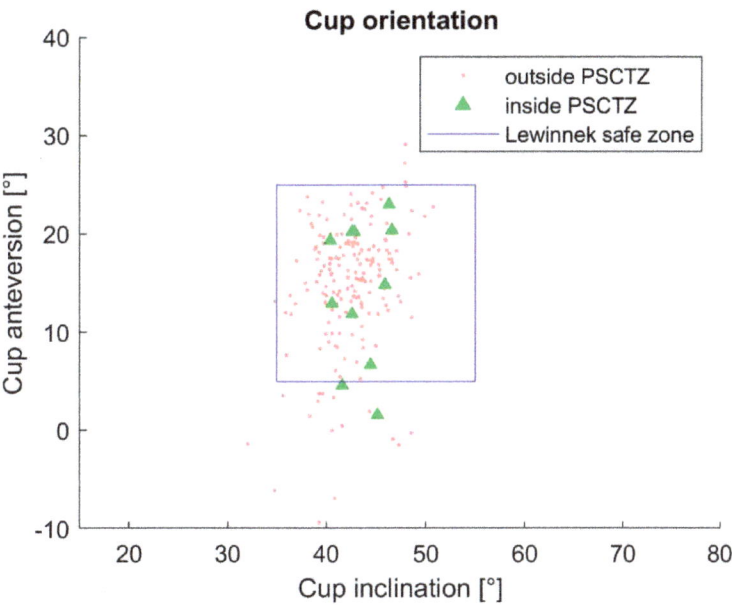

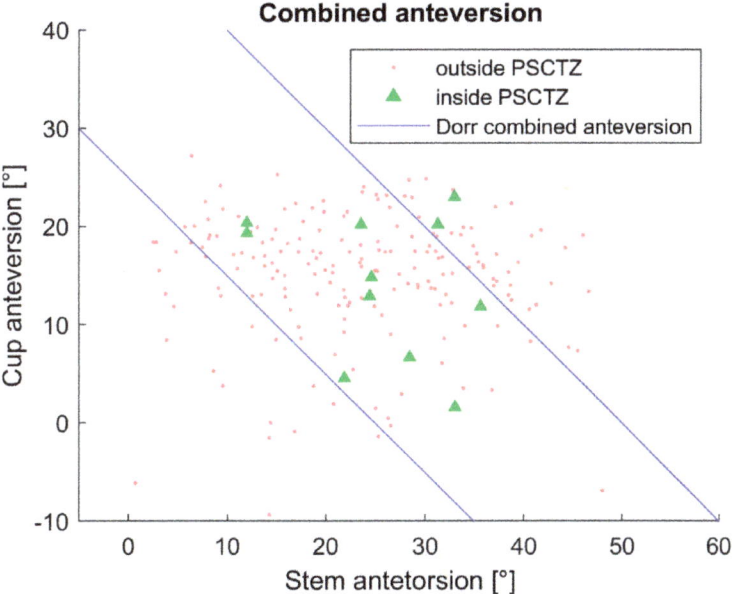

Figure 8. Distribution of the cup orientation and the combined anteversion of the PCSTZ-insiders and outsiders. The conventional safe zones by Lewinnek and Dorr are also visualized.

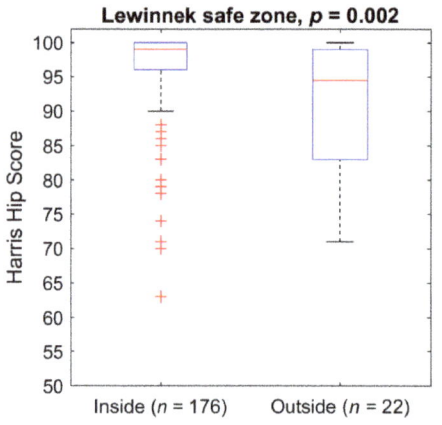
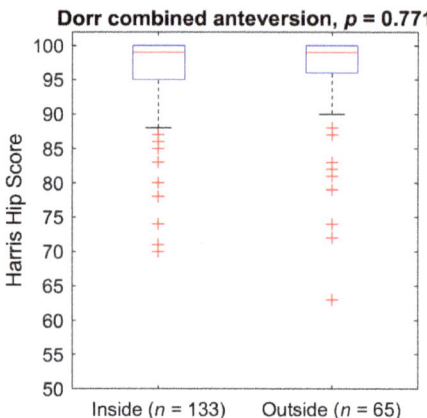

Figure 9. The HHS of the patients divided by the conventional target zones.

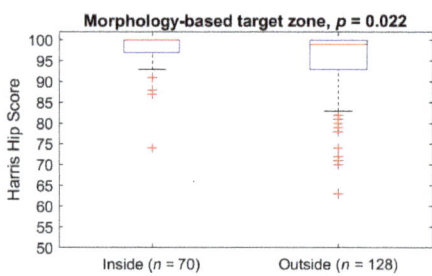

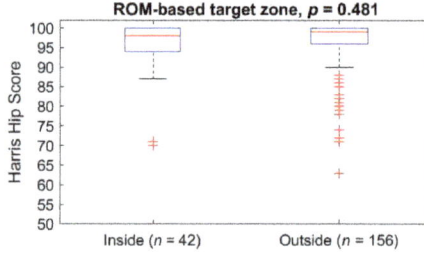
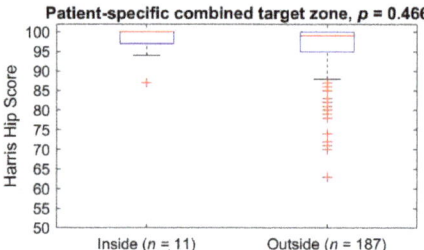

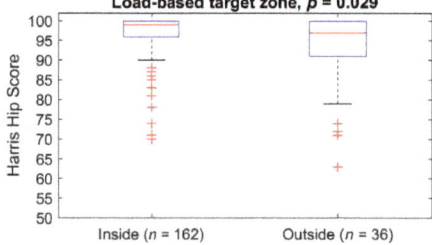

Figure 10. HHS of the patients divided by individual and combined target zones.

4. Discussion

A method for calculating suitable THA implant and implantation parameters for a specific patient considering the most relevant criteria mentioned in the literature was introduced. Additional criteria can be added in a modular fashion. The majority of patients in the cohort show an excellent outcome based on the high median HHS. Fewer patients with an HHS below 95 can be observed inside the PSCTZ. If patients are divided by the individual target zones, the difference is less obvious. Only when all target zones are combined were most outliers with lower scores removed. This stresses the importance of combining all relevant criteria into the planning process. It should be further analyzed how each target zone contributes to the PSCTZ. Only 6% of patients were inside the PSCTZ. More patients inside the PSCTZ might be necessary to detect a significant difference between insiders and outsiders. This could be achieved by a larger cohort or prospective study.

A prospective study would also enable a division of the patients into a treatment and a control group with an even sampling of the cases regarding age, comorbidities and other factors which might affect the postoperative outcome. The current results show that, for some groups, a significant higher HHS coincides with a significantly younger age.

The number of patients inside the Lewinnek safe zone and the Dorr combined anteversion range is very large compared to the number of patients inside the PSCTZ. One reason for the latter might be that not all the criteria used for the PSCTZ were considered during the planning and implantation process, since the commercial planning systems could not offer the method proposed in this paper. Figures 9 and 10 show that the PSCTZ is more conservative than the conventional safe zones. It provides a refined target for the cup orientation and does not violate the recommendation specified by Lewinnek for most of the patients. In the current study, 167 patients were inside the Lewinnek safe zone but outside the PSCTZ. Based on a cohort of 206 patients with dislocations after THA, Abdel et al. showed that 58% of them were within the Lewinnek safe zone [10]. It would be interesting to know whether these patients were inside the PSCTZ. For a related detailed analysis, 3D data of the bony anatomy and implant and implantation parameters of the patients would be required.

Whether the HHS is an adequate score for measuring the clinical outcome of THA is questionable [75]. The HHS reflects certain aspects such as pain and the ability to perform some ADLs. The ROM and anatomical deformities are considered, but have a minor impact on the overall score. Whether a patient had a dislocation is not represented by the score. Mid- and long-term aseptic loosening and wear can be related to resulting hip forces and edge loading, but might be not reflected in a short-term HHS evaluation. Hence, the HHS may not represent all criteria used for PSCTZ calculation. A significant difference in HHS is not necessarily clinically significant. In addition to the HHS, other outcome measures quantifying the quality of life of the patient, such as the Western Ontario and McMaster Universities Osteoarthritis Index (WOMAC) or hip disability and osteoarthritis outcome score (HOOS) might be considered in the future. However, these outcome measures might exhibit the same limitations as mentioned for the HHS.

The cohort contains only Japanese patients. Data of patients from other countries are needed for a further validation of the PSCTZ. The resulting PSCTZ strongly depends on the definition of target ROM and the thresholds of minimal bony coverage, residual bone thickness, maximum anterior cup overhang, distances to impingement and edge loading, and decrease in the resulting hip force. Whether the thresholds are chosen adequately in this study has to be further evaluated. In the future, the thresholds could be defined or adapted according to patient-specific requirements.

The standing pelvic tilt might change after THA [76,77], which changes the functional cup orientation. Using the preoperative pelvic tilt might not reflect the postoperative situation. Especially if the cup orientation is already at the boundary of the PSCTZ, a different pelvic tilt might cause the implant to be outside of the PSCTZ. Therefore, a prediction of the postoperative pelvic tilt from preoperative data as proposed in a recent study of our group could be useful [57]. Other studies recommend the inclusion of additional pelvic tilts, such as sitting, in the ROM and load analysis [47]. Unfortunately, we could only include standing and supine pelvic in the ROM analysis, hence other pelvic tilts were not available for the cohort.

The ROM-based target zone considers only prosthetic and bony impingement. Other planning software also examines bone to implant impingement [78,79]. The approach to detect bony impingent introduced in this study should be compared with other approaches for impingement detection, for instance a collision detection algorithm. The latter also allows for integration of asymmetric cup designs, which is not possible with the prosthetic impingement method used in this study. Osteophytes were not removed from the preoperative pelvic surface models, which might lead to false bony impingement detection in case the osteophytes are resected during THA. These might be reasons for the missing significant difference between in- and outsiders of the ROM-based target zone.

Additional limitations of the study have to be considered. The calculation of the leg length was based on the knee joint, since CT data of the ankle joint was not recorded. The leg length discrepancy might be incorrect if it results from a difference of the lower limbs.

Although different prediction models for the hip force are already commercially used in 2D and 3D preoperative planning of THA [41,80], the validity of the hip force prediction and the contact patch calculation for different bearing surfaces has to be further evaluated [67].

5. Conclusions

Numerous criteria are relevant for THA planning, but conventional planning methods do not systematically consider these together in an integrated approach. The proposed method calculates a PSCTZ including the most relevant criteria. More criteria could and should be added into the modular framework. A retrospective analysis shows that, for a prosthesis implanted in the PSCTZ, a low outcome score of the patient is less likely than using the conventional safe zones. This finding should be further evaluated in a prospective study.

Author Contributions: J.H., M.C.M.F. and K.R. designed the study. K.T. and M.O. collected the clinical data. J.H. and M.C.M.F. processed and analyzed the data and wrote the code. J.H. and M.C.M.F. wrote the manuscript. All authors discussed the results and reviewed the manuscript. All authors have read and agreed to the published version of the manuscript.

Funding: The authors received no specific funding for this work.

Institutional Review Board Statement: The clinical protocol was approved by the Kameda Daiichi Hospital review board. The authors confirm that all methods were performed in accordance with the relevant guidelines and regulations.

Informed Consent Statement: All patients were informed about the use of their anonymized medical data, including medical images, for scientific research and written informed consent was obtained from all patients.

Data Availability Statement: The datasets generated during and/or analyzed in this study are available from the corresponding author upon reasonable requests.

Conflicts of Interest: The authors declare no conflict of interests.

References

1. Bozic, K.J.; Kurtz, S.M.; Lau, E.; Ong, K.; Vail, T.P.; Berry, D.J. The epidemiology of revision total hip arthroplasty in the United States. *J. Bone Jt. Surg.* **2009**, *91*, 128–133. [CrossRef]
2. Pivec, R.; Johnson, A.J.; Mears, S.C.; Mont, M.A. Hip arthroplasty. *Lancet* **2012**, *380*, 1768–1777. [CrossRef]
3. Opperer, M.; Lee, Y.Y.; Nally, F.; Perez, A.B.; Goudarz-Mehdikhani, K.; Della Valle, A.G. A critical analysis of radiographic factors in patients who develop dislocation after elective primary total hip arthroplasty. *Int. Orthop.* **2016**, *40*, 703–708. [CrossRef] [PubMed]
4. Ferguson, R.J.; Palmer, A.J.; Taylor, A.; Porter, M.L.; Malchau, H.; Glyn-Jones, S. Hip replacement. *Lancet* **2018**, *392*, 1662–1671. [CrossRef]

5. Kuijpers, M.F.L.; Hannink, G.; Vehmeijer, S.B.W.; van Steenbergen LNSchreurs, B.W. The risk of revision after total hip arthroplasty in young patients depends on surgical approach, femoral head size and bearing type; an analysis of 19,682 operations in the Dutch arthroplasty register. *BMC Musculoskelet. Disord.* **2019**, *20*, 385. [CrossRef]
6. Corbett, K.L.; Losina, E.; Nti, A.A.; Prokopetz JJZKatz, J.N. Population-based rates of revision of primary total hip arthroplasty: A systematic review. *PLoS ONE* **2010**, *5*, e13520. [CrossRef] [PubMed]
7. Lewinnek, G.E.; Lewis, J.L.; Tarr, R.; Compere CLZimmerman, J.R. Dislocations after total hip-replacement arthroplasties. *J. Bone Jt. Surg.* **1978**, *60*, 217–220. [CrossRef]
8. Callanan, M.C.; Jarrett, B.; Bragdon, C.R.; Zurakowski, D.; Rubash, H.E.; Freiberg, A.A.; Malchau, H. The John Charnley Award: Risk factors for cup malpositioning: Quality improvement through a joint registry at a tertiary hospital. *Clin. Orthop. Relat. Res.* **2011**, *469*, 319–329. [CrossRef]
9. Seagrave, K.G.; Troelsen, A.; Malchau, H.; Husted, H.; Gromov, K. Acetabular cup position and risk of dislocation in primary total hip arthroplasty: A systematic review of the literature. *Acta Orthop.* **2016**, *88*, 10–17. [CrossRef]
10. Abdel, M.P.; Roth, P.; von Jennings, M.T.; Hanssen, A.D.; Pagnano, M.W. What Safe Zone? The Vast Majority of Dislocated THAs Are Within the Lewinnek Safe Zone for Acetabular Component Position. *Clin. Orthop. Relat. Res.* **2016**, *474*, 386–391. [CrossRef]
11. Fackler, C.D.; Poss, R. Dislocation in total hip arthroplasties. *Clin. Orthop. Relat. Res.* **1980**, *151*, 169–178. [CrossRef]
12. Ali Khan, M.A.; Brakenbury, P.H.; Reynolds, I.S. Dislocation following total hip replacement. *J. Bone Jt. Surg.* **1981**, *63*, 214–218. [CrossRef]
13. Dorr, L.D.; Wolf, A.W.; Chandler, R.; Conaty, J.P. Classification and treatment of dislocations of total hip arthroplasty. *Clin. Orthop. Relat. Res.* **1983**, *173*, 151–158. [CrossRef]
14. Kohn, D.; Rühmann, O.; Wirth, C.J. Die Verrenkung der Hüfttotalendoprothese unter besonderer Beachtung verschiedener Zugangswege. *Z. Orthop. Ihre. Grenzgeb.* **1997**, *135*, 40–44. [CrossRef] [PubMed]
15. Biedermann, R.; Tonin, A.; Krismer, M.; Rachbauer, F.; Eibl, G.; Stöckl, B. Reducing the risk of dislocation after total hip arthroplasty. The Effect of Orientation of the Acetabular Component. *J. Bone Jt. Surg.* **2005**, *87*, 762–769. [CrossRef] [PubMed]
16. Masaoka, T.; Yamamoto, K.; Shishido, T.; Katori, Y.; Mizoue, T.; Shirasu, H.; Nunoda, D. Study of hip joint dislocation after total hip arthroplasty. *Int. Orthop.* **2005**, *30*, 26–30. [CrossRef]
17. Dudda, M.; Gueleryuez, A.; Gautier, E.; Busato, A.; Röder, C. Risk factors for early dislocation after total hip arthroplasty: A matched case-control study. *J. Orthop. Surg.* **2010**, *18*, 179–183. [CrossRef]
18. Murphy, W.S.; Kowal, J.H.; Murphy, S.B. The Safe Zone for Acetabular Component Orientation. *Orthop. Proc.* **2013**, *95-B* (Suppl. 28), 44.
19. Danoff, J.R.; Bobman, J.T.; Cunn, G.; Murtaugh, T.; Gorroochurn, P.; Geller, J.A.; Macaulay, W. Redefining the acetabular component safe zone for posterior approach total hip arthroplasty. *J. Arthroplast.* **2016**, *31*, 506–511. [CrossRef]
20. Fujishiro, T.; Hiranaka, T.; Hashimoto, S.; Hayashi, S.; Kurosaka, M.; Kanno, T.; Masuda, T. The effect of acetabular and femoral component version on dislocation in primary total hip arthroplasty. *Int. Orthop.* **2016**, *40*, 697–702. [CrossRef]
21. Ranawat, C.S.; Maynard, M.J. Modern technique of cemented total hip arthroplasty. *Tech. Orthop.* **1991**, *6*, 17–25. [CrossRef]
22. Jolles, B.M.; Zangger, P.; Leyvraz, P.-F. Factors predisposing to dislocation after primary total hip arthroplasty: A multivariate analysis. *J. Arthroplast.* **2002**, *17*, 282–288. [CrossRef]
23. Dorr, L.D.; Malik, A.; Dastane, M.; Wan, Z. Combined anteversion technique for total hip arthroplasty. *Clin. Orthop. Relat. Res.* **2009**, *467*, 119–127. [CrossRef]
24. Jaramaz, B.; DiGioia, A.M., III; Blackwell, M.; Nikou, C. Computer assisted measurement of cup placement in total hip replacement. *Clin. Orthop. Relat. Res.* **1998**, *354*, 70–81. [CrossRef] [PubMed]
25. Barrack, R.L.; Lavernia, C.; Ries, M.; Thornberry, R.; Tozakoglou, E. Virtual reality computer animation of the effect of component position and design on stability after total hip arthroplasty. *Orthop. Clin. N. Am.* **2001**, *32*, 569–577. [CrossRef]
26. Ezquerra, L.; Quilez, M.P.; Pérez, M.Á.; Albareda, J.; Seral, B. Range of Movement for Impingement and Dislocation Avoidance in Total Hip Replacement Predicted by Finite Element Model. *J. Med. Biol. Eng.* **2017**, *37*, 26–34. [CrossRef] [PubMed]
27. Widmer, K.-H. The Impingement-free, Prosthesis-specific, and Anatomy-adjusted Combined Target Zone for Component Positioning in THA Depends on Design and Implantation Parameters of both Components. *Clin. Orthop. Relat. Res.* **2020**, *478*, 1904–1918. [CrossRef] [PubMed]
28. Herrlin, K.; Selvik, G.; Pettersson, H. Space orientation of total hip prosthesis. A method for three-dimensional determination. *Acta Radiol. Diagn.* **1986**, *27*, 619–627. [CrossRef]
29. Hsu, J.; de La Fuente, M.; Radermacher, K. Calculation of impingement-free combined cup and stem alignments based on the patient-specific pelvic tilt. *J. Biomech.* **2019**, *82*, 193–203. [CrossRef]
30. Yoshimine, F. The safe-zones for combined cup and neck anteversions that fulfill the essential range of motion and their optimum combination in total hip replacements. *J. Biomech.* **2006**, *39*, 1315–1323. [CrossRef]
31. Pedersen, D.R.; Callaghan, J.J.; Brown, T.D. Activity-dependence of the "safe zone" for impingement versus dislocation avoidance. *Med. Eng. Phys.* **2005**, *27*, 323–328. [CrossRef]
32. Elkins, J.M.; Callaghan, J.J.; Brown, T.D. The 2014 Frank Stinchfield Award: The 'landing zone' for wear and stability in total hip arthroplasty is smaller than we thought: A computational analysis. *Clin. Orthop. Relat. Res.* **2015**, *473*, 441–452. [CrossRef]
33. Kessler, O.; Patil, S.; Stefan, W.; Mayr, E.; Colwell, C.W., Jr.; D'Lima, D.D. Bony impingement affects range of motion after total hip arthroplasty: A subject-specific approach. *J. Orthop. Res.* **2008**, *26*, 443–452. [CrossRef]

34. Kurtz, W.B.; Ecker, T.M.; Reichmann, W.M.; Murphy, S.B. Factors affecting bony impingement in hip arthroplasty. *J. Arthroplast.* **2010**, *25*, 624–634. [CrossRef] [PubMed]
35. Bunn, A.; Colwell, C.W.; D'lima, D.D. Bony impingement limits design-related increases in hip range of motion. *Clin. Orthop. Relat. Res.* **2012**, *470*, 418–427. [CrossRef] [PubMed]
36. Shoji, T.; Yamasaki, T.; Izumi, S.; Kenji, M.; Sawa, M.; Yasunaga, Y.; Adachi, N. The effect of cup medialization and lateralization on hip range of motion in total hip arthroplasty. *Clin. Biomech.* **2018**, *57*, 121–128. [CrossRef] [PubMed]
37. DiGioia, A.M.; Jaramaz, B.; Blackwell, M.; Simon, D.A.; Morgan, F.; Moody, J.E.; Nikou, C.; Colgan, B.D.; Aston, C.A.; Labarca, R.S.; et al. The Otto Aufranc Award. Image guided navigation system to measure intraoperatively acetabular implant alignment. *Clin. Orthop. Relat. Res.* **1998**, *355*, 8–22. [CrossRef] [PubMed]
38. Widmer, K.-H. Containment versus impingement: Finding a compromise for cup placement in total hip arthroplasty. *Int. Orthop.* **2007**, *31*, 29–33. [CrossRef] [PubMed]
39. Ueno, T.; Kabata, T.; Kajino, Y.; Ohmori, T.; Yoshitani, J.; Tsuchiya, H. Three-Dimensional Host Bone Coverage Required in Total Hip Arthroplasty for Developmental Dysplasia of the Hip and Its Relationship With 2-Dimensional Coverage. *J. Arthroplast.* **2019**, *34*, 93–101. [CrossRef] [PubMed]
40. Fujii, M.; Nakashima, Y.; Nakamura, T.; Ito, Y.; Hara, T. Minimum Lateral Bone Coverage Required for Securing Fixation of Cementless Acetabular Components in Hip Dysplasia. *BioMed Res. Int.* **2017**, *2017*, 4937151. [CrossRef] [PubMed]
41. Pierrepont, J.W.; Stambouzou, C.Z.; Miles, B.P.; O'Connor, P.B.; Walter, L.; Ellis, A.; Molnar, R.; Baré, J.V.; Solomon, M.; McMahon, S.; et al. Patient Specific Component Alignment in Total Hip Arthroplasty. *Recon. Rev.* **2016**, *6*, 25–33. [CrossRef]
42. Mellon, S.J.; Grammatopoulos, G.; Andersen, M.S.; Pandit, H.G.; Gill, H.S.; Murray, D.W. Optimal acetabular component orientation estimated using edge-loading and impingement risk in patients with metal-on-metal hip resurfacing arthroplasty. *J. Biomech.* **2015**, *48*, 318–323. [CrossRef]
43. Clarke, I.; Lazennec, J.-Y. Margin-of-safety Algorithm Used with EOS Imaging to Interpret MHRA Warning for 46-48mm MOM Arthroplasty. *Recon. Rev.* **2015**, *5*, 13–21. [CrossRef]
44. Babisch, J.W.; Layher, F.; Ritter, B.; Venbrocks, R.A. Computer-assisted Biomechanically Based Two-dimensional Planning of Hip Surgery. *Transl. Orthopädische Prax.* **2001**, *37*, 29–38.
45. Maratt, J.D.; Esposito, C.I.; McLawhorn, A.S.; Jerabek, S.A.; Padgett, D.E.; Mayman, D.J. Pelvic tilt in patients undergoing total hip arthroplasty: When does it matter? *J. Arthroplast.* **2015**, *30*, 387–391. [CrossRef] [PubMed]
46. Thelen, T.; Thelen, P.; Demezon, H.; Aunoble, S.; Le Huec, J.-C. Normative 3D acetabular orientation measurements by the low-dose EOS imaging system in 102 asymptomatic subjects in standing position: Analyses by side, gender, pelvic incidence and reproducibility. *Orthop. Traumatol. Surg. Res.* **2017**, *103*, 209–215. [CrossRef] [PubMed]
47. Pierrepont, J.; Hawdon, G.; Miles, B.P.; Connor, B.O.; Baré, J.; Walter, L.R.; Marel, E.; Solomon, M.; McMahon, S.; Shimmin, A.J. Variation in functional pelvic tilt in patients undergoing total hip arthroplasty. *Bone Jt. J.* **2017**, *99*, 184–191. [CrossRef] [PubMed]
48. Dardenne, G.; Dusseau, S.; Hamitouche, C.; Lefèvre, C.; Stindel, E. Toward a dynamic approach of THA planning based on ultrasound. *Clin. Orthop. Relat. Res.* **2009**, *467*, 901–908. [CrossRef] [PubMed]
49. Sutter, E.G.; Wellman, S.S.; Bolognesi, M.P.; Seyler, T.M. A Geometric Model to Determine Patient-Specific Cup Anteversion Based on Pelvic Motion in Total Hip Arthroplasty. *Adv. Orthop.* **2019**, *2019*, 4780280. [CrossRef] [PubMed]
50. Tannast, M.; Langlotz, U.; Siebenrock, K.A.; Wiese, M.; Bernsmann, K.; Langlotz, F. Anatomic referencing of cup orientation in total hip arthroplasty. *Clin. Orthop. Relat. Res.* **2005**, *436*, 144–150. [CrossRef]
51. Babisch, J.W.; Layher, F.; Amiot, L.-P. The rationale for tilt-adjusted acetabular cup navigation. *J. Bone Jt. Surg.* **2008**, *90*, 357–365. [CrossRef] [PubMed]
52. Lembeck, B.; Mueller, O.; Reize, P.; Wuelker, N. Pelvic tilt makes acetabular cup navigation inaccurate. *Acta Orthop.* **2005**, *76*, 517–523. [CrossRef] [PubMed]
53. Jolles, B.M.; Genoud, P.; Hoffmeyer, P. Computer-assisted Cup Placement Techniques in Total Hip Arthroplasty Improve Accuracy of Placement. *Clin. Orthop. Relat. Res.* **2004**, *426*, 174–179. [CrossRef]
54. Osmani, F.A.; Thakkar, S.; Ramme, A.; Elbuluk, A.; Wojack, P.; Vigdorchik, J.M. Variance in predicted cup size by 2-dimensional vs 3-dimensional computerized tomography-based templating in primary total hip arthroplasty. *Arthroplast. Today* **2017**, *3*, 289–293. [CrossRef]
55. Huppertz, A.; Radmer, S.; Asbach, P.; Juran, R.; Schwenke, C.; Diederichs, G.; Hamm, B.; Sparmann, M. Computed tomography for preoperative planning in minimal-invasive total hip arthroplasty: Radiation exposure and cost analysis. *Eur. J. Radiol.* **2011**, *78*, 406–413. [CrossRef]
56. Imai, N.; Ito, T.; Suda, K.; Miyasaka, D.; Endo, N. Pelvic Flexion Measurement From Lateral Projection Radiographs is Clinically Reliable. *Clin. Orthop. Relat. Res.* **2013**, *471*, 1271–1276. [CrossRef]
57. Fischer, M.C.M.; Tokunaga, K.; Okamoto, M.; Habor, J.; Radermacher, K. Preoperative factors improving the prediction of the postoperative sagittal orientation of the pelvis in standing position after total hip arthroplasty. *Sci. Rep.* **2020**, *10*, 15944. [CrossRef]
58. Marques, C.J.; Martin, T.; Fiedler, F.; Weber, M.; Breul, V.; Lampe, F.; Kozak, J. Intra- and Inter-rater Reliability of Navigated Ultrasound in the Assessment of Pelvic Tilt in Symptom-Free Young Adults. *J. Ultrasound Med. Off. J. Am. Inst. Ultrasound Med.* **2018**, *37*, 2333–2342. [CrossRef]

59. Dardenne, G.; Pluchon, J.P.; Letissier, H.; Guezou-Philippe, A.; Gerard, R.; Lefevre, C.; Stindel, E. Accuracy and Precision of an Ultrasound-Based Device to Measure the Pelvic Tilt in Several Positions. *J. Ultrasound Med. Off. J. Am. Inst. Ultrasound Med.* **2020**, *39*, 667–674. [CrossRef] [PubMed]
60. Hartel, M.J.; Petersik, A.; Schmidt, A.; Kendoff, D.; Nüchtern, J.; Rueger, J.M.; Lehmann, W.; Grosserlinden, L.G. Determination of Femoral Neck Angle and Torsion Angle Utilizing a Novel Three-Dimensional Modeling and Analytical Technology Based on CT Datasets. *PLoS ONE* **2016**, *11*, e0149480. [CrossRef] [PubMed]
61. Cyteval, C.; Sarrabère, M.P.; Cottin, A.; Assi, C.; Morcos, L.; Maury, P.; Taourel, P. Iliopsoas Impingement on the Acetabular Component: Radiologic and Computed Tomography Findings of a Rare Hip Prosthesis Complication in Eight Cases. *J. Comput. Assist. Tomogr.* **2003**, *27*, 183–188. [CrossRef]
62. Otomaru, I.; Kobayashi, K.; Okada, T.; Nakamoto, M.; Kagiyama, Y.; Takao, M.; Sugano, N.; Tada, Y.; Sato, Y. Expertise modeling for automated planning of acetabular cup in total hip arthroplasty using combined bone and implant statistical atlases. In *International Conference on Medical Image Computing and Computer-Assisted Intervention*; Springer: Berlin/Heidelberg, Germany, 2009; Volume 2009, pp. 532–539.
63. Kagiyama, Y.; Otomaru, I.; Takao, M.; Sugano, N.; Nakamoto, M.; Yokota, F.; Tomiyama, N.; Tada, Y.; Sato, Y. CT-based automated planning of acetabular cup for total hip arthroplasty (THA) based on hybrid use of two statistical atlases. *Int. J. Comput. Assist. Radiol. Surg.* **2016**, *11*, 2253–2271. [CrossRef]
64. Pathak, P.K.; Gupta, R.K.; Meena, H.S.; Fiske, R. Limb length discrepancy after total hip arthroplasty: A systematic review. *Int. J. Res. Orthop.* **2018**, *4*, 690. [CrossRef]
65. Turley, G.A.; Ahmed, S.M.Y.; Williams, M.A.; Griffin, D.R. Establishing a range of motion boundary for total hip arthroplasty. *Proc. Inst. Mech. Eng. Part H J. Eng. Med.* **2011**, *225*, 769–782. [CrossRef] [PubMed]
66. Sugano, N.; Tsuda, K.; Miki, H.; Takao, M.; Suzuki, N.; Nakamura, N. Dynamic measurements of hip movement in deep bending activities after total hip arthroplasty using a 4-dimensional motion analysis system. *J. Arthroplast.* **2012**, *27*, 1562–1568. [CrossRef] [PubMed]
67. Fischer, M.C.M.; Damm, P.; Habor, J.; Radermacher, K. Effect of the underlying cadaver data and patient-specific adaptation of the femur and pelvis on the prediction of the hip joint force estimated using static models. *J. Biomech.* **2021**, in press. [CrossRef] [PubMed]
68. Imado, K.; Kido, Y.; Miyagawa, H. A method of calculation for contact pressure between femoral head and cup of artificial hip joint. *Tribol. Trans.* **2005**, *48*, 230–237. [CrossRef]
69. Harris, W.H. Traumatic arthritis of the hip after dislocation and acetabular fractures: Treatment by mold arthroplasty. An end-result study using a new method of result evaluation. *J. Bone Jt. Surg.* **1969**, *51*, 737–755. [CrossRef]
70. Fischer, M.C.M.; Krooß, F.; Habor, J.; Radermacher, K. A robust method for automatic identification of landmarks on surface models of the pelvis. *Sci. Rep.* **2019**, *9*, 391. [CrossRef] [PubMed]
71. Fischer, M.C.M.; Grothues, S.A.G.A.; Habor, J.; de La Fuente, M.; Radermacher, K. A robust method for automatic identification of femoral landmarks, axes, planes and bone coordinate systems using surface models. *Sci. Rep.* **2020**, *10*, 20859. [CrossRef] [PubMed]
72. Murray, D.W. The definition and measurement of acetabular orientation. *J. Bone Jt. Surg.* **1993**, *75*, 228–232. [CrossRef] [PubMed]
73. Belzunce, M.A.; Henckel, J.; Di Laura, A.; Hart, A. Uncemented femoral stem orientation and position in total hip arthroplasty: A CT study. *J. Orthop. Res.* **2020**, *38*, 1486–1496. [CrossRef] [PubMed]
74. Habor, J. *The Patient-specific Combined Target Zone for Total Hip Arthroplasty Planning*; Shaker Verlag: Düren, Germany, 2020.
75. Gagnier, J.J.; Huang, H.; Mullins, M.; Marinac-Dabic, D.; Ghambaryan, A.; Eloff, B.; Mirza, F.; Bayona, M. Measurement Properties of Patient-Reported Outcome Measures Used in Patients Undergoing Total Hip Arthroplasty: A Systematic Review. *JBJS Rev.* **2018**, *6*, e2. [CrossRef]
76. Ishida, T.; Inaba, Y.; Kobayashi, N.; Iwamoto, N.; Yukizawa, Y.; Choe, H.; Saito, T. Changes in pelvic tilt following total hip arthroplasty. *J. Orthop. Sci.* **2011**, *16*, 682–688. [CrossRef]
77. Parratte, S.; Pagnano, M.W.; Coleman-Wood, K.; Kaufman, K.R.; Berry, D.J. The 2008 Frank Stinchfield award: Variation in postoperative pelvic tilt may confound the accuracy of hip navigation systems. *Clin. Orthop. Relat. Res.* **2009**, *467*, 43–49. [CrossRef] [PubMed]
78. Shoji, T.; Yamasaki, T.; Izumi, S.; Murakami, H.; Mifuji, K.; Sawa, M.; Yasunaga, Y.; Adachi, N.; Ochi, M. Factors affecting the potential for posterior bony impingement after total hip arthroplasty. *Bone Jt. J.* **2017**, *99*, 1140–1146. [CrossRef] [PubMed]
79. Palit, A.; King, R.; Hart, Z.; Gu, Y.; Pierrepont, J.; Elliott, M.T.; Williams, M.A. Bone-to-Bone and Implant-to-Bone Impingement: A Novel Graphical Representation for Hip Replacement Planning. *Ann. Biomed. Eng.* **2020**, *48*, 1354–1367. [CrossRef]
80. Matziolis, G.; Krakow, L.; Layher, F.; Sander, K.; Bossert, J.; Brodt, S. Patient-Specific Contact Stress Does Not Predict Polyethylene Wear Rate in a Specific Pressfit Cup. *J. Arthroplast.* **2017**, *32*, 3802–3805. [CrossRef]

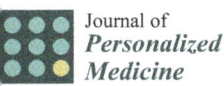

Article

Augmented-Reality-Assisted K-Wire Placement for Glenoid Component Positioning in Reversed Shoulder Arthroplasty: A Proof-of-Concept Study

Klaus Schlueter-Brust [1,*], Johann Henckel [2], Faidon Katinakis [1], Christoph Buken [1], Jörg Opt-Eynde [1], Thorsten Pofahl [3], Ferdinando Rodriguez y Baena [4] and Fabio Tatti [4]

1. Department of Orthopaedic Surgery, St. Franziskus Hospital Köln, 50825 Köln, Germany; Faidon-Ioannis.Katinakis@cellitinnen.de (F.K.); Christoph.Buken@cellitinnen.de (C.B.); info@opti3d.de (J.O.-E.)
2. Institute of Orthopaedics, The Royal National Orthopaedic Hospital, Brockley Hill, Stanmore, London HA7 4LP, UK; johann.henckel@nhs.net
3. Demo Working Group GbR, 50676 Köln, Germany; pofahl@trako.arch.rwth-aachen.de
4. Mechatronics in Medicine Laboratory, Imperial College London, London SW7 2AZ, UK; f.rodriguez@imperial.ac.uk (F.R.y.B.); f.tatti@imperial.ac.uk (F.T.)
* Correspondence: Klaus.schlueter-brust@cellitinnen.de; Tel.: +49-221-5591-1131

Abstract: The accuracy of the implant's post-operative position and orientation in reverse shoulder arthroplasty is known to play a significant role in both clinical and functional outcomes. Whilst technologies such as navigation and robotics have demonstrated superior radiological outcomes in many fields of surgery, the impact of augmented reality (AR) assistance in the operating room is still unknown. Malposition of the glenoid component in shoulder arthroplasty is known to result in implant failure and early revision surgery. The use of AR has many promising advantages, including allowing the detailed study of patient-specific anatomy without the need for invasive procedures such as arthroscopy to interrogate the joint's articular surface. In addition, this technology has the potential to assist surgeons intraoperatively in aiding the guidance of surgical tools. It offers the prospect of increased component placement accuracy, reduced surgical procedure time, and improved radiological and functional outcomes, without recourse to the use of large navigation or robotic instruments, with their associated high overhead costs. This feasibility study describes the surgical workflow from a standardised CT protocol, via 3D reconstruction, 3D planning, and use of a commercial AR headset, to AR-assisted k-wire placement. Post-operative outcome was measured using a high-resolution laser scanner on the patient-specific 3D printed bone. In this proof-of-concept study, the discrepancy between the planned and the achieved glenoid entry point and guide-wire orientation was approximately 3 mm with a mean angulation error of 5°.

Keywords: augmented reality; image-guided surgery; intraoperative imaging; simulation; mixed reality; reversed shoulder arthroplasty; 3D printing; 3D planning

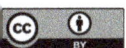

1. Introduction

Early failure rates and sub-optimal performance continue to plague outcomes in reverse shoulder arthroplasty. Whilst the causes of revision surgery and poor function are multifactorial and include patient, implant factors, and surgeon, implant malposition remains a constant. Several computer-assisted strategies and tools are in use with varying outcomes.

Traditional instruments remain the mainstay for the preparation of the glenoid in reverse shoulder arthroplasty, and whilst there are sophisticated 3D planning systems available on the market, delivering these virtual plans remains a challenge even for experienced surgeons [1].

Although not as common as hip or knee arthroplasty, shoulder arthroplasty has become more widely adopted in recent years [2]. Reverse total shoulder arthroplasty (RTSA) is known to be an effective surgical procedure for glenohumeral arthritis, rotator cuff arthropathy, irreparable rotator cuff tears, complex proximal humerus fractures, and failed shoulder prosthesis [3].

The Norwegian Arthroplasty Register reports a 5-year survival rate of 90% for RTSA, a result similar to a 2006 multicentre study by Guery et al. [4,5]. Results from the Register reveal that aseptic loosening of the glenoid component is one of the main causes of early revision surgery. Implant loosening is often due to technical errors, such as the glenoid component being positioned too high and/or in superior inclination [6], which induces severe shear stress, impairing fixation [7,8]. Consequently, precise positioning of the glenoid component is crucial to avoid impingement and premature loosening, and to improve the survival rate [9].

Augmented reality (AR) can be a valuable tool to increase accuracy in both bone preparation and implant placement in surgery. In contrast to virtual reality, which creates a completely virtual environment to the exclusion of the real world, AR overlays virtual information onto a real environment, so that intuitive guidance is provided [10].

Among the various options available, optical-see-through head-mounted-displays (OST-HMD) are the preferable choice for introducing AR in orthopaedic surgery, due to their flexibility and the fact that they allow a natural, unobstructed view of the scene when the AR is switched off [11]. In recent years, several commercial optical see-through products such as the Microsoft HoloLens (Microsoft, Redmond, WA, USA) and Google Glass (Google Inc., Mountain View, CA, USA) have become widely available.

A small number of solutions for AR-based intraoperative surgical guidance have been successfully demonstrated in humans, e.g., for spine [12] and hip [13] surgery. Nevertheless, AR has not been widely adopted and the vast majority of surgeries are still performed manually, without any computer-assisted aids.

To the best of our knowledge, no such solutions exist yet for shoulder arthroplasty, and only one previous study [14] has demonstrated the use of augmented reality for assisted placement of the glenoid component in Total Shoulder Arthroplasty (TSA). This paper presents a proof-of-concept system to provide AR guidance during k-wire placement for glenoid component positioning in reversed shoulder arthroplasty, using the Microsoft HoloLens 2 system. The system was trialled on 3D-printed scapula phantoms derived from real patient anatomy, and the k-wire entry point and orientational errors are reported.

2. Materials and Methods

2.1. Imaging Data

A single CT scan of an osteoarthritic right shoulder was used as reference anatomy for the study. The scan was obtained using the BLUEPRINT™ CT protocol [15], from a 78-year-old female patient with 29.2 BMI, diagnosed with rotator cuff arthropathy, who qualified for reverse shoulder arthroplasty. The scan was completed using a Canon Aquilion 64 scanner, with 0.5 mm collimation width. To improve the image quality and optimise segmentation outcome, a pillow was inserted between the patient's arm and body, to distract the humerus head from the glenoid. The position of the arm was stabilised using a strap. The study had internal institution review board (IRB) approval together with informed consent of the patient. The CT DICOM data were anonymised following standard data protection protocols.

2.2. Procedure Planning

The DICOM CT scan files were imported into the mediCAD® 3D Shoulder software (mediCAD Hectec GmbH, Altdorf/Landshut, Germany) and segmented using an automated procedure provided by the software, followed by manual refinement. A 3D model of the scapula was then reconstructed from the segmented slices.

Surgical planning was performed by loading the CAD model of the implant's glenoid component into the mediCAD software and manually adjusting its position relative to the patient anatomy, to achieve optimal placement. Tornier Aequalis™ Perform™ Reversed implants (Wright Medical Group, Memphis, TN, USA) were used for this study. A 2.5 mm guidance k-wire model was then loaded into the software and positioned using the implant post as reference.

The reconstructed 3D models with and without the planned k-wire position were exported in STL format for use in the subsequent steps of the study.

2.3. Procedure Execution

One experienced shoulder arthroplasty surgeon performed all of the procedures. To avoid learning effects, data analysis was performed after all procedures had been completed, and the surgeon was unaware of the outcome of completed trials when performing subsequent ones.

Nine phantom models of the scapula were produced by 3D printing the exported STL file using a Stratasys Polyjet 3D printer (Stratasys, Eden Prairy, MN, USA). Conventional bone clamps were used to support the phantoms, which were placed in simulated beach chair position during execution of the procedure, as shown in Figure 1A.

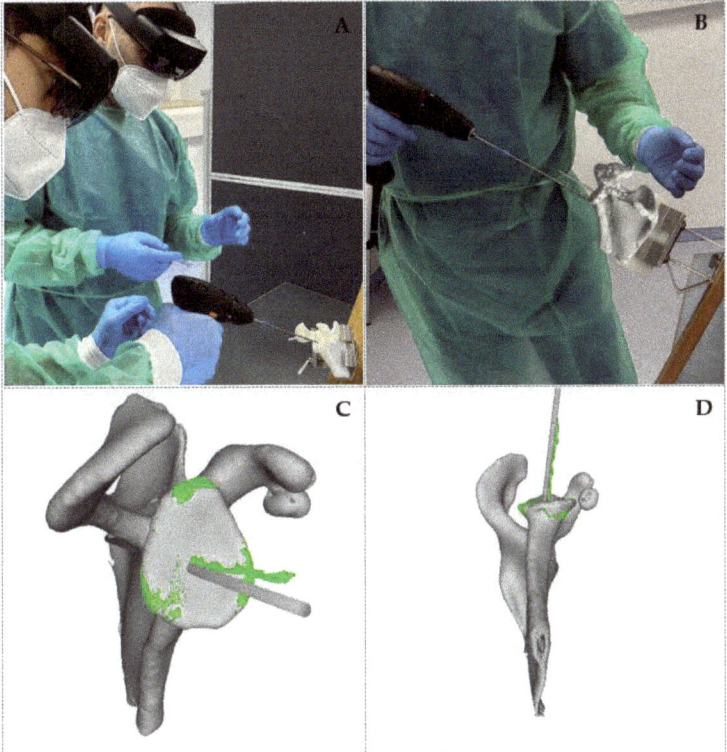

Figure 1. (**A**) Surgical setup and demonstration of the k-wire insertion. (**B**) View of the surgical scene from the HoloLens 2 device, with the AR reference overlaid onto the phantom scapula. (**C,D**) Three-quarter and bottom views of a 3D-scanned phantom (green) registered to the reference anatomy with planned k-wire position (grey). The 3D scan is cropped to include only the glenoid, to optimise registration quality in this area.

AR guidance was provided via a Microsoft HoloLens 2 device worn by the surgeon. The STL model including the planned k-wire position was loaded onto the HoloLens 2 and holographically displayed in front of the surgeon (see Figure 1B), via the mediCAD® MR App (Beta Version). The position of the virtual anatomical model was manually adjusted to match that of the 3D-printed phantom.

Finally, the surgeon inserted a k-wire into the 3D-printed phantom with a standard drill, using the position of the virtual k-wire as a reference.

2.4. Error Measurement

After the k-wire was inserted, the 3D-printed phantoms with the k-wire were digitised using a professional, high-resolution 3D scanner (Artec Space Spyder, Artec3D, Luxembourg).

The model obtained from the 3D scanner was imported into the Blender software (Blender Foundation, Amsterdam, The Netherlands) and co-registered with the preoperative surgical plan by first coarsely aligning the scapula models manually, and then refining the alignment using the iterative closest point (ICP) method [16]. In order to optimise the alignment of the glenoid, points from other regions of the scapula were excluded from the ICP routine (see Figure 1C,D). Once the models were aligned, the orientational error between the planned and achieved k-wire positions was measured by fitting a cylinder to the points corresponding to the planned insertion and scanned drill, respectively, then recording the angular distance between the two as reported by Blender's angular measurement tool. Subsequently, the entry point error was measured by identifying the intersection between the two cylinders and the glenoid surface, and recording their distance, as reported by Blender's distance measurement tool.

3. Results

3.1. Qualitative Results

The addition of preoperative 3D procedure planning increased the overall time required by approximately 5 min. This preoperative stage, however, provided extremely valuable 3D information, with better anatomical orientation, better visualisation, and the possibility to obtain a 3D-printed haptic patient-specific model, for consenting the patient, examining the anatomy, and practicing the surgery. Furthermore, the 3D data could be valuable for surgical education and training.

During the intraoperative stage, both the AR headset and the mediCAD® MR App proved intuitive and easy to use. The headset was comfortable to wear and did not induce any fatigue. The use of AR increased the time required for k-wire insertion by about 3 min. The additional time was primarily required for the manual alignment of the holographic reference anatomy to the phantom scapula.

While inserting the k-wire, it was crucial to minimize head movements in order to maintain optimal alignment between the holographic reference and the phantom. This limited the surgeon's comfort during this stage of the operation, and was highlighted as a challenge to be addressed in order to successfully introduce the technology in an operating theatre.

3.2. Quantitative Results

To evaluate the registration error between the 3D-scanned scapulas and the reference anatomy, we measured the distance of each point in the glenoid region of the scans (green area in Figure 1C,D) to the corresponding nearest neighbour on the reference anatomy. The average distance was around 0.5 mm for all the scapulas, indicating good alignment.

The measured errors between the planned and achieved entry point and k-wire orientation are reported in Table 1, for all the phantoms in the same order in which they were tested. The same results are illustrated graphically in Figure 2. The average ± sd entry-point error was 2.4 ± 0.7 mm, while the average ± sd orientational error was 3.9 ± 2.4°. Table 1 does not highlight evidence of a learning effect.

Table 1. Entry point and orientation errors for all phantoms tested.

Phantom ID	1	2	3	4	5	6	7	8	9
Entry point (mm)	2.8	1.9	1.2	1.8	2.3	2.8	2.3	3.9	2.3
Orientation (°)	9.0	5.3	6.7	2.3	2.1	1.8	4.2	2.2	1.7

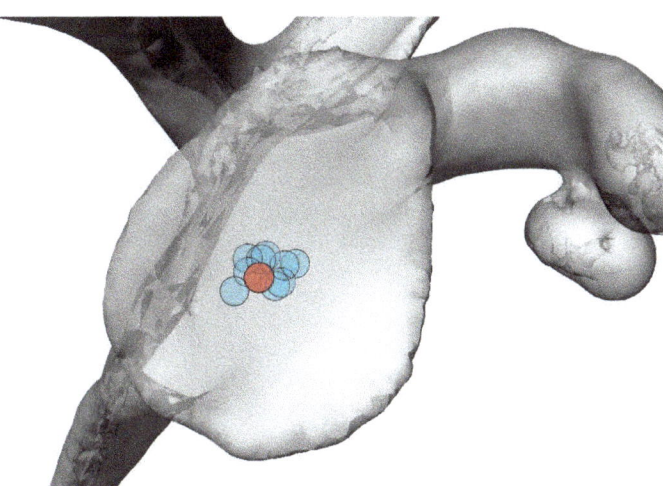

Figure 2. Graphical illustration of the actual entry point for all trials (light blue) relative to the planned entry point (red).

4. Discussion

Our lab results in this proof-of-concept study compare favourably with published data in conventional surgery [17].

The majority of published articles using standard instrumentation techniques reported mean postoperative version errors of 7.1° (min. 3.5° to max. 11.2°), mean postoperative inclination errors of 8.45° (min. 2.8° to max. 11.65°) and mean postoperative positional offset errors of 2.6 mm (min. 1.7 mm to max. 3.4 mm) compared with preoperative plans [17].

The entry-point accuracy measured in this study is comparable to a previously published study demonstrating the use of the HoloLens 1 headset for glenoid component placement, which reported an average entry-point error of 2.3 mm [14]. The study, however, reported a lower average orientational error (2.7°), which might be explained by the use of an automated registration method based on surface scanning of the glenoid.

We have demonstrated the feasibility of replicating the pre-operative CT-based plan in this lab-based study. The use of the high-resolution laser scanner introduced minimal noise to the measurement of the discrepancy between the planned and achieved position and orientation of the guide wire.

Real challenges in the clinical application of this technology in the context of image registration include the presence of residual cartilage on the articular surface in a CT-based planning system. Increased surgical dissection and access are needed and the incision will need to remain distracted to maintain the initial registration until the guide wire is inserted. Blood and residual soft tissues can also obscure the field of view.

Whilst the execution of the plan was the primary objective in this exercise, the challenges of pre-operative surgical planning must not go unmentioned. The quality of the CT scan, including satisfactory distraction of the worn articular surfaces, is needed to facilitate optimal bone segmentation. It can be difficult to assess the bone quality and hence decide upon the ideal position in which to plan and seat the glenoid component. However, the limitations described here are ubiquitous to all image-based Computer-Assisted Surgery (CAS) systems, including Patient-Specific Instrumentation (PSI) jigs, navigation systems, and potential robotic assisted solutions.

Patient specific jig systems are becoming more widely adopted, with many different design strategies in clinical use with varying degrees of radiological measured accuracy. Cabarcas's [17] systematic review of PSI-guided surgery reveals that the results of our pilot study compare favourably with their use.

Because of the increased operative experience of the several senior surgeons who were involved in these above-cited studies, the implant position error was low in comparison to low-volume surgeons. However, the mean errors in our experiment were superior (average ± sd entry-point error was 2.4 ± 0.7 mm, while the average ± sd orientational error was 3.9 ± 2.4°) to those in these studies using standard instrumentation techniques.

Our results cannot be compared directly to studies using PSI for shoulder arthroplasty, but the reported mean postoperative version and inclination errors of 5° or less compared with preoperative plans [17,18] are equal to our results, which were obtained simply using a see-through device (HoloLens 2). This finding suggests that AR-based aid can be particularly advantageous for novice or low-volume shoulder surgeons.

Particular challenges with PSI include the more extensive surgical dissection in order to gain access to seat and secure the bespoke jig to the glenoid. The need for increased surgical releases increases the risk of neuro-vascular injury. Additional challenges in the positioning of the jigs include the presence of unworn cartilage on the periarticular edges of the glenoid leading to poor seating of the guide and the potential for malorientation of the guide wire trajectory. PSI remains a viable option in assisting the surgeon to deliver his/her plan and are relatively inexpensive, costing around 400 € per case.

Computer navigation systems are also in clinical use. They offer greater accuracy and precision in guide wire placement; these systems are relatively expensive, however, in comparison to the results from our AR concept demonstrator, their results are comparable.

Accurate intraoperative landmark registration remains a challenge with greater surgical access needed. Line-of-sight issues with tracking continue to confront the user [19].

Robotic systems for the shoulder are not yet in clinical use; however, the large implant companies are planning to expand into shoulder arthroplasty. They promise sub-millimetre implant accuracy; however, they are very expensive and those in use in hip and knee arthroplasty can cost in excess of 1 million €.

From a technical point of view, the primary challenge that needs to be addressed in order to for AR to become a viable tool for surgery is the accuracy of the calibration between the virtual content displayed by the headset and the real scene. In this proof-of-concept study the operating surgeon was required to align the virtual hologram to the target anatomy manually. Aside from being a laborious operation, the manual alignment is also highly subjective and prone to human error. Future research will therefore look at the incorporation of automated methods for the registration of virtual content onto the target anatomy.

Various methods have been proposed in the literature to automatically align virtual content to a target anatomy. A highly accurate overlay of virtual content was demonstrated in [20], using fiducial markers and a custom head-mounted display. The authors reported an error below 1 mm in a maxillofacial surgical task conducted on plastic bone. While marker-based tracking is an established technology that provides great accuracy, and it is currently the norm for computer-assisted surgical navigation, there are disadvantages to its use in arthroplasty. Indeed, the need to use pins to rigidly attach trackers might increase the risk of complications [21]. In order to remove the need for rigidly attached markers, some groups have developed markerless computer-vision-based solutions that rely on the registration between a preoperative model of the patient anatomy and a 3D model of the same anatomy obtained intraoperatively, either by scanning the surface with a probe (e.g., [14]), or by exploiting the onboard sensors available on the headset (e.g., [10]). While the accuracy of these solutions is currently inferior to marker-based tracking, it is a rapidly expanding research field that holds great promise.

While knowledge of the relative position between the headset and the surgical site is necessary to obtain good alignment, it is not sufficient. Indeed, it is also necessary to account for the optics of the headset and its interaction with the user's eyes. Commercially available general-purpose optical-see-through systems use simple calibration methods whose accuracy is not sufficient for use in surgery, and they generally display the AR content at a fixed focal distance, which introduces perceptual issues for surgical tasks in the peripersonal space. Research in this topic is ongoing, and several methods have been proposed (e.g., [22,23]) to increase the accuracy of general-purpose headsets currently available on the market. Additionally, various companies and research groups have worked on the development of bespoke head-mounted displays, specifically tailored to the needs of intraoperative surgical guidance, e.g., [20,24].

5. Conclusions

The promise of augmented reality to overlay 3D virtual information onto a real scene has vast potential for orthopaedic surgery. AR is, however, a novel technology, still in its infancy, and a number of technical challenges still need to be addressed before it can be considered viable for use in clinical practice. The fast pace at which AR technology is moving and the amount of research interest that it is attracting make us hopeful that AR systems with the required specifications will be available in the future, and that this technology will become part of clinical practice.

Author Contributions: Conceptualization, K.S.-B.; methodology, K.S.-B., F.K. and C.B.; software, K.S.-B., T.P. and J.O.-E.; validation, K.S.-B., F.K. and C.B.; formal analysis, K.S.-B., T.P., J.O.-E. and F.T.; investigation, K.S.-B., T.P., J.O.-E., F.K. and C.B.; resources, K.S.-B.; data curation, K.S.-B., C.B., F.K. and F.T.; writing—original draft preparation, F.T., J.H., F.R.y.B. and K.S.-B.; writing—review and editing, F.T., J.H., K.S.-B. and F.R.y.B.; visualization, K.S.-B., T.P. and J.O.-E.; supervision, F.R.y.B.; K.S.-B., J.H. and F.T.; project administration, K.S.-B. All authors have read and agreed to the published version of the manuscript.

Funding: This research received no external funding.

Institutional Review Board Statement: The study was approved by the Institutional Review Board at St. Franziskus Hospital Köln, 50825 Köln, Germany.

Informed Consent Statement: Informed consent was obtained from all subjects involved in this study.

Data Availability Statement: All data are available upon request.

Conflicts of Interest: Klaus Schlueter-Brust has a consultancy agreement with mediCAD Hectec GmbH, Altdorf/Landshut, Germany. All other authors declare no conflict of interest.

References

1. Olaiya, O.R.; Nadeem, I.; Horner, N.S.; Bedi, A.; Leroux, T.; Alolabi, B.; Khan, M. Templating in shoulder arthroplasty—A comparison of 2D CT to 3D CT planning software: A systematic review. *Shoulder Elb.* **2020**, *12*, 303–314. [CrossRef]
2. Lee, D.H.; Choi, Y.S.; Potter, H.G.; Endo, Y.; Sivakumaran, T.; Lim, T.K.; Chun, T.J. Reverse total shoulder arthroplasty: An imaging overview. *Skelet. Radiol.* **2019**, *49*, 19–30. [CrossRef]
3. Chae, J.; Siljander, M.; Wiater, J.M. Instability in Reverse Total Shoulder Arthroplasty. *J. Am. Acad. Orthop. Surg.* **2018**, *26*, 587–596. [CrossRef] [PubMed]
4. Fevang, B.-T.S.; Lie, S.A.; Havelin, I.L.; Skredderstuen, A.; Furnes, O. Risk factors for revision after shoulder arthroplasty. *Acta Orthop.* **2009**, *80*, 83–91. [CrossRef] [PubMed]
5. Guery, J.; Favard, L.; Sirveaux, F.; Oudet, D.; Mole, D.; Walch, G. Reverse Total Shoulder Arthroplasty. *J. Bone Jt. Surg. Am.* **2006**, *88*, 1742–1747. [CrossRef]
6. Boileau, P. Complications and revision of reverse total shoulder arthroplasty. *Orthop. Traumatol. Surg. Res.* **2016**, *102*, S33–S43. [CrossRef]
7. Wall, B.T.; Mottier, F.; Walch, G. 9: Complications and revision of the reverse prosthesis: A multicenter study of 457 cases. *J. Shoulder Elb. Surg.* **2007**, *16*, e55. [CrossRef]

8. Gutiérrez, S.; Greiwe, R.M.; Frankle, M.; Siegal, S.; Lee, W.E. Biomechanical comparison of component position and hardware failure in the reverse shoulder prosthesis. *J. Shoulder Elb. Surg.* **2007**, *16*, S9–S12. [CrossRef] [PubMed]
9. Chalmers, P.N.; Boileau, P.; Romeo, A.A.; Tashjian, R.Z. Revision Reverse Shoulder Arthroplasty. *J. Am. Acad. Orthop. Surg.* **2019**, *27*, 426–436. [CrossRef]
10. Liu, H.; Auvinet, E.; Giles, J.; Baena, F.R.Y. Augmented Reality Based Navigation for Computer Assisted Hip Resurfacing: A Proof of Concept Study. *Ann. Biomed. Eng.* **2018**, *46*, 1595–1605. [CrossRef]
11. Blackwell, M.; Morgan, F.; DiGioia, A.M. Augmented Reality and Its Future in Orthopaedics. *Clin. Orthop. Relat. Res.* **1998**, *354*, 111–122. [CrossRef] [PubMed]
12. Molina, A.C.; Sciubba, D.M.; Greenberg, J.K.; Khan, M.; Witham, T. Clinical Accuracy, Technical Precision, and Workflow of the First in Human Use of an Augmented-Reality Head-Mounted Display Stereotactic Navigation System for Spine Surgery. *Oper. Neurosurg.* **2021**, *20*, 300–309. [CrossRef] [PubMed]
13. Lane, P.; Murphy, W.; Harris, S.; Murphy, S. Hipinsight: The World's First Augmented Reality-Based Navigation System For Joint Arthroplasty. In *Orthopaedic Proceedings*; The British Editorial Society of Bone & Joint Surgery: London, UK, 2021; Volume 103-B, No. SUPP_9.
14. Kriechling, P.; Roner, S.; Liebmann, F.; Casari, F.; Fürnstahl, P.; Wieser, K. Augmented reality for base plate component placement in reverse total shoulder arthroplasty: A feasibility study. *Arch. Orthop. Trauma Surg.* **2020**. [CrossRef]
15. BLUEPRINT™ Scan Protocol. Available online: https://www.wrightemedia.com/ProductFiles/Files/PDFs/AP-013380_EN_LR_LE.pdf (accessed on 17 May 2021).
16. Besl, P.J.; McKay, N.D. A method for registration of 3-D shapes. *IEEE Trans. Pattern Anal. Mach. Intell.* **1992**, *14*, 239–256. [CrossRef]
17. Cabarcas, B.C.; Cvetanovich, G.L.; Gowd, A.K.; Liu, J.N.; Manderle, B.J.; Verma, N.N. Accuracy of patient-specific instrumentation in shoulder arthroplasty: A systematic review and meta-analysis. *JSES Open Access* **2019**, *3*, 117–129. [CrossRef]
18. Villatte, G.; Muller, A.-S.; Pereira, B.; Mulliez, A.; Reilly, P.; Emery, R. Use of Patient-Specific Instrumentation (PSI) for glenoid component positioning in shoulder arthroplasty. A systematic review and meta-analysis. *PLoS ONE* **2018**, *13*, e0201759. [CrossRef] [PubMed]
19. Schoch, B.S.; Haupt, E.; Leonor, T.; Farmer, K.W.; Wright, T.W.; King, J.J. Computer navigation leads to more accurate glenoid targeting during total shoulder arthroplasty compared with 3-dimensional preoperative planning alone. *J. Shoulder Elb. Surg.* **2020**, *29*, 2257–2263. [CrossRef] [PubMed]
20. Cercenelli, L.; Carbone, M.; Condino, S.; Cutolo, F.; Marcelli, E.; Tarsitano, A.; Marchetti, C.; Ferrari, V.; Badiali, G. The Wearable VOSTARS System for Augmented Reality-Guided Surgery: Preclinical Phantom Evaluation for High-Precision Maxillofacial Tasks. *J. Clin. Med.* **2020**, *9*, 3562. [CrossRef]
21. Smith, T.J.; Siddiqi, A.; Forte, S.A.; Judice, A.; Sculco, P.K.; Vigdorchik, J.M.; Schwarzkopf, R.; Springer, B.D. Periprosthetic Fractures Through Tracking Pin Sites Following Computer Navigated and Robotic Total and Unicompartmental Knee Arthroplasty. *JBJS Rev.* **2021**, *9*, e20.00091. [CrossRef]
22. Hu, X.; Cutolo, F.; Tatti, F.; Baena, F.R.Y. Automatic Calibration of Commercial Optical See-Through Head-Mounted Displays for Medical Applications. In Proceedings of the 2020 IEEE Conference on Virtual Reality and 3D User Interfaces Abstracts and Workshops (VRW), Atlanta, GA, USA, 22–26 March 2020; pp. 755–756. [CrossRef]
23. Hu, X.; Baena, F.R.Y.; Cutolo, F. Alignment-Free Offline Calibration of Commercial Optical See-Through Head-Mounted Displays With Simplified Procedures. *IEEE Access* **2020**, *8*, 223661–223674. [CrossRef]
24. Dibble, C.F.; Molina, C.A. Device profile of the XVision-spine (XVS) augmented-reality surgical navigation system: Overview of its safety and efficacy. *Expert Rev. Med. Devices* **2021**, *18*, 1–8. [CrossRef] [PubMed]

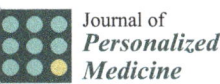 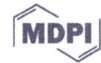

Article

Wear Risk Prevention and Reduction in Total Hip Arthroplasty. A Personalized Study Comparing Cement and Cementless Fixation Techniques Employing Finite Element Analysis

Carlos González-Bravo [1,2,†], Miguel A. Ortega [1,†], Julia Buján [1], Basilio de la Torre [3,4,*,‡] and Loreto Barrios [1,2,‡]

1. Department of Medicine and Medical Specialities, Faculty of Medicine and Health Sciences, Ramón y Cajal Institute of Sanitary Research (IRYCIS), University of Alcalá, Alcalá de Henares, 28034 Madrid, Spain; cgbravo@amasi.es (C.G.-B.); miguel.angel.ortega92@gmail.com (M.A.O.); mjulia.bujan@uah.es (J.B.); loreto@lycea.es (L.B.)
2. A+I Architecture and Engineering Ltd., 28224 Madrid, Spain
3. Department of Surgery, Medical and Social Sciences, Faculty of Medicine and Health Sciences, Ramón y Cajal Institute of Sanitary Research (IRYCIS), University of Alcala, Alcala de Henares, 28034 Madrid, Spain
4. Department of Orthopedic Surgery, University Hospital Ramón y Cajal, 28034 Madrid, Spain
* Correspondence: bjtorre@gmail.com; Tel.: +34-91-885-45-40; Fax: +34-91-885-48-85
† These authors contributed equally to this work.
‡ These authors shared senior authorship in this work.

Citation: González-Bravo, C.; Ortega, M.A.; Buján, J.; Torre, B.d.l.; Barrios, L. Wear Risk Prevention and Reduction in Total Hip Arthroplasty. A Personalized Study Comparing Cement and Cementless Fixation Techniques Employing Finite Element Analysis. *J. Pers. Med.* **2021**, *11*, 780. https://doi.org/10.3390/jpm 11080780

Academic Editor: Maximilian Rudert

Received: 22 July 2021
Accepted: 4 August 2021
Published: 10 August 2021

Publisher's Note: MDPI stays neutral with regard to jurisdictional claims in published maps and institutional affiliations.

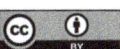

Copyright: © 2021 by the authors. Licensee MDPI, Basel, Switzerland. This article is an open access article distributed under the terms and conditions of the Creative Commons Attribution (CC BY) license (https://creativecommons.org/licenses/by/4.0/).

Abstract: The wear rate on Total Hip Arthroplasty (THA) entails a heavy burden for patients. This becomes more relevant with increased wear risk and its consequences such as osteolysis. In addition, osteolysis has been described in cemented and uncemented acetabular implants, and nowadays, controversy remains as to whether or not to cement the acetabular component. A personalized theoretical study was carried out to investigate which parameters have an influence on wear risk and to determine the best fixation method. Liner wear risk was assessed for two different types of fixation (cemented vs uncemented) through Finite Elements Analysis (FEA). The intraoperative variables used to determine the wear risk (cervical-diaphyseal angle, Center of Rotation positioning -COR-, head material, head size, and liner thickness) are vital parameters in surgical planning. Two types of tridimensional liner models of Ultra High Molecular Weight Polyethene (UHMWPE) were simulated through finite element analysis (FEA—over 216 cases were the core of this research). A significant relationship was found between the cervical-diaphyseal angle and wear risk ($p < 0.0001$), especially in valgus morphology. The acetabular fixation technique ($p < 0.0001$) and liner thickness ($p < 0.0001$) showed a significant relationship with wear risk. According to our study, using a cemented fixation with a thick liner in the right center of rotation appears to be the proper stratagy for preventing polyethylene liner wear.

Keywords: total hip arthroplasty; finite element method; cemented and uncemented acetabular fixation; polyethylene wear patterns; cervical–diaphyseal angle; center of rotation; material head; size head; liner thickness

1. Introduction

THA is an accepted and successful procedure for patients suffering from degenerative hip joint disease. Once the entire joint is replaced with an artificial one, a new variable is introduced in patients' regular activity regardless of age: wear on the polyethylene liners. At present, there seems to be a debate regarding the ideal method of fixation for the liner [1,2]. However, some authors [3] claim that the cemented fixation is the "gold standard" with multiple papers showing a relationship between uncemented cases and an increased wear rate [4–8].

Polyethylene wear is influenced by different parameters such as the center of rotation (COR) location, the femoral head size and material, or the liner thickness. These parameters affect clinical outcomes following hip arthroplasty [4,9].

Cervical–diaphyseal angle (varus or valgus morphology) plays a critical role in the stresses generated at the bearing surfaces [10]. However, studies regarding the role of the cervical–diaphyseal angle on liner wear are absent in the literature.

Nowadays, there is a lack of intensive computational studies and no quantified data on wear risk regarding the aforementioned parameters in cemented or uncemented acetabular fixation. Many studies are limited by the heterogeneity of patients and treatments. This lack of uniformity in clinical studies makes it difficult for surgeons to draw conclusions relevant to their clinical practice.

A personalized study can assess this critical parameter related to specific morphology of the hip joint. The wear risk prevention on the artificial hip joint for these patients could begin with a set of numerical simulations implementing general and particular parameters.

Bearing this in mind, the present research has developed a numerical wear simulation using FEA to check distinct features of wear risk [11–18] with particular focus on the variables that affect the integrity of the liners. One of the most powerful tools in the computational scenario is obtaining an order of magnitude to determine and prevent the causes of wear rate for singular patients and, consequently, to avoid osteolysis progress and failure in THA.

Good decision-making for orthopedic surgeons in a distinctive THA plan is the best wear reduction strategy. The purpose of this study is to quantify the role of previously described parameters in polyethylene wear through a numerical method (FEA).

2. Materials and Methods

For the present study, a set of simulations (216) were carried out over the 3D liners modeled in version 2017 of SOLIDWORKS® (Dassault Systèmes, Vélizy-Villacoubla, France) from real geometry of the Neutral (E1 & ArComXL) G7 acetabular system (in the case of cementless fixation) and Exceed ABT (in the case of cemented fixation) currently marketed by Zimmer Biomet in a Ultra High Molecular Weight Polyethylene (UHMWPE) material. The contact between liner and cup or bone was not assessed in this study and neither was the liner and femoral head contact. However, the last issue was taken into account through the Hertz theory, as shown below. Since the number of possibilities was large, two standard head femoral diameters (32 mm and 36 mm) generally used by surgeons were chosen and, within these, three different thicknesses: one close to the minimum (5.3 mm), the second in the middle range (7.3 mm) and, the last close to maximum (11.3 mm). For a general sketch of variables and values, see Figure 1a,b. Liner material (Table 1 (a)) was considered isotropic as far as its mechanical behavior was concerned. Furthermore, no large displacement was set up in order to obtain the elastic range of results, avoiding nonlinearities in the FEA. With this in mind, a general comparison is possible when it comes to determining the elastic limit (around 25 MPa) of the UHMWPE and, therefore, enabling study of the wear risk in those particular areas of the liner when the von Mises (VM) stress is analyzed, as we will see in the results section.

To simulate a real orientation of the liner inside the acetabulum, 3D models were aligned (Figure 2a) with particular directions of an abduction angle around the H_{AP} axis (40°) and an anatomical orientation in acetabular direction (35°) around the V_{CC}.

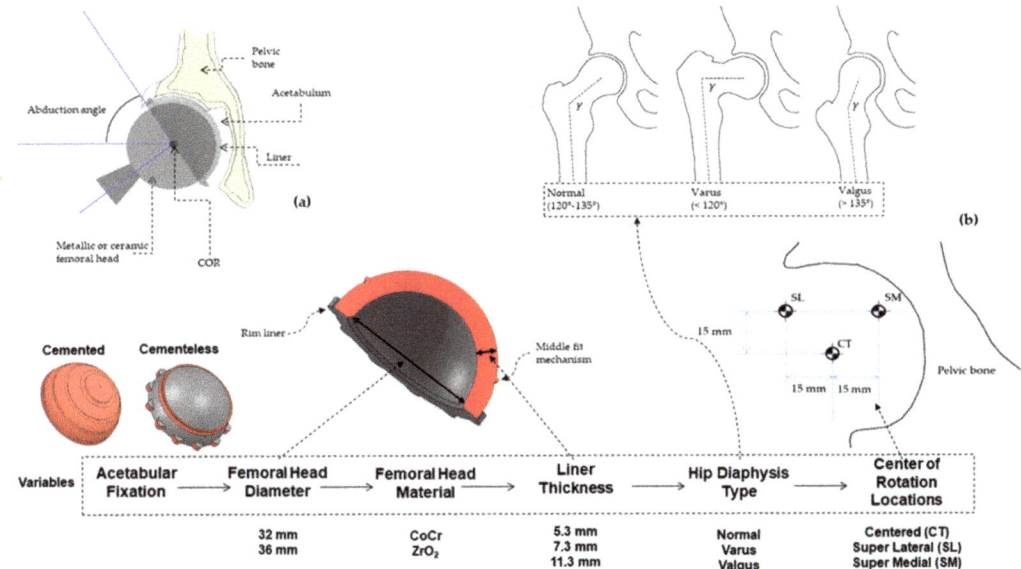

Figure 1. (**a**) Common parts of a Total Hip Arthroplasty (lateral cross-section). (**b**) Summary of parameters and variables analyzed with Cervical-Diaphyseal Angle in Normal, Varus and, Valgus.

Table 1. (**a**) Mechanical properties of UHMWPE liner. (**b**) Mechanical properties of femoral head and equations of contact Hertz theory. (**c**) Biomechanics and geometrical values.

(a)						
E^1 (MPa)	G^2 (MPa)	N^3	F_y^4 (MPa)	f_u^5 (MPa) 2	Strain Max (%)	
940	322	0.46	25	40	500	

[1] Modulus of Elasticity; [2] Modulus of Rigidity; [3] Ratio of Poisson; [4] Yield Strenght; [5] Ultimate Strenght.

(b)				
Material	E^1 (GPa)	ν^2	μ (32)^3	μ (36)^4
CoCr	210	0.30	0.133	0.14
ZrO2	358	0.24	0.096	0.085

[1] Modulus of Elasticity; [2] Ratio of Poisson; [3] Fricction Coeffient for 32 mm of femoral head; [4] Fricction Coeffient for 36 mm of femoral head.

(c)								
Cervical-Diaphyseal Angle	COR^1	a^2 (mm)	b^3 (mm)	h^4 (mm)	α^5 (o)	β^6 (o)	M^7 (N)	R^8 (N)
	SL^9	53	125	45.23	71	13.98	1879.33	2531.98
Normal	CT^{10}	68	110	64.30	71	12.01	1163.38	1819.85
	SM^{11}	83	95	73.79	71	10.72	877.78	1526.77
	SL	65	125	46.34	52	27.98	1834.38	2406.92
Varus	CT	80	110	63.04	52	24.34	1186.83	1772.53
	SM	95	95	69.98	52	21.99	923.15	1517.88
	SL	35	125	29.35	78	9.73	2895.92	3563.87
Valgus	CT	50	110	48.91	78	8.31	1529.42	2199.11
	SM	65	95	58.70	78	7.42	1100.58	1771.38

[1] Center of Rotation; [2] Horizontal distance between COR and vector of gluteus medius; [3] Horizontal distance between COR and body weight vector; [4] Perpendicular distance between COR and vector of gluteus medius; [5] Gluteus medius vector angle with horizontal axis; [6] Total force vector angle with vertical axis; [7] Gluteus medius vector; [8] Total force vector; [9] Super Lateral COR location; [10] Centered COR location; [11] Super Medial COR location.

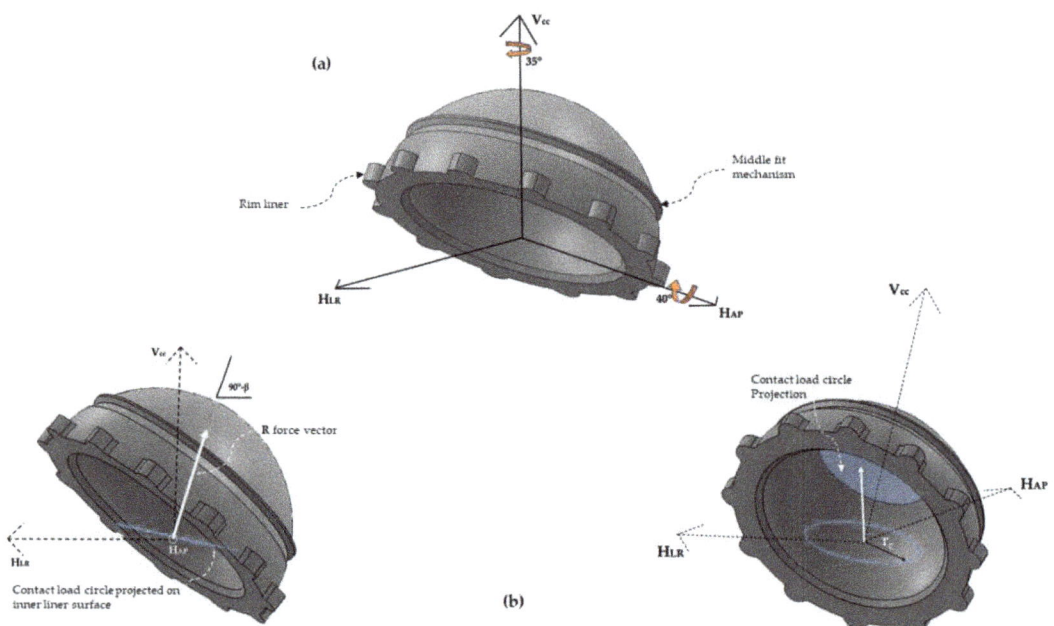

Figure 2. (**a**) 3D liner modeled with its orientation in the three-axis: HLR (Horizontal Left-Right or frontal); HAP (Horizontal Anteroposterior, Sagittal o Dorsoventral); VCC (Vertical Craniocaudal). (**b**) 3D liner with load vector R applied over the contact Hertz theory circle.

The cup angle (40°) was fixed according to the literature [17,19–25] considering that a cup inclination angle greater than 45 degrees is associated with increased wear rates.

As far as Femoral Head Material is concerned, a Contact Hertz Theory [26,27] was used to determine areas of forces contact in both metallic (CoCr) and Ceramic (ZrO$_2$) which have been taken into account in this study by their mechanical properties (Table 2). These properties include friction coefficients for the metal-UHMWPE and ceramic-UHMWPE for each femoral head size taken from previous studies [26,28] and are needed to determine the shear force applied on the spherical surface of the inner liner by means of the contact circle areas (Figure 2b). The contact circle area calculated through Hertz contact theory was projected in the R vector force direction as explained below. Thus, a contact area is created over the inner side of the liner (curve geometry) from a plane circle in the right direction and area location of the force application (R) and with the correct size determined thanks to Hertz theory, as explained below.

Table 2. Mesh liner details for FEA in all geometries.

Liner Thickness (mm)	Femoral Head (mm)	Element Type/ Mesh Quality	Elements Size (mm)	Total Elements	Total Nodes	Element Acept. Ratio < 3 (%)
5.3	32	Solid Tetrahedron/High quality	1.14319	55,010	82,156	99.1
7.3				77,960	113,960	99.1
11.3				137,728	196,708	99.5
5.3	36			66,777	99,442	99.1
7.3				95,977	139,850	99.3
11.3				159,946	228,141	99.5

To calculate the circle area, it was necessary to apply Equations (1) to Equation (3) where r_c (Figure 2b) is the contact radio circle projected in the R force direction that includes the properties of femoral head materials.

$$r_c = \sqrt[3]{\frac{Rr_e}{4E_e}} \qquad (1)$$

$$r_e^{-1} = \frac{1}{r_{fh}} - \frac{1}{r_{ln}} \qquad (2)$$

$$E_e^{-1} = \frac{1-\nu_{fh}}{E_{fh}} - \frac{1-\nu_{ln}}{E_{ln}} \qquad (3)$$

where R is the total force over the hip, re is the equivalent radius equation and E_e is the equivalent elasticity modulus obtained from Equations (2) and (3), respectively. Therefore, E_{fh} and E_{ln} belong to the femoral head and liner elasticity modulus for both materials and, in turn, r_{fh} and r_{ln} correspond to the femoral head and liner radii. Finally, ν_{fh} and ν_{ln} stand for fricction coefficient of the femoral head and liner respectively. The minus sign between fractions is due to the kind of convex–concave (femoral head-liner) contact.

2.1. Load and Boundary Conditions

A different total force vector (R) over the liner geometries was considered for each combination of COR positioning (Center, Super Lateral, and Super Medial) and cervical-diaphyseal angle (varus, valgus or normal).

The body weight (W) was assumed constant with 800 N and used with reduction (W85%), following other authors [29,30]. Values a and b (Figure 3a) were taken from a different set that corresponds with Valgus, Varus, and Normal (Hip Diaphysis Type) and COR positioning (Figure 3b) as Super Lateral (L) Center (CT) and Super Medial (SM).

$$h = a \sin \alpha \qquad (4)$$

$$M = \frac{W_{85\%} b}{h} \qquad (5)$$

$$R = \frac{M \sin \alpha + W_{85\%}}{\cos \beta} \qquad (6)$$

$$\tan \beta = \frac{M \cos \alpha}{M \sin \alpha + W_{85\%}} \qquad (7)$$

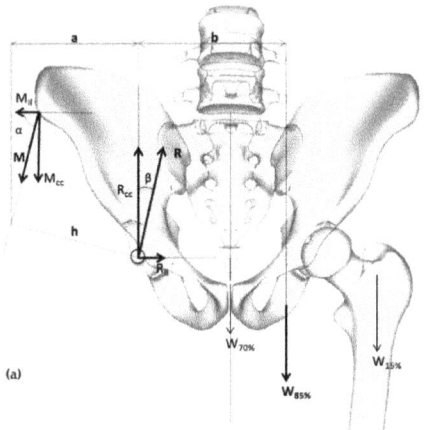 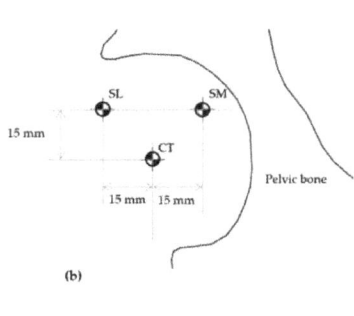

Figure 3. (**a**) Biomechanics diagram forces over hip (frontal projection). (**b**) Displacement for CT, SL, SM as COR positioning.

The Equations (4)–(7) depict the balance of the free body (Figure 3a) with which it is possible to assembly all data (Table 1 (c)). Figure 3b shows the COR location where Superior Lateral (SL) and Medial (SM) locations have both constant vertical value (15 mm) and horizontal constant value (15 mm) from the Center (CT) positioning.

As is shown in Table 1 (c), the gluteus medius vector angle (α) is fixed in each group of values for the three cervical–diaphyseal angles and stems from the geometrical structure of the varus hip (19° below the average value) and valgus hip (7° above the standard value) when the angle is varied [31,32] from 71°.a = 68 mm, given from Le Veau [33].

As aforementioned, specific vector loads were applied over the inner side of the liners depending on their cervical–diaphyseal angle and COR positioning (Table 1 (c)). These loads, which depict the femoral head sphere, were distributed (Figure 2b) all over the circle area, and the dimensions were previously calculated from Hertz contact theory. This area is the contact surface between the ball femoral head and the inner side of the liner and implies a significant reduction of time computed to obtain a desirable order of magnitude in the outcomes.

Finally, a cemented acetabular fixation was configured over the models (ABT geometry) through a complete restriction (Figure 4b) of movements (no displacements on or turns around three spatial axes) of the outer surface including the rim of the liner. The other condition (uncemented) was succeeded by partial rim restriction and the middle fit mechanism on the shell (Figure 4a) with G7 geometry. This kind of restriction avoids nonlinearity created by possible friction contacts if we consider a shell material. To sum up, this research considers the shell and bone mechanical properties, applying these specific boundary conditions over the liner geometry (G7 and ABT). The inner geometry is the same in both cases, but the outer geometry is different.

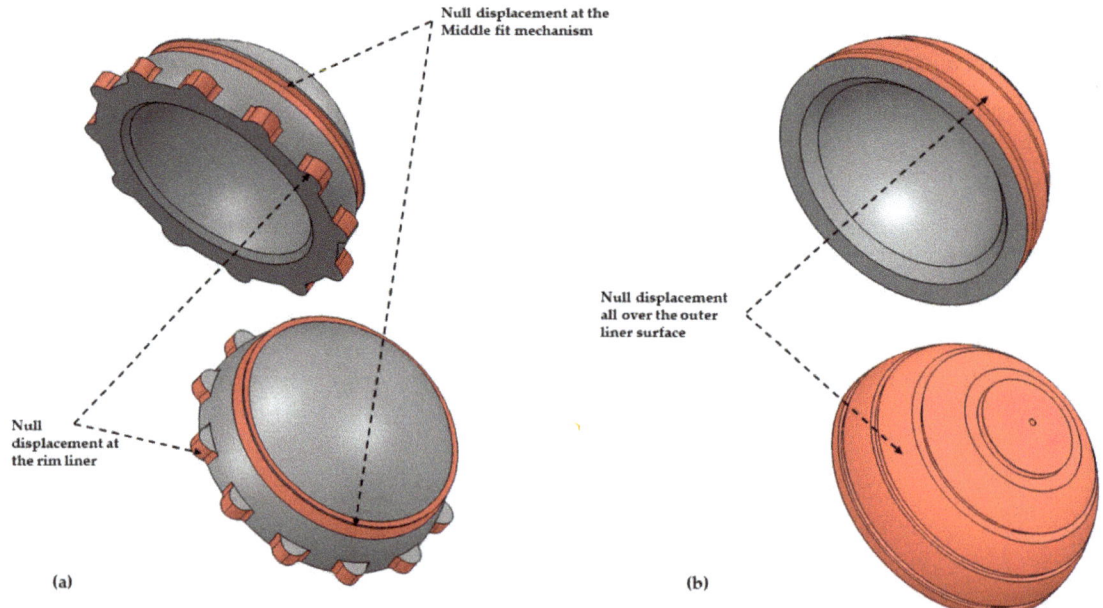

Figure 4. 3D model liner with boundary conditions. (**a**) Cementless acetabular fixation. (**b**) Cemented acetabular.

2.2. FE Modeling and Simulations

Structural static simulations by FEA were carried out over the isotropic behavior of the liner material. This kind of election for the general study is in order to develop a wide range of von Mises results, especially considering the order of magnitude such a numerical tool can give. The simulation software was an iterative solver from SOLIDWORKS 2017. However, results were compared to other software (ANSYS Workbench 19 R2) with equal conditions and parameters (size and kind of elements) with a negligible difference (1.02% using tetrahedron elements and 0.2% using hexahedron elements) as far as the VM stress result is concerned.

Since the number of simulations (216) was extremely high and the results were in a similar order of magnitude between both solvers (SOLIDWORKS and ANSYS Workbench), all simulations were carried out on SOLIDWORKS iterative solver. Other researchers [34] have used the same software as in this research to analyze wear risks in the liner with similar results.

Despite that the size element was the same in all simulations (Table 2), the number of elements (and nodes) was increased from around 55,010 elements in the most miniature liner to 159,946 elements in the biggest liner. On the other hand, the element aspect ratio of values less than 3 was, in all simulations, above 99%.

The election of the solid tetrahedron as a meshing element with an automatic transition to curved shapes over the spherical geometry of liners provides accurate identification of maximum VM points, especially in cementless fixation, since the maximum value was not always in the inner surface of the contact load, as we will discuss in the results.

Finally, to arrive at accurate results, eight Jacobian points were selected in all simulations. The iterative convergence solver spent around 10.4 h of computer time in all simulations using a microprocessor with four cores.

2.3. Wear Risk and Statistical Analyses

VM stress, stress intensity factor (SI) and other results for prediction of wear risk is often used by authors [18,35] as an order of magnitude. VM stress is more reliable as a predictor of wear rate since this kind of criterion comprises the three principal direction stresses in one equation with a long track of approximation to the actual behavior of materials with ductile crack. Therefore, in this research, VM stresses are assumed as a wear risk tester and then contrasted to experimental data from different authors to validate values and locations of maximum points for that kind of stress.

Multiple regression was carried out for statistical analyses running all variables under SPSS software, version 13.0 (SPSS Inc., Chicago, IL, USA). VM Stress was fixed as a dependent variable, and ANOVA analyses were used to determine the *p*-value for all variables. Due to the literature for some variables being quite limited as far as the statistical population is concerned, 1% was considered of statistical significance. However, as mentioned earlier, an order of magnitude was considered to approximate the real significance of all variables.

3. Results

3.1. VM Stress vs. SI Stress

In general, results reveal no difference between VM and SI stresses ($r^2 = 1$) when we analyze outcomes as a whole. In a more particular view and taking into account the acetabular fixation, we can observe that the correlation between both types of stresses (WM and SI) depicts a slight difference. VM stress (Figure 5a) is a little lower (8.19%) than SI stress (Figure 5b) even in terms of wear risk probability. The equivalent is tangible when we analyze the acetabular fixation's general behavior in any parameter (cervical–diaphyseal angle, COR positioning, liner thickness, femoral head material, or femoral head size).

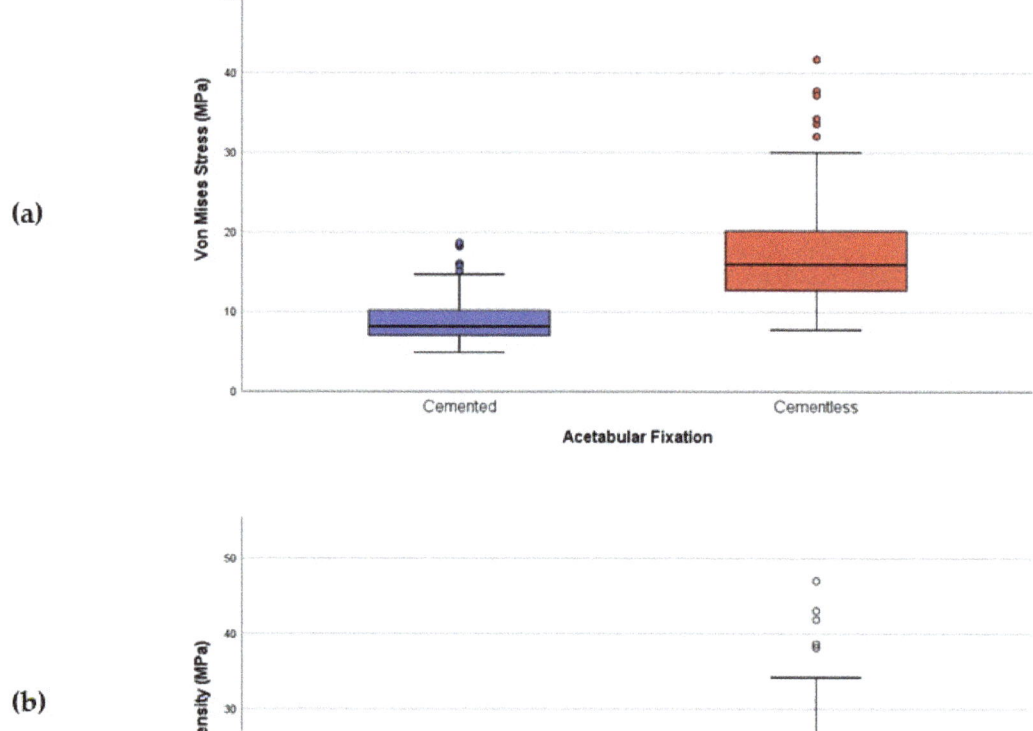

Figure 5. Acetabular Fixation wear risk based on stresses; (**a**) VM Stress; (**b**) SI stress.

3.2. General Analyses of the Parameters

Considering a summary of statistical parameters, VM Stress as a variable dependent displays a r^2 = 0.570 (Table 3 (a)) and its statistical significance is recorded through a *p*-value < 0.0001 (Table 3 (b)).

Table 3. (a) Statistical summary for VM Stress variable dependent. (b) ANOVA Analyses for VM Stress dependent variable (MPa). (c) Statistical coefficients for VM Stress dependent variable.

(a)				
	R	R Square	Adjusted R Square	Std. Error of the Estimate
	0.755	0.570	0.558	4.409221380

(b)					
	Sum of Squares	df	Mean Square	F	p-value
Regression	5394.873	6	899.146	46.249	<0.0001
Residual	4063.218	209	19.441	-	-
Total	9458.091	215	-	-	-

(c)					
	B	Std. Error	Beta	t	p-value
(Constant)	23.240	5.417		4.290	<0.0001
Acetabular Fixation	8.303	0.600	0.627	13.837	<0.0001
Cervical-Diaphyseal Angle	1.711	0.367	0.211	4.656	<0.0001
Thickness Liner	−2.321	0.367	−0.286	−6.317	<0.0001
COR	−0.986	0.367	−0.122	−2.684	0.008
Head Material	−1.521	0.600	−0.115	−2.536	0.012
Head Diameter	−0.493	0.150	−0.149	−3.287	0.001

Results for valgus show a p-value < 0.0001 (Table 3 (c)) as the statistical significance between cervical–diaphyseal angle and wear risk.

The same is true for both acetabular fixation and thickness parameters with a p-value < 0.0001. Head Diameter showed a lesser significance (p-value = 0.001). The p-value for COR (p-value = 0.008) and head material (p-value = 0.012) showed a weaker relationship between those two parameters and wear risk.

On the other hand, a graphical comparative for all parameters shows the general behavior comparing cemented and uncemented acetabular fixation in which there is a lesser wear risk for cement fixation than for cementless. Besides, this tendency is common in all parameters since a low decrease is observed from values for cemented fixation, while, in comparison, the cementless has a more pronounced decrease of its sub-parameters.

In the cervical–diaphyseal angle variable (Figure 6), valgus was more than 20 MPa for cementless fixation, which doubled the cemented model (around 10 MPa), being the highest values for each type in comparison with varus (15 MPa for cementless and 8 MPa for cemented).

As far as COR parameter (Figure 7a) is concerned, a mean VM Stress graph shows that Superior and Lateral (SL) location consistently exhibits the most significant value (over 18 MPa). An intermediate value is found for the Center (CT) location (12.50 MPa), and the lowest value is found on all occasions in Superior and Medial (SM) position (10.15 MPa).

Both femoral head material and size parameters (Figure 7b,c) manifest the same stress behavior with an insignificant difference between them. Nonetheless, there is a significant variation between cemented and uncemented fixation. The values for cemented fixation are much lower (below 10 MPa) than for cementless fixation (above 15 MPa).

Finally, VM Stress increased with a decrease in the liner thickness (Figure 7d) for uncemented fixation. However, VM stress remained nearly constant for the three different liner thicknesses for cemented fixation.

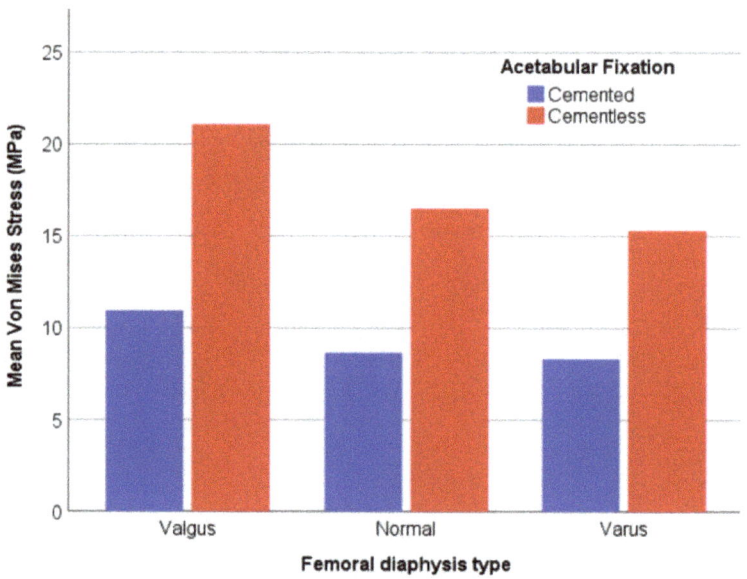

Figure 6. Bar graph with the relationship between VM Stress (MPa) and the femoral diaphysis type.

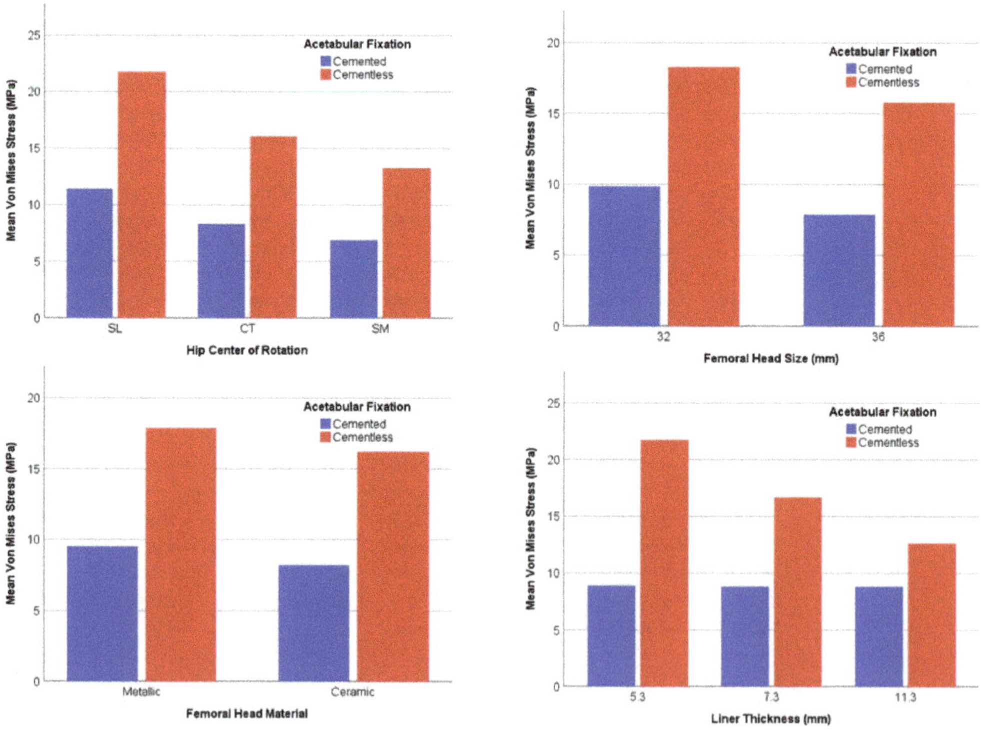

Figure 7. Bar graph with the relationship between variables and VM Stress (MPa); (**a**) VM Stress and Hip Center of Rotation; (**b**) VM Stress and Femoral Head Material; (**c**) VM Stress and Femoral Head Size; (**d**) VM Stress and Liner Thickness.

3.3. Stress Distribution over the Liner

The comparative analysis of stress distribution over the inner and outer surface of the liner (Figure 8) in cemented and cementless fixation depicts a particular stress map of each acetabular fixation with its stress range values in MPa. In order to apply the render in a specific case, a 32 mm head size was chosen made of CoCr with a thickness liner of 5.3 mm, located at Super Lateral COR position and with valgus cervical–diaphyseal morphology. Nonetheless, the general distribution of all liners analyzed follow the same stress map.

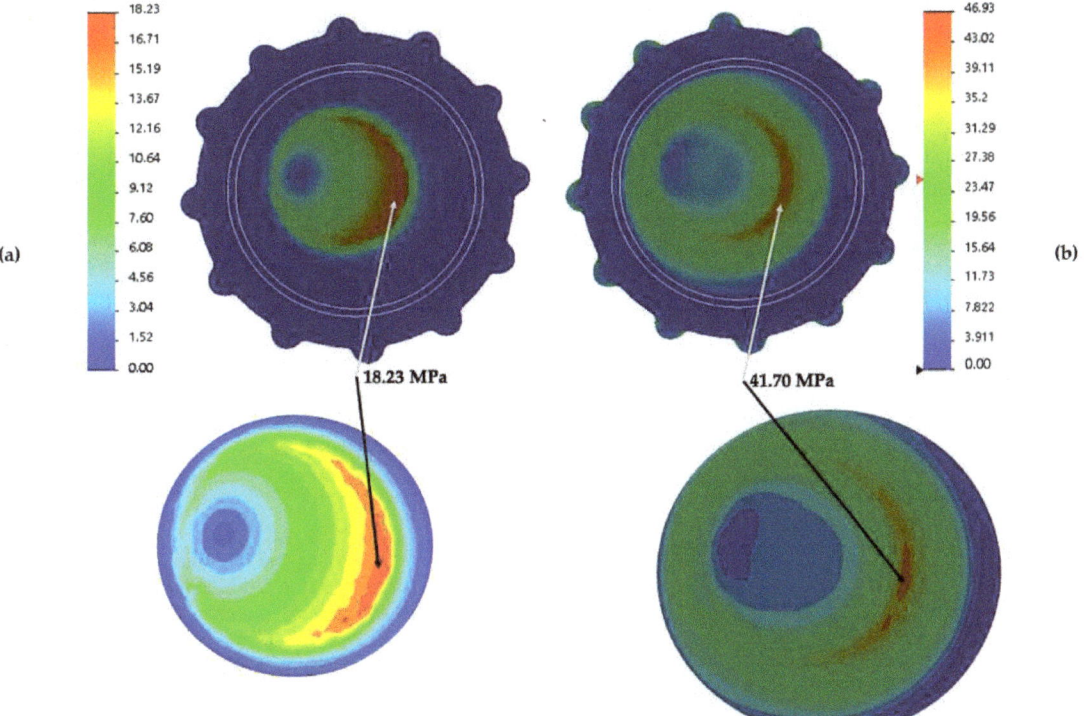

Figure 8. FEA results in images; (**a**) VM Stress cemented fixation of the inner liner surface; (**b**) VM Stress uncemented fixation of the inner liner surface.

The inner surface of liners exhibits how the stress area changes from a more intensive location (Figure 8a) in cemented fixation to a more widespread distribution in cementless (Figure 8b). However, while the location of the stresses for cemented is entirely concentrated, its maximum value (the maximum of the whole liner) is shorter (18.23 MPa) than the uncemented fixation (41.70 MPa). In other words, on that side of the liner, the cement fixation is 43.72% of that of the cementless.

These values are in the same area in both types of fixation, but the cementless is not the area of maximum VM Stress value. A glance at the outer side of both sorts of fixation shows the same area of maximum VM Stress value for the cementless fixation.

The study of the outer surface (Figure 9) shows different VM Stress behavior. Cemented fixation (Figure 9a) develops a slight distribution in a half-moon shape with a maximum VM Stress in the middle of that shape (5.57 MPa), whereas the cementless (Figure 9b) has three different areas of VM stress.

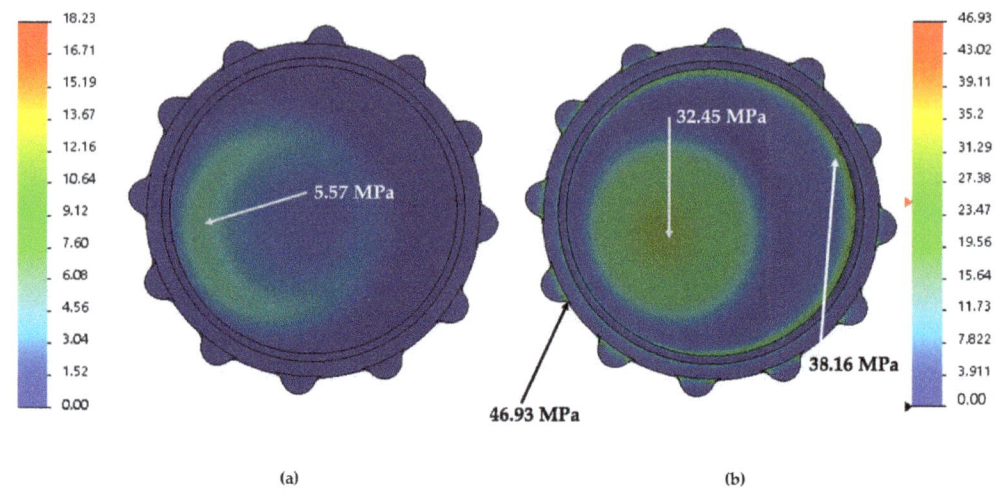

Figure 9. FEA results in images; (**a**) VM Stress cemented fixation of the outer liner surface; (**b**) VM Stress uncemented fixation of the outer liner surface.

The first stress area is located on the top of the liner (32.35 MPa) with a circle shape at the exact location where cemented fixation depicts a half-moon shape. The second area (38.16 MPa) matches a circle made in the liner and is responsible for its fitting assembly with the cup fixed on the pelvic bone. Finally, the third area (46.43 MPa) is located on the rim of the liner.

4. Discussion

Despite the general fact that THA is a well-accepted and reliable surgical procedure to return patients to proper function, aseptic loosening of implants, mainly of the acetabular component, due to polyethylene wear, continues to be a concern among orthopedic surgeons. A personalized theoretical study focused on cervical–diaphyseal morphology was run to obtain detailed results of these specific variables and of wear risk in patients who underwent a hip replacement.

This constitutes the first particularized study that quantifies the wear risk of polyethylene in Primary Hip Arthroplasty. Moreover, it guides the ideal reconstruction of the acetabular component, taking into account the different anatomical aspects of the patient. The results obtained are not intended to be an axiom in the surgical decision, but rather a reference for the hip surgeon regarding surgical planning.

Our findings roughly correlate with previous studies regarding the role of the type of fixation (cemented vs uncemented), COR positioning, femoral head size and material and liner thickness in wear risk. To the best of our knowledge, no previous studies have assessed the role of cervical–diaphyseal morphology in liner wear.

Several critical reviews have led to controversy regarding best acetabular fixation method. Nevertheless, three thorough reviews [1–3] suggested that a higher annual wear rate may be encountered in uncemented acetabular components when compared to cemented components. Moreover, according to Hartofilakidi et al., lytic lesions associated with uncemented acetabular components seemed to be more aggressive than those associated with cemented components [36]. This study confirms, from simulations and numerical data, that wear rate increases in UHMWPE liners with uncemented acetabular fixation.

The location of the osteolysis described for uncemented cups in previous studies [7,9,37] seems to have a similar distribution as the areas of stress described in our study (Figures 8 and 9) for uncemented fixation. These areas are concentrated in the outer area of the liner, mostly in the liner-shell interface. This could be due to the high stress suffered by UHMWPE in contact with the metallic cup [13,38].

The significant difference between cemented and cementless fixations might be explained, from a contact mechanics perspective, due to both kinds of fixations' specific boundary conditions. Stress distribution in each type of fixation is quite different, hence the strains along the liner thickness.

As regards the COR, several prior studies [18,39–41] have linked the elevation and lateralization positioning of the COR, with the failure of THA. For uncemented cups, Georgiades et al set the probability value for statistical significance at 5% [39]. They reported both parameters, lateral ($p = 0.001$) and superior ($p = 0.049$) positioning of the COR, as the responsible cause of wear rate and osteolysis around the acetabular component. Likewise, Hirakawa et al. drew a similar scenario in 2001 [19] with $p < 0.0001$ in lateral positioning and only $p = 0.39$ for superior positioning as statistical significance. Although we have analyzed superior positioning combined with lateral and medial displacement of COR, the statistical significance reached ($p = 0.008$) coinciding with previous clinical studies (Table 4). Our results suggest an increment (40%) of wear risk in SL positioning when compared to SM positioning (Figure 7a), while CT shows intermediate values.

Table 4. Comparative of statistical influence (p-value) among several authors. COR (L) values for Lateral positioning; COR (S) values for Superior positioning.

Author	COR (L)	COR (S)	Thickness	Head Size	Head Material
Gerogiades, 2010	0.001	0.049	-	-	-
Hirakawa, 2001	<0.0001	0.39	-	-	-
Sato, 2012	-	-	-	-	0.45
Garvin, 2015	-	-	-	-	0.58
Gwynne-Jones, 2009	-	-	-	0.21	0.6
Bragdon, 2012	-	-	-	0.23–0.90	-
Lachiewicz, 2016	-	-	-	0.593	-
Teeter, 2018	-	-	-	<0.001/0.055	0.316
Astion, 1996	-	-	0.03	-	-
Shen, 2011	-	-	0.17	0.19–0.64	-
Current study			<0.0001	0.001	0.012

This aspect is highly relevant in two particular clinical settings. It is essential to perform the acetabular reconstruction in the proper anatomical COR in patients with high hip dislocation sequelae, avoiding the superior placement. Likewise, in patients with hypertrophic arthritis of the hip, with a large medial osteophyte, it is necessary to ream in a medial direction to avoid the acetabular component's superior and lateral placement.

With regard to the head material we find values close to 5% in the statistical significance, although prior studies such as Sato with $p = 0.45$ [42], Garvin with $p = 0.58$ [43], or Teeter with $p = 0.32$ [44] do not suggest a relationship between this variable and wear risk. Our results seem to suggest that there is less wear risk in ceramic head material than in metallic. However, Figure 7b provides a graphical analysis of the difference found in our study between CoCr an ZrO_2, which hardly reached 8%.

Another ongoing debate in the literature is the relationship between the head size (diameter) and the wear rate. Again, Teeter declared an unequal distribution (between head size and wear risk) of femoral head size across all groups [42] studied in his research ($p < 0.001$ for ceramic CoCr and $p = 0.055$ for OxZr-CoCr). Other authors such as Bragdon with p-value in the range from $p = 0.23$ to $p = 0.90$ [45] and Lachiewicz with $p = 0.593$ [46] stated similar conclusions. Our research has studied size for 32 mm and 36 mm. We are under the impression that our results are easier to interpret with the help of bar graphs (Figure 7c) in which only a slight difference can be appreciated (15%–17%) between both diameters. Our findings do not support the general idea that a larger head size increases wear rate. These results have clinical relevance when a surgeon decides to use a large-diameter head to achieve a greater range of motion and stability. However, we must consider that this lack of difference found in our study regarding the head size could be explained due to the static structural analyses, in which there are no sliding distance considerations.

The correlation of liner thickness and wear rate has been the subject of many previous studies. Berry suggested that the use of thin liners along with uncemented cups and an acetabular abduction angle of more than 45° was a risk factor for polyethylene wear [4]. Astion [9] found an increase in stress contact ($p = 0.03$) related to decrease of liner thickness. Muratoglu [47], pointing in the same direction, recommended liners thicker than 5 mm. Shen reported an apparent contradiction between his data [35] from the FEA study (an increase of stress with a decrease of liner thickness) and his data from the hip simulator (apparently no significance stress-thickness with $p = 0.17$). Finally, Bartel suggested, after a FEA, that minimum plastic thickness of 4–6 mm should be maintained [38].

Surprisingly, our results point to no relationship between liner thickness and wear risk when it comes to cemented fixation. On the contrary, our results with cementless fixation resemble those previously cited. Considering this, using a cemented fixation could constitute a strategy to minimize the effect between both parameters (liner thickness and wear risk), as may be suggested by the findings showed in Figure 7d.

One of the main novelties of our study is the assessment of the role of the cervical–diaphyseal angle in wear risk. This parameter is usually treated as an inherent parameter for each patient in the literature. However, this parameter is influenced by surgeon decision making medializing or lateralizing the femur by using a standard or high-offset stem. Indeed, our results show that the higher the cervical–diaphyseal angle, the more wear risk. A 31% decrease in wear rate was found when comparing valgus hips (maximum values for cervical–diaphyseal angle) with varus hips (minimum values for cervical–diaphyseal angle). This finding may have relevance in clinical practice as patients with coxa valgus, prevalent in the sequela of hip dysplasia, may benefit from the use of "high offset" stems in order to reduce the wear risk of polyethylene.

Our study has several limitations that warrant consideration. Firstly, FEA modeling focused on wear prediction under a normal walking condition, but it did not evaluate other daily activities. Secondly, our study did not consider the dynamic aspect of the acetabular orientation since pelvic tilt, lumbo–pelvic kinematics and spine–hip relationship-adjusted cup alignment were not assessed. Lastly, wear FEA analysis of the liner simulated the dry contact between bearing surfaces, not taking into account the lubrication that exist under physiological conditions.

Despite these limitations, this study provides a quantification of the relationship between wear risk and five parameters closely correlated with polyethylene wear in previously conducted clinical studies. It also provides the first evidence that cervical–diaphyseal angle may affect polyethylene liner wear.

5. Conclusions

In conclusion, although this is a theoretical study, it constitutes a personalized approach to quantifying the effects of many variables on the wear polyethylene risk probability, especially concerning cervical–diaphyseal angle morphology and the two widespread currently acetabular fixations. It provides guidance for the orthopedic surgeon to plan the acetabular reconstruction in THA, preventing and reducing wear risk by the use of a cemented fixation with high polyethylene liner thickness, a femoral head equal to or greater than 32 mm, and a high-offset femoral stem.

Author Contributions: Conceptualization, C.G.-B., B.d.l.T., L.B.; methodology, C.G.-B., M.A.O., B.d.l.T.; software, C.G.-B., L.B.; validation, C.G.-B., J.B., B.d.l.T., L.B.; formal analysis, C.G.-B., M.A.O., B.d.l.T.; investigation, C.G.-B., M.A.O., J.B., B.d.l.T., L.B.; resources, J.B., B.d.l.T.; data curation, C.G.-B., L.B.; writing—original draft preparation, C.G.-B., M.A.O., B.d.l.T.; writing—review and editing, C.G.-B., M.A.O., J.B., B.d.l.T.; supervision, J.B., B.d.l.T.; project administration, M.A.O., J.B.; funding acquisition, J.B., B.d.l.T. All authors have read and agreed to the published version of the manuscript.

Funding: This work was supported by grants from Community of Madrid (B2017/BMD-3804 MITIC-CM).

Institutional Review Board Statement: Not applicable.

Informed Consent Statement: Not applicable.

Data Availability Statement: The data used to support the findings of the present study are available from the corresponding author upon request.

Conflicts of Interest: The authors declare no conflict of interest.

References

1. Pakvis, D.; Van Hellemondt, G.; De Visser, E.; Jacobs, W.; Spruit, M. Is there evidence for a superior method of socket fixation in hip arthroplasty? A systematic review. *Int. Orthop.* **2011**, *35*, 1109–1118. [CrossRef]
2. Van Der Veen, H.C.; Van Jonbergen, H.P.W.; Poolman, R.W.; Bulstra, S.K.; Van Raay, J.J.A.M. Is there evidence for accelerated polyethylene wear in uncemented compared to cemented acetabular components? A systematic review of the literature. *Int. Orthop.* **2013**, *37*, 9–14. [CrossRef]
3. Clement, N.D.; Biant, L.C.; Breusch, S.J. Total hip arthroplasty: To cement or not to cement the acetabular socket? A critical review of the literature. *Arch. Orthop. Trauma Surg.* **2012**, *132*, 411–427. [CrossRef]
4. Berry, D.J.; Barnes, C.L.; Scott, R.D.; Cabanela, M.E.; Poss, R. Catastrophic failure of the polyethylene liner of uncemented acetabular components. *J. Bone Jt. Surg.* **1994**, *76*, 575–578. [CrossRef]
5. Harris, W.H. The problem is osteolysis. *Clin. Orthop. Relat. Res.* **1995**, *311*, 46–53.
6. Yamaguchi, T.; Naito, M.; Asayama, I.; Shiramizu, K. Cementless total hip arthroplasty using an autograft of the femoral head for marked acetabular dysplasia: Case series. *J. Orthop. Surg. Hong Kong* **2004**, *12*, 14–18. [CrossRef]
7. Gwynne-Jones, D.P.; Garneti, N.; Wainwright, C.; Matheson, J.A.; King, R. The Morscher Press Fit acetabular component: A NINE- TO 13-YEAR REVIEW. *J. Bone Jt. Surg.* **2009**, *91-B*, 859–864. [CrossRef] [PubMed]
8. Busch, V.; Klarenbeek, R.; Slooff, T.; Schreurs, B.W.; Gardeniers, J. Cemented hip designs are a reasonable option in young patients. *Clin. Orthop. Relat. Res.* **2010**, *468*, 3214–3220. [CrossRef] [PubMed]
9. Astion, D.J.; Saluan, P.; Stulberg, B.N.; Rimnac, C.M.; Li, S. The porous-coated anatomic total hip prosthesis: Failure of the metal-backed acetabular component. *JBJS* **1996**, *78*, 755–766. [CrossRef] [PubMed]
10. Pauwels, F. *Biomechanics of the Normal and Diseased Hip*; Springer: Berlin/Heidelberg, Germany, 1976.
11. Barbour, P.S.M.; Barton, D.C.; Fisher, J. The influence of contact stress on the wear of UHMWPE for total replacement hip prostheses. *Wear* **1995**, *181–183*, 250–257. [CrossRef]
12. Bevill, S.L.; Bevill, G.R.; Penmetsa, J.R.; Petrella, A.J.; Rullkoetter, P.J. Finite element simulation of early creep and wear in total hip arthroplasty. *J. Biomech.* **2005**, *38*, 2365–2374. [CrossRef]
13. Kurtz, S.M.; Edidin, A.A.; Bartel, D.L. The role of backside polishing, cup angle, and polyethylene thickness on the contact stresses in metal-backed acetabular components. *J. Biomech.* **1997**, *30*, 639–642. [CrossRef]
14. Liu, F.; Leslie, I.; Williams, S.; Fisher, J.; Jin, Z. Development of computational wear simulation of metal-on-metal hip resurfacing replacements. *J. Biomech.* **2008**, *41*, 686–694. [CrossRef] [PubMed]
15. Maxian, T.A.; Brown, T.D.; Pedersen, D.R.; Callaghan, J.J. A sliding-distance-coupled finite element formulation for polyethylene wear in total hip arthroplasty. *J. Biomech.* **1996**, *29*, 687–692. [CrossRef]
16. Munro, J.T.; Anderson, I.A.; Walker, C.G.; Shim, V.B. Finite element analysis of retroacetabular osteolytic defects following total hip replacement. *J. Biomech.* **2013**, *46*, 2529–2533. [CrossRef]
17. Nadzadi, M.E.; Pedersen, D.R.; Yack, H.J.; Callaghan, J.J.; Brown, T.D. Kinematics, kinetics, and finite element analysis of commonplace maneuvers at risk for total hip dislocation. *J. Biomech.* **2003**, *36*, 577–591. [CrossRef]
18. Wang, L.; Yang, W.; Peng, X.; Li, D.; Dong, S.; Zhang, S.; Zhu, J.; Jin, Z. Effect of progressive wear on the contact mechanics of hip replacements—Does the realistic surface profile matter? *J. Biomech.* **2015**, *48*, 1112–1118. [CrossRef] [PubMed]
19. Hirakawa, K.; Mitsugi, N.; Koshino, T.; Saito, T.; Hirasawa, Y.; Kubo, T. Effect of Acetabular Cup Position. *Clin. Orthop. Relat. Res.* **2001**, *388*, 135–142. [CrossRef]
20. Udomkiat, P.; Dorr, L.D.; Wan, Z. Cementless hemispheric porous-coated sockets implanted with press-fit technique without screws: Average ten-year follow-up. *J. Bone Jt. Surg. Ser. A* **2002**, *84*, 1195–1200. [CrossRef] [PubMed]
21. Bobman, J.T.; Danoff, J.R.; Babatunde, O.M.; Zhu, K.; Peyser, K.; Geller, J.A.; Gorroochurn, P.; Macaulay, W. Total Hip Arthroplasty Functional Outcomes Are Independent of Acetabular Component Orientation When a Polyethylene Liner Is Used. *J. Arthroplast.* **2016**, *31*, 830–834.e3. [CrossRef] [PubMed]
22. Del Schutte, H.J.; Lipman, A.J.; Bannar, S.M.; Livermore, J.T.; Ilstrup, D.; Morrey, B.F. Effects of acetabular abduction on cup wear rates in total hip arthroplasty. *J. Arthroplast.* **1998**, *13*, 621–626. [CrossRef]
23. Esposito, C.I.; Gladnick, B.P.; Lee, Y.; Lyman, S.; Wright, T.M.; Mayman, D.J.; Padgett, D.E. Cup position alone does not predict risk of dislocation after hip arthroplasty. *J. Arthroplast.* **2015**, *30*, 109–113. [CrossRef] [PubMed]
24. Kennedy, J.G.; Rogers, W.B.; Soffe, K.E.; Sullivan, R.J.; Griffen, D.G.; Sheehan, L.J. Effect of acetabular component orientation on recurrent dislocation, pelvic osteolysis, polyethylene wear, and component migration. *J. Arthroplast.* **1998**, *13*, 530–534. [CrossRef]

25. Nishii, T.; Sakai, T.; Takao, M.; Sugano, N. Fluctuation of Cup Orientation During Press-Fit Insertion: A Possible Cause of Malpositioning. *J. Arthroplast.* **2015**, *30*, 1847–1851. [CrossRef]
26. Farhoudi, H.; Oskouei, R.H.; Jones, C.F.; Taylor, M. A novel analytical approach for determining the frictional moments and torques acting on modular femoral components in total hip replacements. *J. Biomech.* **2015**, *48*, 976–983. [CrossRef]
27. Johnson, K.L.; Johnson, K.L. *Contact Mechanics*; Cambridge University Press: Cambridge, UK, 1987; ISBN 0521347963.
28. Bishop, N.E.; Hothan, A.; Morlock, M.M. High friction moments in large hard-on-hard hip replacement bearings in conditions of poor lubrication. *J. Orthop. Res.* **2013**, *31*, 807–813. [CrossRef]
29. Bergmann, G.; Deuretzabacher, G.; Heller, M.; Graichen, F.; Rohlmann, A. Hip forces and gait patterns from routine activities. *J. Biomech.* **2001**, *34*, 859–871. [CrossRef]
30. Simpson, D.J.; Monk, A.P.; Murray, D.W.; Gill, H.S. Biomechanics in orthopaedics: Considerations of the hip and knee. *Surgery* **2010**, *28*, 478–482. [CrossRef]
31. Gottschalk, F.; Kourosh, S.; Leveau, B. The functional anatomy of tensor fasciae latae and gluteus medius and minimus. *J. Anat.* **1989**, *166*, 179. [PubMed]
32. Inman, V.T. Functional aspects of the abductor muscles of the hip. *JBJS* **1947**, *29*, 607–619.
33. Le Veau, B.; Williams, M.; Lissner, H.R. *Biomecanichs of Human Motion*; Mexico-Trillas: Mexico City, Mexico, 1991; ISBN 9682433088.
34. Wong, C.; Stilling, M. Polyethylene wear in total hip arthroplasty for suboptimal acetabular cup positions and for different polyethylene types: Experimental evaluation of wear simulation by finite element analysis using clinical radiostereometric measurements. In *Tribology in Total Hip Arthroplasty*; Springer: Berlin/Heidelberg, Germany, 2011; pp. 135–158.
35. Shen, F.-W.; Lu, Z.; McKellop, H.A. Wear versus thickness and other features of 5-Mrad crosslinked UHMWPE acetabular liners. *Clin. Orthop. Relat. Res.* **2011**, *469*, 395–404. [CrossRef] [PubMed]
36. Hartofilakidis, G.; Georgiades, G.; Babis, G.C. A comparison of the outcome of cemented all-polyethylene and cementless metal-backed acetabular sockets in primary total hip arthroplasty. *J. Arthroplast.* **2009**, *24*, 217–225. [CrossRef] [PubMed]
37. Harris, W.H. Results of uncemented cups: A critical appraisal at 15 years. *Clin. Orthop. Relat. Res.* **2003**, 121–125. [CrossRef]
38. Bartel, D.L.; Burstein, A.H.; Toda, M.D.; Edwards, D.L. The effect of conformity and plastic thickness on contact stresses in metal-backed plastic implants. *J. Biomech. Eng.* **1985**, *107*, 193–199. [CrossRef]
39. Georgiades, G.; Babis, G.C.; Kourlaba, G.; Hartofilakidis, G. Effect of cementless acetabular component orientation, position, and containment in total hip arthroplasty for congenital hip disease. *J. Arthroplast.* **2010**, *25*, 1143–1150. [CrossRef] [PubMed]
40. Gallo, J.; Havranek, V.; Zapletalova, J. Risk factors for accelerated polyethylene wear and osteolysis in ABG i total hip arthroplasty. *Int. Orthop.* **2010**, *34*, 19–26. [CrossRef] [PubMed]
41. Karydakis, G.; Karachalios, T. Comparative In Vivo Wear Measurement of Conventional and Modern Bearing Surfaces in Total Hip Replacements by the Use of POLYWARE®Computerized System. In *Tribology in Total Hip Arthroplasty*; Springer: Berlin/Heidelberg, Germany, 2011; pp. 217–228.
42. Sato, T.; Nakashima, Y.; Akiyama, M.; Yamamoto, T.; Mawatari, T.; Itokawa, T.; Ohishi, M.; Motomura, G.; Hirata, M.; Iwamoto, Y. Wear resistant performance of highly cross-linked and annealed ultra-high molecular weight polyethylene against ceramic heads in total hip arthroplasty. *J. Orthop. Res.* **2012**, *30*, 2031–2037. [CrossRef]
43. Garvin, K.L.; White, T.C.; Dusad, A.; Hartman, C.W.; Martell, J. Low Wear Rates Seen in THAs With Highly Crosslinked Polyethylene at 9 to 14 Years in Patients Younger Than Age 50 Years. *Clin. Orthop. Relat. Res.* **2015**, *473*, 3829–3835. [CrossRef]
44. Teeter, M.G.; MacLean, C.J.; Somerville, L.E.; Howard, J.L.; McCalden, R.W.; Lanting, B.A.; Vasarhelyi, E.M. Wear performance of cobalt chromium, ceramic, and oxidized zirconium on highly crosslinked polyethylene at mid-term follow-up. *J. Orthop.* **2018**, *15*, 620–623. [CrossRef]
45. Bragdon, C.R.; Doerner, M.; Martell, J.; Jarrett, B.; Palm, H.; Multicenter Study Group; Malchau, H. The 2012 John Charnley Award: Clinical multicenter studies of the wear performance of highly crosslinked remelted polyethylene in THA. *Clin. Orthop. Relat. Res.* **2013**, *471*, 393–402. [CrossRef]
46. Lachiewicz, P.F.; Soileau, E.S.; Martell, J.M. Wear and Osteolysis of Highly Crosslinked Polyethylene at 10 to 14 Years: The Effect of Femoral Head Size. *Clin. Orthop. Relat. Res.* **2016**, *474*, 365–371. [CrossRef] [PubMed]
47. Muratoglu, O.K.; Bragdon, C.R.; O'Connor, D.; Perinchief, R.S.; Estok, D.M.; Jasty, M.; Harris, W.H. Larger diameter femoral heads used in conjunction with a highly cross-linked ultra-high molecular weight polyethylene: A new concept. *J. Arthroplast.* **2001**, *16*, 24–30. [CrossRef] [PubMed]

Article

Patient Satisfaction, Functional Outcomes, and Implant Survivorship in Patients Undergoing Customized Unicompartmental Knee Arthroplasty

Cyrus Anthony Pumilia [1,*,†], Lennart Schroeder [2,†], Nana O. Sarpong [3] and Gregory Martin [4]

1. College of Medicine, University of Central Florida, Orlando, FL 32816, USA
2. Department of General, Trauma and Reconstructive Surgery, University Hospital, Ludwig Maximilians University, 81377 Munich, Germany; lennartschroeder@gmx.de
3. Columbia University Medical Center, Department of Orthopedic Surgery, New York—Presbyterian Hospital, Columbia University, New York, NY 10032, USA; nosarp1@gmail.com
4. Department of Orthopedic Surgery, Personalized Orthopaedics of the Palm Beaches, Boynton Beach, FL 33437, USA; gm277@yahoo.com

* Correspondence: c.pumilia22@gmail.com
† These authors contributed equally to this article.

Abstract: Customized unicompartmental knee arthroplasty (C-UKA) utilizes implants manufactured on an individual patient basis, derived from pre-operative computed tomography images in an effort to more closely approximate the natural anatomy of the knee. The outcomes from 349 medial and lateral fixed-bearing C-UKA were reviewed. Implant survivorship analysis was conducted via retrospective chart review, and follow-up analysis was conducted via a single postoperative phone call or email. The rate of follow-up was 69% (242 knees). The average age at surgery was 71.1 years and the average body mass index was 28.8 kg/m^2. Seven revision arthroplasties (2.1%) had knowingly been performed at an average of 1.9 years postoperatively (range: 0.1–3.9 years), resulting in an implant survivorship of 97.9% at an average follow-up of 4.2 years (range: 0.1–8.7) and 97.9% at an average of 4.8 years (range: 2.0–8.7) when knees with less than two years of follow-up were excluded. The reasons for revision were implant loosening (one knee), infection (two knees), progression of osteoarthritis (two knees), and unknown reasons (two knees). The average KOOS, JR. interval score was 84 (SD: 14.4). Of those able to be contacted for follow-up analysis, 67% were "very satisfied," 26% were "satisfied," 4% were "neutral," 2% were "dissatisfied," and 1% were "very dissatisfied." When asked if the knee felt "natural," 60% responded with "always," 35% responded with "sometimes," and 5% responded with "never." After analyzing a large cohort of C-UKA, we found favorable rates of survivorship, satisfaction, and patient-reported functional outcomes.

Keywords: patient-specific; individualized; 3D-printing; unicondylar knee arthroplasty; unicompartmental knee replacement; unicondylar knee replacement; partial knee arthroplasty; partial knee replacement; UKA; UKR

1. Introduction

Unicompartmental knee arthroplasty (UKA) was first pioneered in the 1940s and 1950s by Campbell, McKeever, and MacIntosh using interpositional tibial plateau prostheses [1–3]. Their original reports demonstrated improvements in pain and function through prosthetic replacement of degenerated joint compartments and correction of varus or valgus deformities. Presently, UKA serves as a viable surgical alternative to total knee arthroplasty (TKA) when joint degeneration is limited to either the medial or lateral tibiofemoral compartment. Though UKA has undergone periods of criticism since its inception, namely, questioning its survival in comparison to TKA [4,5], it may offer faster recovery [6–8], reduced complication rates [7–10], improved patient-reported functional outcomes [11–13], and a more normal feeling knee [14,15] in appropriately selected patients. The importance of continuing to study UKA and its technological developments is highlighted by the significant and increasing healthcare burden that osteoarthritis (OA) poses across the world and the increasing number of patients with OA-related knee disorders who seek to maintain a high level of activity [16–19].

One of the more recent technological developments in arthroplasty has been the introduction of customized, or patient-specific, implants. In contrast to the traditional method of selecting implant size and geometry from an available set of options, these implants are manufactured on an individual basis from a three-dimensional rendering of pre-operative computed tomography (CT) imaging. Their development originated from the high variability seen in distal femoral and proximal tibial bone geometry [16–19], as well as the increasing focus on restoring the natural knee anatomy with arthroplasty in recent years [20,21]. In theory, a closer approximation of the natural anatomy would provide for improved kinematics, as shown in customized TKA (C-TKA) [22,23]. Since first appearing in the literature in 2009 [24], C-UKA has shown some potential improvements over conventional UKA, though kinematic studies have not been conducted. Namely, C-UKA has shown improved fit of the tibial component [25,26] and reduced contact stress on the opposite tibiofemoral compartment [27].

To date, there are only limited data on the clinical outcomes of C-UKA. Previous studies have shown satisfactory radiographic outcomes [28], as well as satisfactory short-term clinical results [26,29]. Only one study, to the best of the authors' knowledge, has investigated the outcomes of C-UKA at the mid-term follow-up [30]. The aim of the present study was to retrospectively analyze patient satisfaction, PROMs, and implant survivorship in a large patient cohort with C-UKA at the mid-term follow-up.

2. Materials and Methods

After obtaining approval from the institutional review board, all patients who had undergone fixed-bearing C-UKA (iUni, ConforMIS, Billerica, MA, USA) by a single surgeon between March 2010 and August 2017 were identified. Surgery was performed using customized, or patient-specific, cutting guides provided by the manufacturer. Either a medial or lateral parapatellar approach was utilized. Patient selection for UKA began with four-view plain radiographs of the knee (weightbearing anteroposterior, weightbearing lateral, Rosenberg, and Sunrise views). If joint degeneration appeared to be contained to solely the medial or lateral tibiofemoral compartment, the patient was considered for UKA and further evaluated with a computed topography arthrogram (CT-arthrogram). If the CT-arthrogram confirmed unicompartmental disease and the patient met the indications, UKA was offered. The indications in our patient cohort included an intact anterior cruciate ligament, a body mass index (BMI) below 40, non-inflammatory arthritis, a correctable varus deformity of less than 10 degrees or a correctable valgus deformity of less than 5 degrees, a flexion contracture less than 15 degrees, and a range of motion greater than 90 degrees, some of which were described by Scott et al. [31–34]. No age minimum was utilized. There were no significant changes to the selection or surgical protocols during the time period of the study. Approximately 20–25% of the surgeon's yearly knee arthroplasty collective consisted of UKA.

Patient demographics, surgical variables, and intra- and postoperative complications, as well as re-operations, were recorded from electronic medical records. To assess patient satisfaction, functional outcomes, and implant survivorship, a single postoperative follow-up questionnaire was administered by phone. Patients who were unable to be contacted by phone were contacted by email, through which questionnaires were administered. If contact could not be established after three attempts, the patient was classified as non-contactable.

The KOOS, JR. [35] questionnaire was administered during follow-up to evaluate PROMs. This seven-item PROM combines questions on pain, symptoms, and functional limitations to provide a single score ranging from 0 to 100, with higher scores representing a healthier knee. To assess patient satisfaction, the study subjects were asked to respond to the question "Are you satisfied with your knee replacement?" on a five-item word rating scale of very satisfied, satisfied, neutral, dissatisfied, and very dissatisfied. To survey patient-perceived feelings of the C-UKA, the study participants were asked if their replaced knee felt "natural," with answer choices including "always," "sometimes," or "never." The average time of follow-up was determined after all patients were contacted by phone or classified as non-contactable.

Two separate patient cohort analyses were performed: A follow-up analysis and an implant survivorship analysis. Patients who had died were excluded from both analyses. Follow-up analysis consisted of questionnaire data obtained from contactable patients. In the contactable patients, implant survivorship analysis was performed by asking if revision had been performed during the follow-up phone call. The time point at which the phone call was conducted was considered the follow-up length. In non-contactable patients, implant survivorship analysis was performed by chart abstraction to identify if revision surgery had been recorded in the EMR. The last documented clinic visit without recorded revision surgery, as confirmed by patient history, examination, and imaging, was considered the follow-up length. Implant survivorship analysis was divided into two groups based upon follow-up length. One group consisted of all implanted knees and the other consisted of only knees with greater than or equal to two years of follow-up. Component revision for any reason in both contactable and non-contactable patients was defined as the implant survival endpoint. Patients who underwent revision, did not consent to participation, were non-contactable, or were confirmed as deceased were excluded from the follow-up analysis.

To examine the significance of contingencies, Fisher's exact test was performed and Student's *t*-test was used to determine nonrandom associations between the analyzed variables.

3. Results

The study population consisted of 297 patients (349 knees), of which 118 (40%) were female. The average age at surgery was 71.1 years (SD: 9.2 years) with a mean BMI of 28.8 kg/m^2 (SD: 4.7) (Table 1). Of the total C-UKA, 287 (82%) were implanted medially and 62 (18%) laterally. At the time of follow-up, 12 patients (13 knees) (3.7%) had died and were therefore excluded from the survivorship and follow-up analyses. One patient died shortly after the UKA procedure, presumably from cardiopulmonary arrest. Death notice for the remaining 11 patients was received during attempted phone contact with no further investigation conducted. At the time of follow-up, seven revision arthroplasties (2.1%) had knowingly been performed at an average of 1.9 years postoperatively (range of 0.1–3.9 years). The reasons for revision were implant loosening (one knee), infection (two knees), progression of osteoarthritis leading to the implantation of a total knee replacement (two knees), and unknown reasons (two knees). This resulted in an implant survivorship of 97.9% at the time of phone follow-up or last documented clinic visit in all knees (Figure 1). When all knees with less than two years of follow-up were excluded from the implant survivorship analysis, 304 knees (87.1%) were left with an average follow-up length of 4.8 years (range of 2.0–8.7 years). Thirteen of these knees (3.7%) were known to be deceased. This left 291 knees (83.4%) remaining, upon which six revisions were reported (2.1%), also resulting in an implant survivorship of 97.9%.

Table 1. Patient demographics.

Number of Knees Included in Revision Rate Analysis	n = 349 (287 medial, 62 lateral)
Number of knees available for follow-up and outcome analysis	n = 242
Average time to follow-up	4.2 years (range of 0.1–8.7)
Gender	40% female 60% male
Age at surgery	71.1 years (SD: 9.2)
Body mass index (BMI)	28.8 kg/m^2 (SD: 4.7)

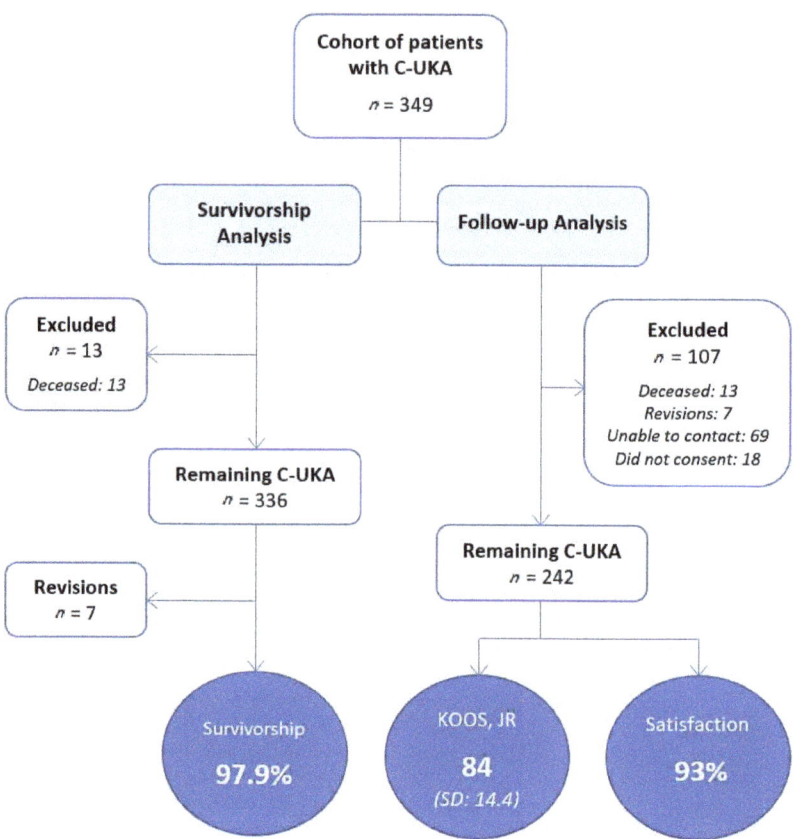

Figure 1. Flowchart of survivorship and follow-up analyses.

Of the 349 knees enrolled, 242 (69%) were able to be contacted, consented for participation, and were therefore included in the follow-up analysis (Figure 1). Of those not included in the follow-up analysis, 79% (69) were unable to be contacted and 21% (18) did not consent to participation. The average follow-up, as determined by the time from preoperative hospital admission to follow-up contact or last documented clinic visit, was found to be 4.2 years (range of 0.1–8.7 years). Medical records revealed two postoperative complications related to the UKA procedure. One patient developed a hematoma postoperatively and was brought back to the operating room for wound irrigation, debridement, and tibial liner exchange. The other patient was brought back to the operating room for wound irrigation, debridement, and primary closure after a fall causing wound dehiscence at five weeks postoperation.

The evaluation of functional outcomes, as measured by the KOOS, JR, showed an average score of 84 (SD: 14.4). When assessing patient satisfaction, 67% of patients were "very satisfied," 26% were "satisfied," 4% were "neutral," 2% were "dissatisfied," and 1% were "very dissatisfied" (Figure 2). When asked if the knee felt "natural," 60% of the study participants responded that their knee "always" felt natural, 35% responded that their knee "sometimes" felt natural, and 5% responded that their knee "never" felt natural (Figure 3).

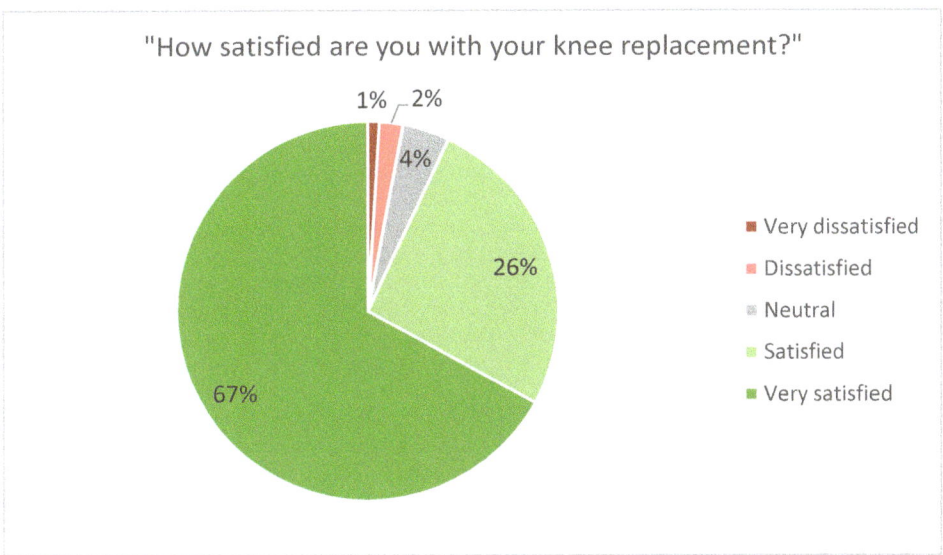

Figure 2. Patient satisfaction with C-UKA.

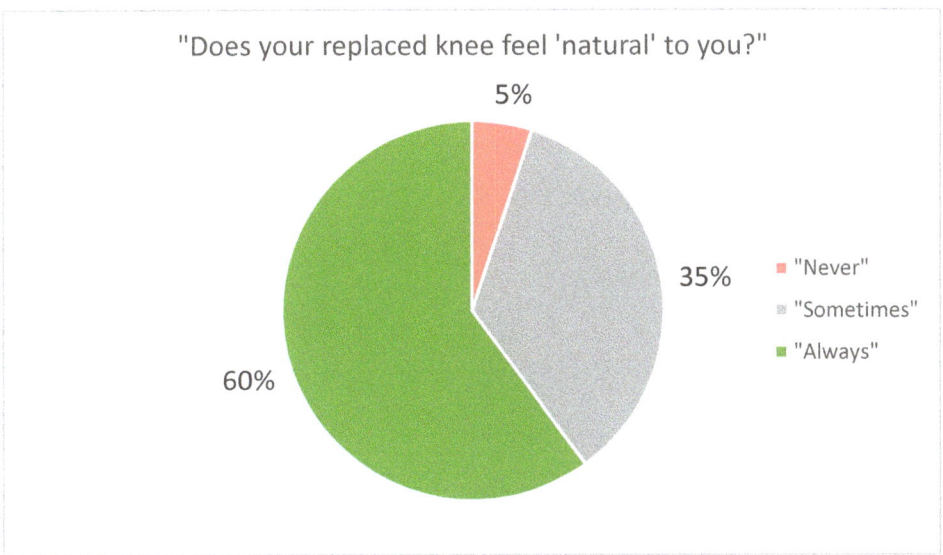

Figure 3. Responses to "Does your replaced knee feel 'natural' to you?"

4. Discussion

Innovation in prosthesis design and implantation has long been the norm in arthroplasty. In recent years, numerous new UKA technologies, such as customized implantation, have been developed and are becoming increasingly reported in the literature [36]. Though C-UKA has demonstrated favorable characteristics, such as improved component fit [25,26] and reduced opposite compartment contact stress [27], its clinical outcomes have yet to be established at mid- or long-term follow-up. To the best of the authors' knowledge, this patient cohort is the largest to be studied after C-UKA. We retrospectively analyzed the survival, satisfaction, and PROMs of 349 knees at an average follow-up of 4.2 years.

Implant survivorship is one of the most common concerns with UKA. Data from the Australian Orthopaedic Association National Joint Replacement Registry show revision rates of 5.2% at three years and 7.5% at five years in fixed-bearing UKA [37], similar to those of the National Joint Registry for England, Wales, and Northern Ireland at 3.43% and 5.36%, respectively [38]. Data from the New Zealand Joint Registry show a revision rate of 4.4% at four years [39]. The data available in the literature for the revision rate of fixed-bearing UKA (combined medial and lateral) include 10% at 5.5 years from Middleton et al. [40], 7.8% at 5.7 years from Biswal et al. [41], and 4% at five years from Whittaker et al. [42]. Though accurate comparison of data is not feasible, especially considering our retrospective study design, as well as the potential variance in the surgeon threshold for revision, an implant survivorship of 97.9% was observed in our cohort of C-UKA at follow-up of 4.2 years.

Survivorship in C-UKA has only been reported by two previous studies. In 2018, Talmo et al. [30] found a revision rate of 25.2% in a retrospective analysis of 115 medial C-UKAs at follow up of 4.5 years (average time to implant failure of 2.8 years). These findings were not echoed by our study, or by Demange et al. [26], who found a rate of 3% at 3.1 years in a prospective cohort of 33 lateral C-UKAs. The most common reason for revision reported by Talmo et al. [30] was aseptic loosening (75.9%), which was a less common reason for revision in our study (14%). Their data do not suggest a clear reason for this discrepancy. Though the average age in their study was much lower (54 vs. 71 years), Demange et al. [26] mirrored our findings with a similarly low average age of 59 years. The average BMI of all studies was similar, ranging from 28.7 to 29 kg/m^2. The selection criteria of Talmo et al. [30] were not reported and therefore may have differed. Furthermore, patient activity levels were not reported and may have also contributed to the discrepancy in survival if their cohort was significantly more active than ours or that of Demange et al. [26]. Comparison between studies is further limited in that both consist of single-surgeon C-UKA data. The reported technique did not differ substantially between surgeons, and the data of Talmo et al. [30] suggest that surgeon experience did not contribute (as evidenced by substantial surgeon experience in UKA and no clear downward trend in the failure rate as experience with C-UKA increased). Nevertheless, there is a possibility that minor differences in utilization of the customized implantation contributed to the discrepancy in the results.

To the best of the authors' knowledge, the satisfaction rates in C-UKA have not previously been reported in the literature. Satisfaction rates have been reported in C-TKA, though with Reimann et al. [43] showing a significant increase in comparison to conventional TKA. Previous studies investigating conventional, fixed-bearing UKA have reported similar satisfaction rates to those of the present study. Biswal et al. [41] reported a satisfaction rate of 92% in a cohort of 128 medial and lateral UKAs at follow-up of 5.7 years. Middleton et al. [40] reported the same satisfaction rate of 92% in a cohort of 129 medial and lateral UKAs at follow-up of 5.5 years. We report a satisfaction rate of 93% at follow-up of 4.2 years.

Superior functional outcomes, as assessed by PROMs, have often been cited as an advantage of UKA over TKA [11,12]. Functional outcomes were assessed in our study using the KOOS, JR., a validated PROM in joint replacement [35], resulting in an average interval score of 84 out of 100 (SD: 14.4). Though no previous studies have reported KOOS, JR. scores after UKA, normative data collected for subjects aged 18–64 years with healthy knees show a mean score of 92.3 (SD: 11.7) that decreases with age and female sex to 91.5 (SD: 12.1) in 56–64-year-old males and 86.6 (SD: 14.6) in 56–64-year-old females [44]. Further reference may be provided by converting KOOS, JR. scores to equivalent Oxford Knee Scores (OKS) [45] using the PROM crosswalk created by Polascik et al. [46]. In their study, they provided a conversion table and demonstrated similar sample means and distributions between the true and derived PROM scores. It is important to note that this conversion may be limited in converting sample means, as opposed to individual scores, and that it has only been validated in a single study population. Nonetheless, it may be able to provide context for the results of the present study when one is not familiar with the KOOS, JR. Accordingly, the mean KOOS, JR. score of 84 in our study equates to an OKS of 44 (out of 48). For reference, Middleton et al. [40] reported a mean OKS of 38 in 129 fixed-bearing UKAs at 5.5 years, Pandit et al. [47] reported a mean OKS of 41.3 in 1000 mobile-bearing UKAs at 5.6 years, and the New Zealand Joint Registry reported a mean OKS of 41.65 in a cohort of 3112 mixed mobile- and fixed-bearing UKAs at five years [39]. Direct comparison of C-UKA and conventional UKA in future studies may provide more insight into the effects of C-UKA on functional outcomes.

Future studies that directly compare C-UKA to conventional UKA may also provide insight into where C-UKA could be able to provide advantages, if any, in the decision making between UKA and TKA. The primary concern in the use of UKA over TKA is implant survivorship. For UKA to be worthwhile in any individual patient, it must provide a large enough margin of benefit over TKA for a long enough period of time, as revision to TKA comes at a cost to the patient and may have slightly inferior outcomes to that of primary TKA [48,49]. With UKA often being selected for improved functional outcomes [11–13] and a more normal feeling knee [14,15], the theorized closer anatomic approximation and more natural kinematics in C-UKA may be able to provide said margin of benefit if its theory translates into long-term clinical results. Kinematics have yet to be investigated in C-UKA, though they have been investigated in C-TKA, demonstrating improved femoral rollback and improved femoral internal rotation at full extension (i.e., the "screw-home" mechanism) over conventional TKA [22,23]. A large percentage of patients in our study (95%) reported that their knee "always" or "sometimes" felt "natural," though without comparison to another patient cohort, conclusions are difficult to draw. However, the direction of the results may indicate a successful restoration of patients' perceived natural feelings of the knee, which may have been a contributing factor for the high satisfaction rate observed. C-UKA may also have an impact on how long the benefits of UKA can be provided, given its potential effects on two of the most common causes of implant failure in UKA: Progression of osteoarthritis and aseptic loosening [50,51]. Biomechanical analysis of medial C-UKA has shown reduced contact stress on the lateral compartment [27], suggesting possible reductions in progression of osteoarthritis. Anatomic studies in C-UKA have shown significantly greater tibial component coverage of the cortical rim [25,26], which may reduce risk for component loosening via tibial bone resorption [52,53], as the component can rely more on the strength of cortical bone as compared to that of weaker, cancellous bone. Though the survivorship shown in our study was favorable, imaging studies were not included in our analysis, and therefore, the above two causes of implant failure cannot be assessed. Clinical investigation and longer-term follow-up of the potential benefits described above will be needed to draw concrete conclusions.

Multiple limitations of the present study must be addressed. Without a control group, direct comparison of C-UKA to conventional UKA in our cohort was not possible, thereby limiting conclusions. Furthermore, the inherent shortcomings in the retrospective design of this study may have limited the findings. Though the retrospective design allowed for a larger cohort than would have otherwise been possible, loss to follow-up may have introduced attrition bias, should those subjects have had different outcomes than those analyzed. This effect would likely be more pronounced in the follow-up analysis, as 31% of the subjects were unable to be contacted. The survivorship analysis accounted for 96% of subjects (the remaining being deceased) and was conducted from either phone follow-up or chart documentation, with the follow-up length recorded as either the time of the phone follow-up or the last documented clinic visit. Nevertheless, the possibility exists that non-contactable patients in this analysis who were only analyzed via internal medical records may have sought care elsewhere after their last documented clinic visit. It is unknown whether the loss to follow-up seen in this study was due to subject unwillingness to accept contact or if contact never reached those subjects. The average age in our cohort was 71.1 years, so it may be likely that a significant portion of uncontactable patients were unknowingly deceased or had outdated contact information. Furthermore, the large range of follow-up lengths (0.1–8.7 years) may be seen as a potential limitation to the survivorship analysis. This study was carried out in this fashion so as to avoid any exclusion bias, especially that of missing early revisions, as demonstrated by our average time to revision of 1.9 years.

Additionally, our data were only that of a single surgeon, whose patient selection process, experience in UKA, and surgical volume may have played a large role in the results [34,54–56]. Specifically, the surgeon in the present study utilized a CT arthrogram in the selection process, which may not be used at all institutions. The yearly volume was greater than 50 UKAs and previous experience with the studied C-UKA implantation system was high. Though our patient-reported outcomes were good, the threshold for revision to TKA may vary among surgeons and has the potential to have contributed to the observed survivorship rates. Furthermore, the patient population that commonly presents to this center and their level of medical comorbidities, as well as administration of PROMs over the phone, may have influenced outcomes and could limit comparison to other studies.

5. Conclusions

After retrospectively analyzing a large cohort of customized unicompartmental knee arthroplasties, we found favorable rates of survivorship, satisfaction, and patient-reported functional outcomes. Though our cohort showed favorable results, these findings may have been limited by the retrospective study design and do not provide insight into how customized unicompartmental knee arthroplasty may compare to other methods. Future studies may be able to provide longer follow-up times, a broader range of patient populations and surgeons, and control groups consisting of traditional implantation in order to truly determine the effects of customized implantation on unicompartmental knee arthroplasty.

Author Contributions: Conceptualization, C.A.P., L.S., N.O.S. and G.M.; methodology, C.A.P. and G.M.; software, L.S.; validation, C.A.P., N.O.S. and G.M.; formal analysis, L.S.; investigation, C.A.P.; resources, L.S. and G.M.; data curation, C.A.P. and L.S.; writing—original draft preparation, C.A.P. and L.S.; writing—review and editing, C.A.P., L.S., N.O.S. and G.M.; visualization, C.A.P. and L.S.; supervision, L.S., N.O.S. and G.M.; project administration, G.M.; funding acquisition, G.M. All authors have read and agreed to the published version of the manuscript.

Funding: Research support was provided by Conformis Inc to cover the costs associated with patient follow-up and medical chart review.

Institutional Review Board Statement: This study was conducted according to the guidelines of the Declaration of Helsinki, and approved by the Western Institutional Review Board® (protocol number, 20170307; date of approval, 22 February 2017).

Informed Consent Statement: Informed consent was obtained from all subjects involved in the study.

Data Availability Statement: Data sharing is not applicable to this article. All data and findings have been presented in the above paper.

Conflicts of Interest: Cyrus Anthony Pumilia reports grants from Conformis during completion of the study. Schroeder reports personal fees from Conformis Inc., during the conduct of the study. Nana Sarpong has no conflicts of interest. Gregory M Martin: IP royalties; Paid consultant; Paid presenter or speaker; Research support; provide Publishing royalties, financial or material support.

References

1. Campbell, W.C. Interposition of vit allium plates in arthroplasties of the knee: Preliminary report. *Am. J. Surg.* **1940**, *47*, 639–641. [CrossRef]
2. MacIntosh, D. Hemiarthroplasty of the knee using space occupying prosthesis for painful varus and valgus deformities. *J. Bone Jt. Surg.* **1958**, *40*, 1431.
3. McKeever, D.C. Tibial Plateau Prosthesis. *Clin. Orthop. Relat. Res.* **1960**, *18*, 86–95.

4. Johal, S.; Nakano, N.; Baxter, M.; Hujazi, I.; Pandit, H.; Khanduja, V. Unicompartmental Knee Arthroplasty: The Past, Current Controversies, and Future Perspectives. *J. Knee Surg.* **2018**, *31*, 992–998. [CrossRef] [PubMed]
5. Jamali, A.A.; Scott, R.D.; Rubash, H.E.; Freiberg, A.A. Unicompartmental knee arthroplasty: Past, present, and future. *Am. J. Orthop.* **2009**, *38*, 17–23. [PubMed]
6. Lombardi, A.V., Jr.; Berend, K.R.; Walter, C.A.; Aziz-Jacobo, J.; Cheney, N.A. Is recovery faster for mobile-bearing unicompartmental than total knee arthroplasty? *Clin. Orthop. Relat. Res.* **2009**, *467*, 1450–1457. [CrossRef]
7. Kulshrestha, V.; Datta, B.; Kumar, S.; Mittal, G. Outcome of Unicondylar Knee Arthroplasty vs Total Knee Arthroplasty for Early Medial Compartment Arthritis: A Randomized Study. *J. Arthroplast.* **2017**, *32*, 1460–1469. [CrossRef]
8. Liddle, A.D.; Pandit, H.; Judge, A.; Murray, D.W. Patient-reported outcomes after total and unicompartmental knee arthroplasty: A study of 14,076 matched patients from the National Joint Registry for England and Wales. *Bone Jt. J.* **2015**, *97-b*, 793–801. [CrossRef]
9. Ode, Q.; Gaillard, R.; Batailler, C.; Herry, Y.; Neyret, P.; Servien, E.; Lustig, S. Fewer complications after UKA than TKA in patients over 85 years of age: A case-control study. *Orthop. Traumatol. Surg. Res. OTSR* **2018**, *104*, 955–959. [CrossRef]
10. Lim, J.W.; Cousins, G.R.; Clift, B.A.; Ridley, D.; Johnston, L.R. Oxford unicompartmental knee arthroplasty versus age and gender matched total knee arthroplasty—Functional outcome and survivorship analysis. *J. Arthroplast.* **2014**, *29*, 1779–1783. [CrossRef]
11. Wilson, H.A.; Middleton, R.; Abram, S.G.F.; Smith, S.; Alvand, A.; Jackson, W.F.; Bottomley, N.; Hopewell, S.; Price, A.J. Patient relevant outcomes of unicompartmental versus total knee replacement: Systematic review and meta-analysis. *BMJ* **2019**, *364*, l352. [CrossRef]
12. Casper, D.S.; Fleischman, A.N.; Papas, P.V.; Grossman, J.; Scuderi, G.R.; Lonner, J.H. Unicompartmental Knee Arthroplasty Provides Significantly Greater Improvement in Function than Total Knee Arthroplasty Despite Equivalent Satisfaction for Isolated Medial Compartment Osteoarthritis. *J. Arthroplast.* **2019**, *34*, 1611–1616. [CrossRef]
13. Noticewala, M.S.; Geller, J.A.; Lee, J.H.; Macaulay, W. Unicompartmental knee arthroplasty relieves pain and improves function more than total knee arthroplasty. *J. Arthroplast.* **2012**, *27*, 99–105. [CrossRef] [PubMed]
14. Kim, M.S.; Koh, I.J.; Choi, Y.J.; Lee, J.Y.; In, Y. Differences in Patient-Reported Outcomes Between Unicompartmental and Total Knee Arthroplasties: A Propensity Score-Matched Analysis. *J. Arthroplast.* **2017**, *32*, 1453–1459. [CrossRef]
15. Peersman, G.; Verhaegen, J.; Favier, B. The forgotten joint score in total and unicompartmental knee arthroplasty: A prospective cohort study. *Int. Orthop.* **2019**, *43*, 2739–2745. [CrossRef]
16. Meric, G.; Gracitelli, G.C.; Aram, L.J.; Swank, M.L.; Bugbee, W.D. Variability in Distal Femoral Anatomy in Patients Undergoing Total Knee Arthroplasty: Measurements on 13,546 Computed Tomography Scans. *J. Arthroplast.* **2015**, *30*, 1835–1838. [CrossRef]
17. Weinberg, D.S.; Streit, J.J.; Gebhart, J.J.; Williamson, D.F.; Goldberg, V.M. Important Differences Exist in Posterior Condylar Offsets in an Osteological Collection of 1,058 Femurs. *J. Arthroplast.* **2015**, *30*, 1434–1438. [CrossRef] [PubMed]
18. Meier, M.; Zingde, S.; Steinert, A.; Kurtz, W.; Koeck, F.; Beckmann, J. What Is the Possible Impact of High Variability of Distal Femoral Geometry on TKA? A CT Data Analysis of 24,042 Knees. *Clin. Orthop. Relat. Res.* **2019**, *477*, 561–570. [CrossRef]
19. Meier, M.; Zingde, S.; Best, R.; Schroeder, L.; Beckmann, J.; Steinert, A.F. High variability of proximal tibial asymmetry and slope: A CT data analysis of 15,807 osteoarthritic knees before TKA. *Knee Surg. Sports Traumatol. Arthrosc. Off. J. ESSKA* **2020**, *28*, 1105–1112. [CrossRef]
20. Takahashi, T.; Ansari, J.; Pandit, H.G. Kinematically Aligned Total Knee Arthroplasty or Mechanically Aligned Total Knee Arthroplasty. *J. Knee Surg.* **2018**, *31*, 999–1006. [CrossRef]
21. Leyvraz, P.F.; Rakotomanana, L. The anatomy and function of the knee–the quest for the holy grail? *J. Bone Jt. Surg. Br. Vol.* **2000**, *82*, 1093–1094. [CrossRef]
22. Patil, S.; Bunn, A.; Bugbee, W.D.; Colwell, C.W., Jr.; D'Lima, D.D. Patient-specific implants with custom cutting blocks better approximate natural knee kinematics than standard TKA without custom cutting blocks. *Knee* **2015**, *22*, 624–629. [CrossRef]
23. Zeller, I.M.; Sharma, A.; Kurtz, W.B.; Anderle, M.R.; Komistek, R.D. Customized versus Patient-Sized Cruciate-Retaining Total Knee Arthroplasty: An In Vivo Kinematics Study Using Mobile Fluoroscopy. *J. Arthroplast.* **2017**, *32*, 1344–1350. [CrossRef]
24. Fitz, W. Unicompartmental knee arthroplasty with use of novel patient-specific resurfacing implants and personalized jigs. *J. Bone Jt. Surg. Am. Vol.* **2009**, *91* (Suppl. 1), 69–76. [CrossRef] [PubMed]
25. Carpenter, D.P.; Holmberg, R.R.; Quartulli, M.J.; Barnes, C.L. Tibial plateau coverage in UKA: A comparison of patient specific and off-the-shelf implants. *J. Arthroplast.* **2014**, *29*, 1694–1698. [CrossRef] [PubMed]
26. Demange, M.K.; Von Keudell, A.; Probst, C.; Yoshioka, H.; Gomoll, A.H. Patient-specific implants for lateral unicompartmental knee arthroplasty. *Int. Orthop.* **2015**, *39*, 1519–1526. [CrossRef]
27. Kang, K.T.; Son, J.; Suh, D.S.; Kwon, S.K.; Kwon, O.R.; Koh, Y.G. Patient-specific medial unicompartmental knee arthroplasty has a greater protective effect on articular cartilage in the lateral compartment: A Finite Element Analysis. *Bone Jt. Res.* **2018**, *7*, 20–27. [CrossRef]
28. Koeck, F.X.; Beckmann, J.; Luring, C.; Rath, B.; Grifka, J.; Basad, E. Evaluation of implant position and knee alignment after patient-specific unicompartmental knee arthroplasty. *Knee* **2011**, *18*, 294–299. [CrossRef]
29. Arnholdt, J.; Holzapfel, B.M.; Sefrin, L.; Rudert, M.; Beckmann, J.; Steinert, A.F. Individualized unicondylar knee replacement: Use of patient-specific implants and instruments. *Oper. Orthop. Traumatol.* **2017**, *29*, 31–39. [CrossRef] [PubMed]
30. Talmo, C.T.; Anderson, M.C.; Jia, E.S.; Robbins, C.E.; Rand, J.D.; McKeon, B.P. High Rate of Early Revision After Custom-Made Unicondylar Knee Arthroplasty. *J. Arthroplast.* **2018**, *33*, S100–S104. [CrossRef]

31. Kozinn, S.C.; Marx, C.; Scott, R.D. Unicompartmental knee arthroplasty. A 4.5-6-year follow-up study with a metal-backed tibial component. *J. Arthroplast.* **1989**, *4*, S1–S9. [CrossRef]
32. Kozinn, S.C.; Scott, R. Unicondylar knee arthroplasty. *J. Bone Jt. Surg. Am. Vol.* **1989**, *71*, 145–150. [CrossRef]
33. Deshmukh, R.V.; Scott, R.D. Unicompartmental knee arthroplasty: Long-term results. *Clin. Orthop. Relat. Res.* **2001**, *392*, 272–278. [CrossRef]
34. Scott, R.D. Unicondylar arthroplasty: Redefining itself. *Orthopedics* **2003**, *26*, 951–952. [CrossRef]
35. Lyman, S.; Lee, Y.Y.; Franklin, P.D.; Li, W.; Cross, M.B.; Padgett, D.E. Validation of the KOOS, JR: A Short-form Knee Arthroplasty Outcomes Survey. *Clin. Orthop. Relat. Res.* **2016**, *474*, 1461–1471. [CrossRef]
36. Aydemir, A.N.; Yucens, M. Trends in unicompartmental knee arthroplasty. *Acta Ortop. Bras.* **2020**, *28*, 19–21. [CrossRef] [PubMed]
37. *Hip, Knee & Shoulder Arthroplasty Annual Report 2019*; Australian Orthopaedic Association National Joint Replacement Registry, AOANJRR: Adelaide, South Australia. Available online: https://aoanjrr.sahmri.com/documents/10180/668596/Hip%2C+Knee+%26+Shoulder+Arthroplasty/c287d2a3-22df-a3bb-37a2-91e6c00bfcf0 (accessed on 28 May 2020).
38. National Joint Registry for England Wales and Northern Ireland 16th Annual Report. Available online: https://reports.njrcentre.org.uk/Portals/0/PDFdownloads/NJR%2016th%20Annual%20Report%202019.pdf (accessed on 28 May 2020).
39. *Twenty Year Report, January 1999 to December 2018*; New Zealand Joint Registry: Auckland, New Zealand. Available online: https://nzoa.org.nz/system/files/DH8328_NZJR_2019_Report_v4_7Nov19.pdf (accessed on 28 May 2020).
40. Middleton, S.W.F.; Schranz, P.J.; Mandalia, V.I.; Toms, A.D. The largest survivorship and clinical outcomes study of the fixed bearing Stryker Triathlon Partial Knee Replacement—A multi-surgeon, single centre cohort study with a minimum of two years of follow-up. *Knee* **2018**, *25*, 732–736. [CrossRef] [PubMed]
41. Biswal, S.; Brighton, R.W. Results of unicompartmental knee arthroplasty with cemented, fixed-bearing prosthesis using minimally invasive surgery. *J. Arthroplast.* **2010**, *25*, 721–727. [CrossRef]
42. Whittaker, J.P.; Naudie, D.D.; McAuley, J.P.; McCalden, R.W.; MacDonald, S.J.; Bourne, R.B. Does bearing design influence midterm survivorship of unicompartmental arthroplasty? *Clin. Orthop. Relat. Res.* **2010**, *468*, 73–81. [CrossRef]
43. Reimann, P.; Brucker, M.; Arbab, D.; Lüring, C. Patient satisfaction—A comparison between patient-specific implants and conventional total knee arthroplasty. *J. Orthop.* **2019**, *16*, 273–277. [CrossRef]
44. Raja, A.; Williamson, T.; Horst, P.K. Extrapolation of Normative KOOS, JR Data for the Young Patient Population Undergoing Knee Arthroplasty Procedures. *J. Arthroplast.* **2018**, *33*, 3655–3659. [CrossRef]
45. Dawson, J.; Fitzpatrick, R.; Murray, D.; Carr, A. Questionnaire on the perceptions of patients about total knee replacement. *J. Bone Jt. Surg. Br. Vol.* **1998**, *80*, 63–69. [CrossRef]
46. Polascik, B.A.; Hidaka, C.; Thompson, M.C.; Tong-Ngork, S.; Wagner, J.L.; Plummer, O.; Lyman, S. Crosswalks Between Knee and Hip Arthroplasty Short Forms: HOOS/KOOS JR and Oxford. *J. Bone Jt. Surg. Am. Vol.* **2020**. [CrossRef]
47. Pandit, H.; Jenkins, C.; Gill, H.S.; Barker, K.; Dodd, C.A.; Murray, D.W. Minimally invasive Oxford phase 3 unicompartmental knee replacement: Results of 1000 cases. *J. Bone Jt. Surg. Br. Vol.* **2011**, *93*, 198–204. [CrossRef]
48. Sun, X.; Su, Z. A meta-analysis of unicompartmental knee arthroplasty revised to total knee arthroplasty versus primary total knee arthroplasty. *J. Orthop. Surg. Res.* **2018**, *13*, 158. [CrossRef] [PubMed]
49. Lim, J.B.T.; Pang, H.N.; Tay, K.J.D.; Chia, S.L.; Lo, N.N.; Yeo, S.J. Clinical outcomes and patient satisfaction following revision of failed unicompartmental knee arthroplasty to total knee arthroplasty are as good as a primary total knee arthroplasty. *Knee* **2019**, *26*, 847–852. [CrossRef]
50. Epinette, J.A.; Brunschweiler, B.; Mertl, P.; Mole, D.; Cazenave, A. Unicompartmental knee arthroplasty modes of failure: Wear is not the main reason for failure: A multicentre study of 418 failed knees. *Orthop. Traumatol. Surg. Res. OTSR* **2012**, *98*, S124–S130. [CrossRef] [PubMed]
51. van der List, J.P.; Zuiderbaan, H.A.; Pearle, A.D. Why Do Medial Unicompartmental Knee Arthroplasties Fail Today? *J. Arthroplast.* **2016**, *31*, 1016–1021. [CrossRef]
52. Chau, R.; Gulati, A.; Pandit, H.; Beard, D.J.; Price, A.J.; Dodd, C.A.F.; Gill, H.S.; Murray, D.W. Tibial component overhang following unicompartmental knee replacement—Does it matter? *Knee* **2009**, *16*, 310–313. [CrossRef]
53. Gudena, R.; Pilambaraei, M.A.; Werle, J.; Shrive, N.G.; Frank, C.B. A Safe Overhang Limit for Unicompartmental Knee Arthroplasties Based on Medial Collateral Ligament Strains: An In Vitro Study. *J. Arthroplast.* **2013**, *28*, 227–233. [CrossRef]
54. Badawy, M.; Espehaug, B.; Indrekvam, K.; Havelin, L.I.; Furnes, O. Higher revision risk for unicompartmental knee arthroplasty in low-volume hospitals. *Acta Orthop.* **2014**, *85*, 342–347. [CrossRef] [PubMed]
55. Badawy, M.; Fenstad, A.M.; Bartz-Johannessen, C.A.; Indrekvam, K.; Havelin, L.I.; Robertsson, O.; W-Dahl, A.; Eskelinen, A.; Mäkelä, K.; Pedersen, A.B.; et al. Hospital volume and the risk of revision in Oxford unicompartmental knee arthroplasty in the Nordic countries-an observational study of 14,496 cases. *BMC Musculoskelet. Disord.* **2017**, *18*, 388. [CrossRef]
56. Baker, P.; Jameson, S.; Critchley, R.; Reed, M.; Gregg, P.; Deehan, D. Center and surgeon volume influence the revision rate following unicondylar knee replacement: An analysis of 23,400 medial cemented unicondylar knee replacements. *J. Bone Jt. Surg. Am. Vol.* **2013**, *95*, 702–709. [CrossRef] [PubMed]

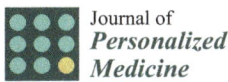

Article

Patient-Specific Implants for Pelvic Tumor Resections

Kevin Döring, Kevin Staats, Stephan Puchner and Reinhard Windhager *

Division of Orthopaedics, Department of Orthopaedics and Trauma Surgery, Medical University of Vienna, 1090 Vienna, Austria; kevin.doering@meduniwien.ac.at (K.D.); kevin.staats@meduniwien.ac.at (K.S.); stephan.puchner@meduniwien.ac.at (S.P.)
* Correspondence: reinhard.windhager@meduniwien.ac.at

Abstract: Introduction Limb salvage surgery for periacetabular malignancies is technically demanding and associated with a considerable likelihood of postoperative complications and surgical revision. Reconstruction using custom-made implants represents the treatment of choice. This study was conducted to analyze treatment outcomes of custom-made implants in a single orthopaedic tumor center. Patients and Methods Twenty patients with a histologically verified periacetabular malignancy and a median follow up time of 5 (1–17) years were included. Results The median number of revision surgeries per patient was 1.5 (0–7). Complications were dislocations in 3 patients, aseptic loosening in 4 patients, deep infections in 9 patients, thromboembolic events in 5 patients and sciatic nerve lesions in 4 patients. Overall survival was 77% after one year, 69% after two years and 46% after five years. Median Harris Hip Score was 81 (37–92) points at last follow up. Conclusion Although internal hemipelvectomy and reconstruction using custom-made implants is linked with a high risk of postoperative complications, good functional outcomes can be regularly achieved. This information may help treating surgeons to find adequate indications, as eligible patients need to be critically selected and integrated into the decision-making process.

Keywords: pelvic tumors; 3D printed prostheses; computer aided design pelvic reconstruction; arthroplasty; complications; bone tumor; pelvis

1. Introduction

Limb sparing surgery of primary malignant pelvic tumors has become the treatment of choice over the last decade, mainly due to improvement in surgical technique, imaging and perioperative management [1,2]. However, limb-sparing surgery remains challenging with respect to defect reconstruction and management of complications [3]. Among the three types of resections and reconstructions described by Enneking and Dunham in 1978, involvement of the acetabulum (Type 2) remains the most challenging area, whereas Type 1, resection involving the ileum and Type 3, resection involving the pubis and ischium require less or only minimal reconstruction [4]. Several methods have been applied for reconstruction of the acetabulum, such as iliofemoral arthrodesis or pseudarthrosis, allograft reconstruction, irradiated, autoclaved or frozen autografts, femoral neck autografts and allograft-prosthetic composites, all of them being associated with a higher complication rate than simple excision arthroplasty or transposition of the hip [2,5–7]. Thus, low complication rates and a possible fast recovery with satisfactory functional outcomes are important factors influencing the decision-making process with patients.

Endoprosthetic replacement bears the advantage of immediate stability and allows early weight bearing, which is of utmost importance in this mainly young patient group. Among the endoprosthetic replacement, custom-made endoprostheses have been used even in the last three decades and still represent the technique of choice due to high variability in pelvic anatomy [8]. In cases when part of the iliac crest can be spared, other implants like saddle prostheses or ice-cream cone endoprostheses have been applied [9,10]. These endoprostheses offer the advantage of immediate availability but come with the

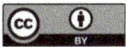

drawback of limited adaptability during the procedure. Three-dimensional (3D) printing has revolutionized the production of custom-made implants. While in the beginning, 3D models have been produced with the help of CAD techniques by milling or laser printing of raisin which served as templates to produce the endoprosthesis, 3D printing of metal not only allows to speed up the manufacturing process but also enables the creation of rough surfaces at the bone interface for rapid and long-lasting osseointegration. [2] One of the big advantages of this process was the improved visualization of the complex and variable pelvic anatomy, which significantly improve the accuracy of resection margins and thus help to improve local tumor control. [11] Another significant improvement was the introduction of patient specific jigs to exactly define resection planes, which is a prerequisite for a perfect match between osteotomy and custom implant [12]. This technique of thorough planning made the procedure more straight forward and reduced surgery time.

Nevertheless, the complication rate and especially the deep infection risk of custom-made implants is significantly higher in the pelvic region compared to reconstructions of other regions, which dampened enthusiasm about this type of reconstruction [13,14]. Furthermore, as pelvic reconstruction using custom-made implants is only rarely necessary, follow up data on this type of reconstruction are rare. Thus, we conducted this study to analyze the outcome of custom-made prostheses in a single center setting over a follow-up period of three decades.

For this, we asked the following questions:

(1) What where complication rates and revision free survivals following reconstruction with pelvic custom-made implants?
(2) What was the oncological survival after extensive pelvic tumor resection?
(3) What were functional outcomes and physical limitations?

2. Materials and Methods

2.1. Study Design

This study was conducted as a retrospective analysis of the Vienna Bone and Soft Tissue Tumor Registry at the orthopedic department of the Medical University of Vienna analyzing patients who were treated for malign pelvic bone tumors using custom made prostheses between 1990 and 2000.

2.2. Patients

Between (1) 1990 and 2000, 26 patients underwent resection of (2) pelvic malign bone tumors at a single center in Austria and (3) received reconstruction using custom made pelvic prostheses; those patients were considered potentially eligible for this retrospective study. Except of oncological survival analyses, 6 of these 26 patients were excluded due to a follow up below one year and, thus, no possibility of an adequate prosthesis assessment regarding function and complications. The median (range) age at surgery was 25 (13–63) years, the median follow-up after surgery was 5 (1–17) years. A total of 9 of the 20 patients were men and 11 were women. Twelve patients received postoperative chemotherapy. The median tumor size was 343 (22–3600) cm^3 (Table 1). Because patients excluded from retrospective analyses often fare worse than patients included, we wished to analyze whether patients excluded from this study differed in important aspects. For this reason, a comparison between groups was performed. In general, patients excluded from this study due to low follow up time showed worse oncological outcomes, as all patients excluded died of disease in the year after primary resection ($p = 0.005$), but no other differences were found (Table 2). Follow-up examinations were performed in our outpatient clinic by clinical joint and radiographic assessment.

Table 1. Demographic data.

Parameter	Patients (n = 20)	RFS
Median age at surgery	25 (13–63) years	0.9 [T]
Median follow up after surgery	5 (1–17) years	0.7 [T]
Sex		
Male/Female	9/11	0.7 [*]
Primary tumor size and localization		
Median tumor size	343 (min = 22, max = 3600) cm^3	0.9 [T]
Ilium	19	0.3 [*]
Pubis	1	
Tumor entity		
Chondrosarcoma	8	0.5 [*]
Ewing sarcoma	5	0.7 [*]
Osteosarcoma	4	0.6 [*]
PNET	2	0.2 [*]
Hemangiopericytoma	1	
Grade		
Low (G1–G2)	5	0.5 [*]
High (G3–G4)	14	0.3 [*]
N/A	1	

RFS = Revision free survival. [T] = T-test, [*] = Log-rank test

Table 2. Demographic statistics of patients included and lost to follow up.

Parameter	Included (n = 20)	Lost to Follow Up (n = 6)	p
Median Age at surgery	25 (13–63) years	40 (10–61) years	0.7 [T]
Follow up after surgery	5 (1–17) years	3 (0–8) months	0.007 [T]
Sex			
Male/Female	9/11	2/4	0.6 [#]
Oncological status			
No evidence of disease	12 (60%)	0 (0%)	0.01 [#]
Dead of disease	7 (35%)	6 (100%)	0.005 [#]
Dead of other cause	1 (5%)	0 (0%)	
Conversion to hemipelvectomy	3 (15%)	3 (50%)	0.07 [#]
Infection	9 (45%)	3 (50%)	0.8 [#]
Thromboembolic event	5 (25%)	2 (33%)	0.7 [#]
Conservative/surgical treatment	2/3	0/2	

Differences between groups tested via, [T] = T-test, [#] = Chi-square-test.

2.3. Surgical Approach and Extend of Reconstruction

Thorough preoperative planning is obligatory to attain a well-directed identification of patients eligible for an extensive resection and reconstruction linked to a potentially high level of postoperative complications. To achieve this, computer tomography (CT) and magnetic resonance imaging (MRI) were used in combination of a complete staging and assessment of relevant comorbidities. Before surgery, bowel preparation and ureter catheterization are performed. In surgery, the patient is placed in a mobile lateral position to allow for flexible intraoperative patient rearrangements. Depending on tumor extension, a ventral or combined ventral and dorsal approach, as proposed by Windhager et al., is used [11]. This type of approach allows a good intraoperative visualization of osteotomies and controlled fixation of porously coated fixation sites. Custom-made endoprostheses were provided either as single or split designs, depending on resection size and form. The extend of the pelvic resection and reconstruction was grouped according to the Enneking and Dunham classification of internal hemipelvectomies depending on resection involvement of the iliac, pubic, or ischial bone [4] (Figure 1). Custom-made prostheses were planned using computer tomography (CT) and thereafter constructed into real size planning models, on which resection lines were defined by the surgeon (Figure 2). Thereafter, the definitive individualized prosthesis (Howmedica, Kiel, Germany) was produced and implanted. Wide resection margins were achieved in 18 patients, while one patient had marginal resection. One resection was histologically deemed intralesional. Patients typically received a hip to leg plaster cast in the surgical theater until 6 weeks after surgery. Afterwards, patients were mobilized under guidance of a hip brace and subsequent weight bearing increase for another 6 weeks. Orthoses were removed 4 to 6 months after surgery.

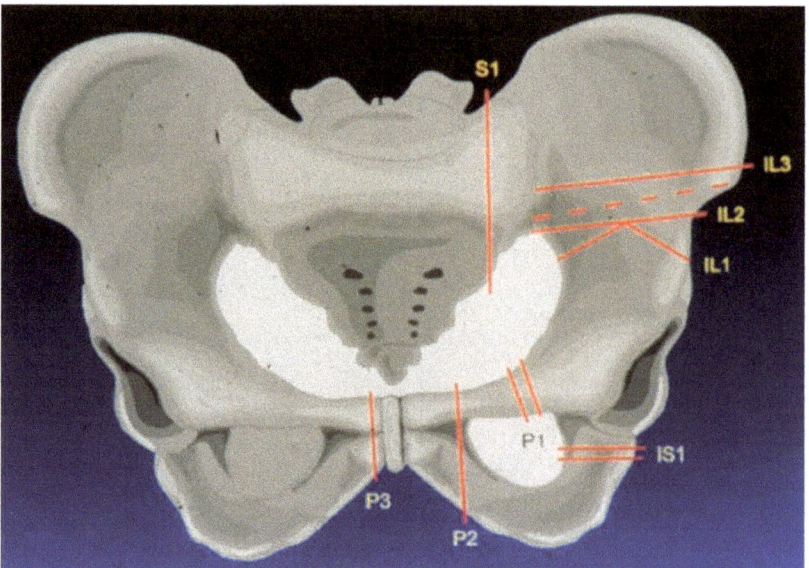

Figure 1. Most frequent resection lines in our cohort according to the Enneking and Dunham classification.

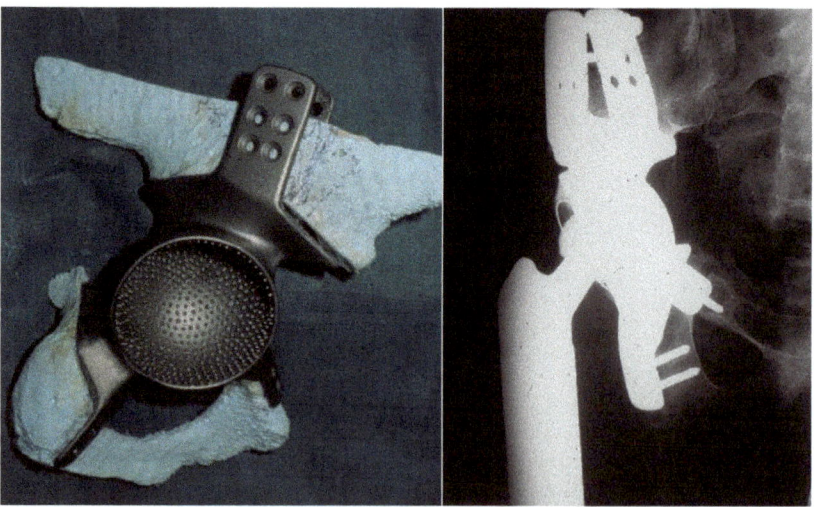

Figure 2. Real-size planning model for preoperative prosthesis and osteotomy planning.

2.4. Primary and Secondary Study Objectives

This studies' primary goal was to assess prosthesis survival and postoperative complications after implantation of pelvic custom-made prostheses. To achieve this, surgical protocols, outpatient visits and discharge letters were screened for complications and revisions. Complications following custom made prosthesis implantation were grouped according to the ISOLS classification of endoprosthetic failure by Henderson et al. into type I or soft-tissue failure and dislocation, type II or aseptic loosening, type III or structural failure with periprosthetic fractures or implant breaking, type IV or deep infection or periprosthetic joint infection (PJI), and type V or tumor progression and prosthesis contamination [15]. Our secondary study objectives were the assessment of patient survival and functional outcomes. The Harris Hip Score (HHS) was used to determine functional outcomes [16].

2.5. Ethical Approval

Ethical approval for this study was obtained from the Ethics commission of the Medical University of Vienna.

2.6. Statistical Analysis

Descriptive statistics were used to detect frequencies, medians and ranges of postoperative complications. After assessment of relevant demographic and surgery related variables, we used Kaplan Meier survival analyses and log rank testing to determine revision free and total oncological survivals. To further distinguish complications regarding different reasons for revision, we differentiated complications according to the ISOLS classification to process revision specific survival analyses. We further analyzed "prosthesis explantation", "thromboembolic events" and "sciatic nerve lesions" as additional parameters due to high prevalence. As all patients who were excluded due to low follow up died of disease in the year after surgery, these patients were included in the oncological survival calculations. Relevant parameters, such as surgical approach, extend of resection, type of femoral stem or pelvic cup and postoperative complications, were reviewed in univariate analyses using independent T-Tests to screen for a possible impact on HHS. The statistical analysis was performed with IBM SPSS version 26 (IBM). A p value < 0.05 was considered significant.

3. Results

3.1. Complications Following Pelvic Reconstruction

Patients were likely to require surgical revision after implantation of custom-made implants. At the time of last follow up, four patients had no surgical revision after prosthesis implantation, while 16 patients had at least one revision (Table 3). The median number of revision surgeries per patient was 1.5 (0–7). The first surgical revision was performed with a median of 27 (0 days–6 years) days after surgery. No surgical parameters influencing revision free survival were found (Table 4). Regarding type I complications according to the ISOLS classification by Henderson et al., we found a revision free survival of 90% after one year and 84% after two and five years. Type I complications occurred in three patients suffering from dislocation of their pelvic prosthesis, which required surgical revision after a median of 5 months (14 days–20 months) after surgery. Two of these patients received open reduction, while one patient had a femoral stem change. Dislocations did not recidivate after surgical revision. Type II complications or aseptic loosening showed a revision free survival of 95% after one year, 89% after two years and 78% after five years. Aseptic loosening occurred in four patients after a median of 38.5 (10–80) months. One of these patients required stem change to a KMFTR proximal femoral modular endoprosthesis and needed two additional revisions for aseptic loosening thereafter. Type IV complications or deep infections were the most prevalent surgical complications, with 9 out of 20 patients suffering from infections which needed surgical revision after a median of 86 days (13 days–5 years) after primary prosthesis implantation. Although most of these infections could be treated with debridement and antibiotic therapy, three patients required implant removal due to otherwise uncontrollable infections after a median of 15 months (95 days–16 years) after surgery. There were no revisions due to type III complications or periprosthetic fractures, as well as type V complications or tumor progression in this study. Four patients suffered from sciatic nerve lesions, of whom two received singular surgical neurolysis with a median of 26 (24–28) months after surgery. Thromboembolic events were frequently observed after surgery, with 5 out of 20 patients suffering from thromboses. Three of these patients required immediate revision surgery at the day of prosthesis implantation, while two patients were successfully treated conservatively.

Table 3. Complications leading to surgical revisions.

Surgical Complications	Patients ($n = 20$)	Median Time to Revision
Median sum surgical revisions per patient	1.5 (0–7)	
Prosthesis explantation	3	15 months (95 days–16 years)
Deep infection	9	86 days (13 days–5 years)
Aseptic loosening	4	38.5 (10–80) months
Dislocation	3	5 months (14 days–20 months)
Sciatic nerve lesions	4	26 (24–28) months
Conservative/surgical treatment	2/2	
Thromboembolic event	5	0 (0–0) days
Conservative/surgical treatment	2/3	

3.2. Oncological Survival after Extensive Pelvic Tumor Resection and Reconstruction

By including all patients with adequate follow up and patients with a follow up under one year due to death by disease, we found an overall survival of 77% after one year, 69% after two years and 46% after five years (Figure 3). Eight patients suffered from metastatic lesions, which occurred in the lung ($n = 5$), brain ($n = 2$), liver ($n = 2$), peritoneum ($n = 1$) and spleen ($n = 1$). Three of these patients received lobectomy, while one patient had resection of his brain metastasis.

3.3. Functional Outcomes and Physical Limitations

Fifteen patients with a minimum follow up of one year could be functionally assessed, while a complete Harris Hip Score could be retrieved in 11 patients, showing good results with a median score of 81 (37–92) points at time of last follow up visit at the outpatient clinic. Six patients were able to walk without walking aid and six patients needed one walking stick, while three patients were mobilized with two crutches. No information regarding walking limitations could be assessed in five patients (Table 4). We found that patients which were surgically revised for infections showed a worse HHS than patients who had no revision due to infection (59.6 versus 84.2 points, $p = 0.033$).

Table 4. Surgical parameters.

Parameter	Patients ($n = 20$)	RFS
Surgical approach		
Ventral + Dorsal	12	0.9 *
Ventral	7	0.5 *
N/A	1	
Type of internal hemipelvectomy (Enneking/Dunham)		
I–IV	8	0.6 *
I, II, III	3	0.6 *
I, II	3	0.5 *
II, III	2	0.8 *

Table 4. *Cont.*

Parameter	Patients (*n* = 20)	RFS
I, II, IV	2	0.7 *
N/A	2	0.5 *
Femoral stem		
Zweymueller	12	0.7 *
Austroprosthesis	3	0.5 *
N/A	5	0.9 *
Cemented Polyethylene Cup		
Brunswick	9	0.4 *
N/A	9	0.9 *
Mueller	2	0.3 *
Surgical margin		
Negative	19	0.6 *
Positive	1	
Oncologic status at final follow up		
No evidence of disease	12	0.7 *
Dead of disease	7	0.3 *
Dead of other cause	1	
Functional status at final follow up		
Median Harris Hip Score (*n* = 11)	81 (37–92) points	
Mobilized with hip orthosis	4	0.2 *
Walking without aid	6	0.4 *
Walking with a walking stick	6	0.98 *
Walking with two crutches	3	0.1 *
No information	5	0.93 *

RFS = Revision free survival. * = Log-rank test

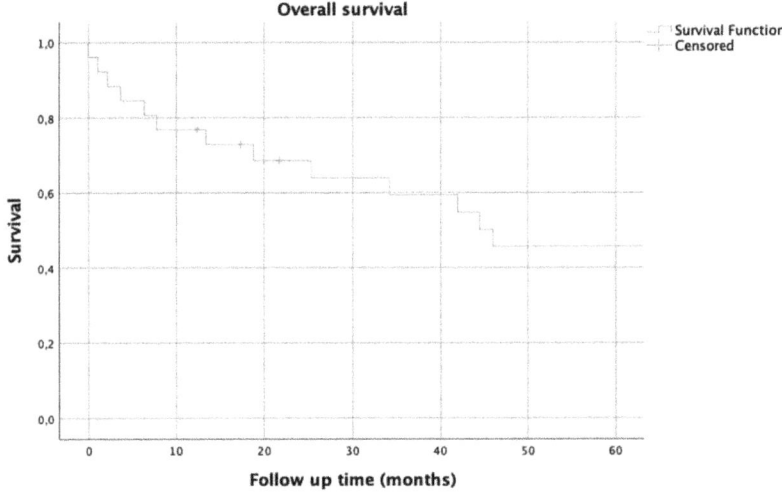

Figure 3. Kaplan–Meier survival analysis for overall oncological survival.

4. Discussion

Defect reconstruction using extensive custom-made pelvic implants after tumor resection is an effective but risky surgery reserved for suitable patients with large periacetabular tumors. Due to the rare indication, relatively little is known at medium- to long-term follow up. We found that postsurgical complications, such as deep infections, were very common and linked to potential prosthesis explantation with concomitant severe functional losses. We further found that patients had, in consideration of the reconstruction extend, comparatively good functional results (Figure 4). This information should promote the use of limb salvage surgery using custom-made prostheses in otherwise unsalvageable limbs and provide a scientific basis for complication and function comparisons of future custom-made prosthesis design models, such as 3D-printed custom-made prostheses.

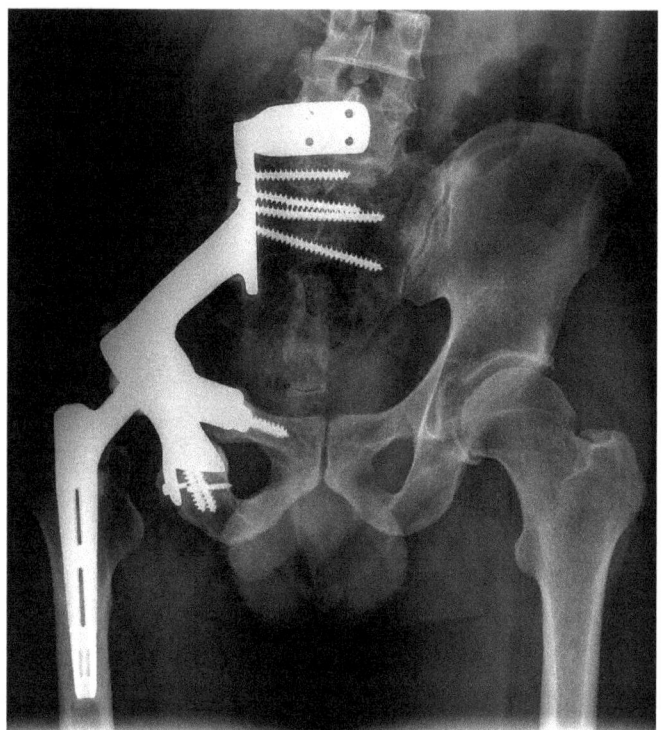

Figure 4. Patient 1 suffered from Ewing's sarcoma and received wide resection via a type I and II internal hemipelvectomy through a combined ventral and dorsal approach with implantation of a 3D custom made prosthesis and articulating austroprosthesis stem in 1991. The picture shows the patient with no subjective physical limitations and walking without aid at a 19 year follow up.

4.1. Limitations

As a retrospective study, potential biases of this study type need to be disclosed.

As surgeries were performed between 1990 and 2000, not only implant types, but also surgical techniques, as well as anesthesia [17] and oncological therapies, evolved to the present date. However, indications for custom-made prostheses may still be found. Due to the lack of differentiated data, especially with regard to complications on this type of pelvic reconstruction, we nonetheless believe that this studies' results are of importance, in particular as a potential baseline for emerging custom-made prosthesis designs and as a field report for treating surgeons.

No detailed influences on revision- or overall oncological survivals were given in statistical analyses due to low power linked to low patient numbers ($n = 20$). Although this limitation may have hampered the breakdown of more intricate findings, such as parameters related to a diminished prosthesis survival, this study aimed to give a more generalized and descriptive outlook on experiences with a rare kind of extensive pelvic reconstruction.

As only patients treated due to malignant tumors were included in this study, this studies' results are limited and need to be considered exclusively in this patient collective. This is especially important with a recent emerge of studies describing the use of custom-made pelvic implants and components in revision arthroplasty settings, as this patient collective comes with different demographics and functional status [18–20].

Due to this studies' limitation to custom-made pelvic reconstruction, no direct comparison of surgical outcomes regarding alternative reconstruction strategies can be made. As patients with periacetabular tumors receiving endoprosthetic reconstruction might differ from patients treated with biologic reconstruction, such as iliofemoral or ischiofemoral arthrodeses or coaptations, allograft reconstruction or ablation in terms of expected survival, functional outcomes and the range and frequencies of postoperative complications, results of this study should be limited to patients with presumably large and highly malignant acetabular tumors treated with custom-made endoprostheses [11].

Missing data need to be disclosed due to the potential long follow up period, as preoperative imaging was not available in every case. In cases when MRI or CT were missing, radiologic reports created by radiologic specialists were used for tumor size quantifications and localization assessments. Detailed functional scores were sometimes unavailable.

4.2. Complications after Extensive Pelvic Reconstructions

Although the use of custom-made prostheses led to primary stable reconstructions, complications were very common at medium- to long-term follow ups. Thus, especially in reflection of a high postoperative prosthesis morbidity with potentially devastating complications, patients need to be carefully selected, thoroughly educated and integrated into the decision-making process (Figure 5).

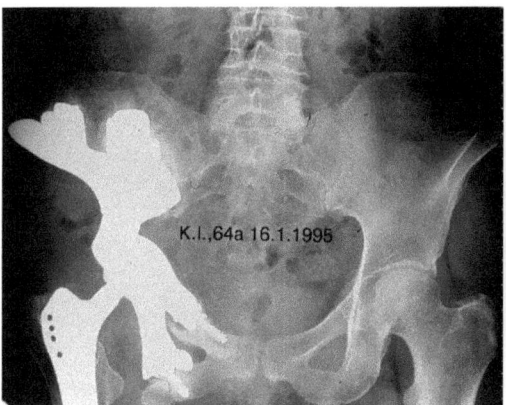 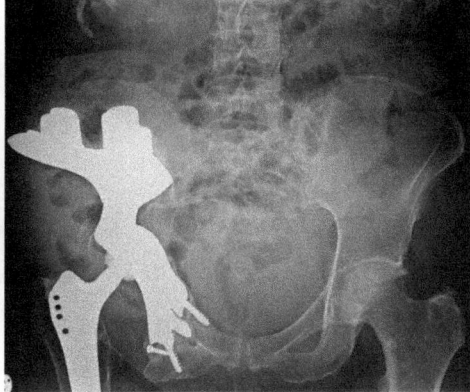

Figure 5. Patient 2 suffered from a periacetabular chondrosarcoma and received wide resection by a type II, III internal hemipelvectomy through a combined ventral and dorsal approach and subsequent reconstruction with a custom-made pelvic implant articulating with a Zweymueller stem in 1992. The patient suffered from aseptic loosening of the implant six years after primary surgery, which was addressed by accretion of iliac crest autograft bone. A deep vein thrombosis was treated conservatively. The X-ray, which was taken 20 years after primary surgery, shows good hip function, and the patient can walk with a walking stick and has an HHS of 89 points.

Deep infection was the most prevalent complication after implantation, with 9 out of 20 patients (45%) experiencing this complication type, followed by aseptic prosthesis loosening in 4 out of 20 patients (20%) and dislocations with need of surgical revision in 3 out of 20 patients (15%). Thromboembolic events were particularly threatening and required immediate surgical revision in 3 out of 20 patients (15%). These results are similar to those of other studies describing outcomes after implantation of extensive custom-made prostheses, with an especially high prevalence of deep infections and aseptic loosening described in literature [21–23]. Although complications were frequent, literature shows acceptable but developable implant survival times of pelvic custom-made endoprostheses. Witte et al. presented a 3-year implant survival rate of 61.4%, while Holzapfel et al. showed an implant survival of 77% at five years [24,25]. At our institution, these high complication numbers led to a diminished use of custom-made endoprostheses at the expense of saddle endoprostheses or ice-cone shaped endoprostheses in the last decades [26,27]. These types of implants come with the inherent advantages of immediate availability, in comparison to a mandatory planning period for custom-made prostheses. However, not all types of periacetabular tumors may be addressed with saddle- or ice-cone shaped endoprostheses, as enough iliac bone is required for implant fixation.

We believe that emerging 3D-printed custom-made prostheses show great promise in reconstruction of extensive periacetabular tumors due to a potential reduction of duration of surgery and thus postoperative complications, a higher prosthesis survival and stability and better availability due to a fast 3D-printing process (Figures 6 and 7) [2,28]. Current, early studies show favorable results of 3D-printed implants, as Wang et al. reported no deep infection in 13 patients and Jovicic et al. showed no deep infections in 11 patients [2,29]. Additionally, modern concepts of osseointegration, such as osteoconductive, alveolar structures as well as improved porous surfaces between the implant-bone interface may easily be implemented in 3D-printed implants [8]. Another important aspect of 3D-printed implants is an advancement in dead space management, as 3D-printed design structures may lead to an improved soft tissue attachment and thus less soft tissue pouches.

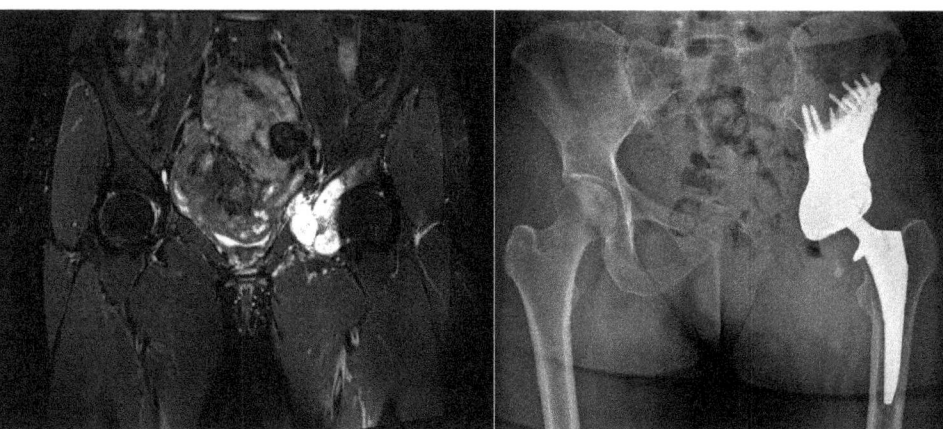

Figure 6. The patient suffered from chondrosarcoma (**left**) and received type II and III wide resection and implantation of a 3D-printed custom-made prosthesis with an Avantage cup (Zimmer Biomet, Warsaw, IN, USA) and Actis femoral stem (DePuy Synthes, Raynham, MA, USA) in August 2020. One year after surgery, the 50-year-old patient can walk for an hour with crutches, while smaller distances can be completed without walking aid. (**right**).

4.3. Overall Oncological Survival after Resection of Extensive Pelvic Tumors

In relation to the necessary extend of resection and reconstruction required for wide resection margins and the median tumor size before resection, overall survival was acceptable with rates of 77% after one year, 69% after two years and 46% after five years. Although oncological survival comparisons after endoprosthetic pelvic reconstructions need to be cautiously evaluated due to high heterogeneity of underlying tumor entities and usually small patient numbers in other studies, these studies' numbers went according with literature, as Wilson et al. reported a pooled mean 5-year patient survival of 55% (37.5–72%) in a recent systematic review [3]. Due to these numbers and a possibly high follow up period, we think that indications for custom-made reconstruction may be found especially in young and otherwise fit patients, due to functional demands and a higher probability to survive extensive pelvic surgeries.

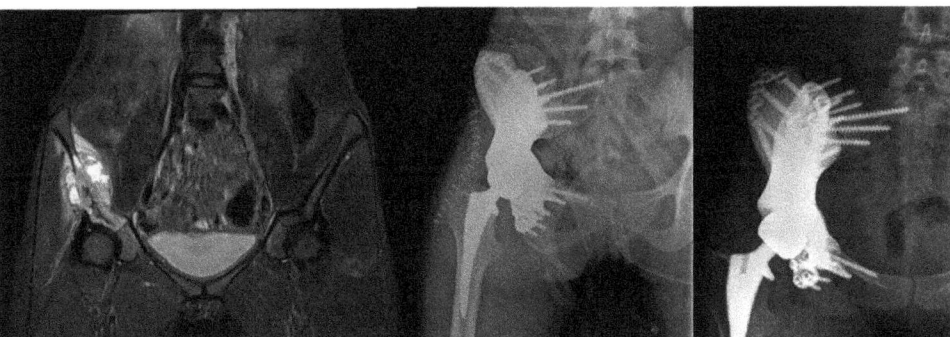

Figure 7. The patient suffered from an osteosarcoma (**left**) and received a type I and II wide resection and implantation of a 3D-printed Materialise custom-made prosthesis (Materialise, Gilching, GER). In this patient, a cemented Durasul inlay (Zimmer Biomet, Warsaw, IN, USA) articulates with an Actis femoral stem (DePuy Synthes, Raynham, MA, USA). (**middle**) Wound dehiscence led to surgical debridement four months after prosthesis implantation. Two years after surgery, the 24-year-old patient is pain free and has a moderate limb walk with no walking aid required. (**right**).

4.4. Functional Results of Patients Mobilized with Custom-Made Prostheses

In frontiers of limb salvage surgery, functional outcomes are of particular importance to justify invasive and complication-ridden procedures. In this context, this study showed good functional results, with a median HHS of 81 (37–92) points at time of last follow up. More than half of all patients showed a high weight bearing capability, as six patients walked without walking aid and six other patients only needed one walking stick. Reports of acceptable to good functional results after extensive pelvic reconstruction are common in the literature. In a retrospective case series, Abudu et al. reported a mean MSTS-93 score of 21 out of 30 points in 35 patients, while Jaiswal et al. showed a mean TESS of 59.4% in 98 patients [22,30]. These results underline the need of stable pelvic constructs, as functional outcomes are good and desirable in oncologic patients surviving their disease.

5. Conclusions

Internal hemipelvectomy and reconstruction using custom-made implants comes with a high risk for postoperative complications. However, good functional outcomes can be regularly achieved. This information may help treating surgeons to find adequate indications, as eligible patients need to be critically selected. Future studies evaluating new generations of 3D-printed custom-made pelvic implants are needed to determine their clinical value.

Author Contributions: Conceptualization, K.D., K.S., S.P., R.W.; methodology, K.D., R.W.; validation, K.D., K.S., S.P., R.W., formal analysis, K.D., K.S.; investigation, K.D., S.P., R.W.; resources, K.D., S.P.; data curation, K.D., K.S., S.P.; writing—original draft preparation, K.D., K.S., S.P., R.W.; writing—review and editing, S.P., R.W., visualization, K.D., R.W.; supervision, R.W.; project administration, K.D., R.W. All authors have read and agreed to the published version of the manuscript.

Funding: This research received no external funding.

Institutional Review Board Statement: The study was conducted according to the guidelines of the Declaration of Helsinki, and approved by the Ethics Committee of the Medical University of Vienna (protocol code 767/2008).

Informed Consent Statement: Not applicable.

Data Availability Statement: The datasets used for this study are available from the corresponding author on reasonable request.

Conflicts of Interest: R.W. reports grants from De Puy Synthes, personal fees from Johnson & Johnson Medical Limited, grants from Johnson & Johnson Medical Limited, personal fees from Stryker European Operations Limited, outside the submitted work. The authors declare no other conflict of interest. The funders had no role in the design of the study; in the collection, analyses, or interpretation of data; in the writing of the manuscript, or in the decision to publish the results.

References

1. Pant, R.; Moreau, P.; Ilyas, I.; Paramasivan, O.N.; Younge, D. Pelvic limb-salvage surgery for malignant tumors. *Int. Orthop.* **2001**, *24*, 311. [CrossRef]
2. Wang, J.; Min, L.; Lu, M.; Zhang, Y.; Wang, Y.; Luo, Y.; Zhou, Y.; Duan, H.; Tu, C. What are the Complications of Three-dimensionally Printed, Custom-made, Integrative Hemipelvic Endoprostheses in Patients with Primary Malignancies Involving the Acetabulum, and What is the Function of These Patients? *Clin. Orthop. Relat. Res.* **2020**, *478*, 2487. [CrossRef]
3. Wilson, R.J.; Freeman, T.H., Jr.; Halpern, J.L.; Schwartz, H.S.; Holt, G.E. Surgical Outcomes After Limb-Sparing Resection and Reconstruction for Pelvic Sarcoma: A Systematic Review. *JBJS Rev.* **2018**, *6*, e10. [CrossRef] [PubMed]
4. Enneking, W.F.; Dunham, W.K. Resection and reconstruction for primary neoplasms involving the innominate bone. *J. Bone Jt. Surg. Am.* **1978**, *60*, 731. [CrossRef]
5. Campanacci, D.; Chacon, S.; Mondanelli, N.; Beltrami, G.; Scoccianti, G.; Caff, G.; Frenos, F.; Capanna, R. Pelvic massive allograft reconstruction after bone tumour resection. *Int. Orthop.* **2012**, *36*, 2529. [CrossRef] [PubMed]
6. Gebert, C.; Wessling, M.; Hoffmann, C.; Roedl, R.; Winkelmann, W.; Gosheger, G.; Hardes, J. Hip transposition as a limb salvage procedure following the resection of periacetabular tumors. *J. Surg. Oncol.* **2011**, *103*, 269. [CrossRef]
7. Donati, D.; Di Bella, C.; Frisoni, T.; Cevolani, L.; DeGroot, H. Alloprosthetic composite is a suitable reconstruction after periacetabular tumor resection. *Clin. Orthop. Relat. Res.* **2011**, *469*, 1450. [CrossRef]
8. Wang, J.; Min, L.; Lu, M.; Zhang, Y.; Wang, Y.; Luo, Y.; Zhou, Y.; Duan, H.; Tu, C. Three-dimensional-printed custom-made hemipelvic endoprosthesis for primary malignancies involving acetabulum: The design solution and surgical techniques. *J. Orthop. Surg. Res.* **2019**, *14*, 389. [CrossRef]
9. Donati, D.; D'Apote, G.; Boschi, M.; Cevolani, L.; Benedetti, M.G. Clinical and functional outcomes of the saddle prosthesis. *J. Orthop. Traumatol.* **2012**, *13*, 79. [CrossRef]
10. Fisher, N.E.; Patton, J.T.; Grimer, R.J.; Porter, D.; Jeys, L.; Tillman, R.M.; Abudu, A.; Carter, S.R. Ice-cream cone reconstruction of the pelvis: A new type of pelvic replacement: Early results. *J. Bone Jt. Surg. Br.* **2011**, *93*, 684. [CrossRef]
11. Windhager, R.; Karner, J.; Kutschera, H.P.; Polterauer, P.; Salzer-Kuntschik, M.; Kotz, R. Limb salvage in periacetabular sarcomas: Review of 21 consecutive cases. *Clin. Orthop. Relat. Res.* **1996**, *331*, 265. [CrossRef]
12. Khan, F.A.; Lipman, J.D.; Pearle, A.D.; Boland, P.J.; Healey, J.H. Surgical technique: Computer-generated custom jigs improve accuracy of wide resection of bone tumors. *Clin. Orthop. Relat. Res.* **2013**, *471*, 2007. [CrossRef]
13. Windhager, R.; Leithner, A.; Hochegger, M. Revision of tumour endoprostheses around the knee joint. Review and own results. *Orthopade* **2006**, *35*, 176. [CrossRef]
14. Puchner, S.E.; Funovics, P.T.; Böhler, C.; Kaider, A.; Stihsen, C.; Hobusch, G.M.; Panotopoulos, J.; Windhager, R. Oncological and surgical outcome after treatment of pelvic sarcomas. *PLoS ONE* **2017**, *12*, e0172203. [CrossRef]
15. Henderson, E.R.; O'Connor, M.I.; Ruggieri, P.; Windhager, R.; Funovics, P.T.; Gibbons, C.L.; Guo, W.; Hornicek, F.J.; Temple, H.T.; Letson, G.D. Classification of failure of limb salvage after reconstructive surgery for bone tumours: A modified system Including biological and expandable reconstructions. *Bone Jt. J.* **2014**, *96*, 1436. [CrossRef]
16. Harris, W.H. Traumatic arthritis of the hip after dislocation and acetabular fractures: Treatment by mold arthroplasty. An end-result study using a new method of result evaluation. *J. Bone Jt. Surg. Am.* **1969**, *51*, 737. [CrossRef]
17. Chua, A.W.; Chua, M.J.; Kam, P.C.; Broekhuis, D.; Karunaratne, S.; Stalley, P.D. Anaesthetic challenges for pelvic reconstruction with custom three-dimensional-printed titanium implants: A retrospective cohort study. *Anaesth. Intensive Care* **2019**, *47*, 368. [CrossRef] [PubMed]
18. Fröschen, F.S.; Randau, T.M.; Hischebeth, G.T.R.; Gravius, N.; Gravius, S.; Walter, S.G. Mid-term results after revision total hip arthroplasty with custom-made acetabular implants in patients with Paprosky III acetabular bone loss. *Arch. Orthop. Trauma Surg.* **2020**, *140*, 263. [CrossRef] [PubMed]
19. Burastero, G.; Cavagnaro, L.; Chiarlone, F.; Zanirato, A.; Mosconi, L.; Felli, L.; de Lorenzo, F.D.R. Clinical study of outcomes after revision surgery using porous titanium custom-made implants for severe acetabular septic bone defects. *Int. Orthop.* **2020**, *44*, 1957. [CrossRef] [PubMed]
20. Chiarlone, F.; Zanirato, A.; Cavagnaro, L.; Alessio-Mazzola, M.; Felli, L.; Burastero, G. Acetabular custom-made implants for severe acetabular bone defect in revision total hip arthroplasty: A systematic review of the literature. *Arch. Orthop. Trauma Surg.* **2020**, *140*, 415. [CrossRef]
21. Dai, K.R.; Yan, M.N.; Zhu, Z.A.; Sun, Y.H. Computer-aided custom-made hemipelvic prosthesis used in extensive pelvic lesions. *J. Arthroplast.* **2007**, *22*, 981. [CrossRef]
22. Abudu, A.; Grimer, R.J.; Cannon, S.R.; Carter, S.R.; Sneath, R.S. Reconstruction of the hemipelvis after the excision of malignant tumours. Complications and functional outcome of prostheses. *J. Bone Jt. Surg. Br.* **1997**, *79*, 773. [CrossRef]

23. Ozaki, T.; Hoffmann, C.; Hillmann, A.; Gosheger, G.; Lindner, N.; Winkelmann, W. Implantation of hemipelvic prosthesis after resection of sarcoma. *Clin. Orthop. Relat. Res.* **2002**, *396*, 197. [CrossRef]
24. Holzapfel, B.M.; Pilge, H.; Prodinger, P.M.; Toepfer, A.; Mayer-Wagner, S.; Hutmacher, D.W.; von Eisenhart-Rothe, R.; Rudert, M.; Gradinger, R.; Rechl, H. Customised osteotomy guides and endoprosthetic reconstruction for periacetabular tumours. *Int. Orthop.* **2014**, *38*, 1435. [CrossRef]
25. Witte, D.; Bernd, L.; Bruns, J.; Gosheger, G.; Hardes, J.; Hartwig, E.; Lehner, B.; Melcher, I.; Mutschler, W.; Schulte, M.; et al. Limb-salvage reconstruction with MUTARS hemipelvic endoprosthesis: A prospective multicenter study. *Eur. J. Surg. Oncol.* **2009**, *35*, 1318. [CrossRef]
26. Barrientos-Ruiz, I.; Ortiz-Cruz, E.J.; Peleteiro-Pensado, M. Reconstruction After Hemipelvectomy With the Ice-Cream Cone Prosthesis: What Are the Short-term Clinical Results? *Clin. Orthop. Relat. Res.* **2017**, *475*, 735. [CrossRef]
27. Jansen, J.A.; van de Sande, M.A.J.; Dijkstra, P.D.S. Poor long-term clinical results of saddle prosthesis after resection of periacetabular tumors. *Clin. Orthop. Relat. Res.* **2013**, *471*, 324. [CrossRef]
28. Wang, B.; Hao, Y.; Pu, F.; Jiang, W.; Shao, Z. Computer-aided designed, three dimensional-printed hemipelvic prosthesis for peri-acetabular malignant bone tumour. *Int. Orthop.* **2018**, *42*, 687. [CrossRef] [PubMed]
29. Jovičić, M.S.; Vuletić, F.; Ribičić, T.; Šimunić, S.; Petrović, T.; Kolundžić, R. Implementation of the three-dimensional printing technology in treatment of bone tumours: A case series. *Int. Orthop.* **2021**, *45*, 1079. [CrossRef] [PubMed]
30. Jaiswal, P.K.; Aston, W.J.; Grimer, R.J.; Abudu, A.; Carter, S.; Blunn, G.; Briggs, T.W.; Cannon, S. Peri-acetabular resection and endoprosthetic reconstruction for tumours of the acetabulum. *J. Bone Jt. Surg. Br.* **2008**, *90*, 1222. [CrossRef] [PubMed]

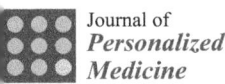

Article

True Kinematic Alignment Is Applicable in 44% of Patients Applying Restrictive Indication Criteria—A Retrospective Analysis of 111 TKA Using Robotic Assistance

Kim Huber [1], Bernhard Christen [1], Sarah Calliess [1,2] and Tilman Calliess [1,*]

1. articon Spezialpraxis für Gelenkchirurgie, 3013 Berne, Switzerland; kimihuber@hotmail.com (K.H.); b.christen@articon.ch (B.C.); s.calliess@articon.ch (S.C.)
2. Campusradiologie Bern, Engeried-Spital, 3012 Berne, Switzerland
* Correspondence: t.calliess@articon.ch; Tel.: +41-31-337-8924

Abstract: Introduction: Image-based robotic assistance appears to be a promising tool for individualizing alignment in total knee arthroplasty (TKA). The patient-specific model of the knee enables a preoperative 3D planning of component position. Adjustments to the individual soft-tissue situation can be done intraoperatively. Based on this, we have established a standardized workflow to implement the idea of kinematic alignment (KA) for robotic-assisted TKA. In addition, we have defined limits for its use. If these limits are reached, we switch to a restricted KA (rKA). The aim of the study was to evaluate (1) in what percentage of patients a true KA or an rKA is applicable, (2) whether there were differences regarding knee phenotypes, and (3) what the differences of philosophies in terms of component position, joint stability, and early patient outcome were. Methods: The study included a retrospective analysis of 111 robotic-assisted primary TKAs. Based on preoperative long leg standing radiographs, the patients were categorized into a varus, valgus, or neutral subgroup. Initially, all patients were planned for KA TKA. When the defined safe zone had been exceeded, adjustments to an rKA were made. Intraoperatively, the alignment of the components and joint gaps were recorded by robotic software. Results and conclusion: With our indication for TKA and the defined boundaries, "only" 44% of the patients were suitable for a true KA with no adjustments or soft tissue releases. In the varus group, it was about 70%, whereas it was 0% in the valgus group and 25% in the neutral alignment group. Thus, significant differences with regard to knee morphotypes were evident. In the KA group, a more physiological knee balance reconstructing the trapezoidal flexion gap (+2 mm on average laterally) was seen as well as a closer reconstruction of the surface anatomy and joint line in all dimensions compared to rKA. This resulted in a higher improvement in the collected outcome scores in favor of KA in the very early postoperative phase.

Keywords: individualized alignment; restricted kinematic alignment; robotic-assisted TKA; MAKO; safe zone; total knee arthroplasty

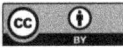

1. Introduction

In the effort to improve total knee arthroplasty (TKA), there is a growing interest in customizing alignment to the patient's individual anatomy and soft-tissue balance. This is discussed as an alternative to the established standard mechanical alignment (MA) that has the same target for everybody. However, this individualized alignment is often not clearly defined, and a multitude of different philosophies, approaches, and terms can be found in the literature [1]. The clearest defined concept with the best clinical evidence available is the kinematic alignment (KA) approach [2]. The defined primary aim of KA is to reconstruct the individual joint surface of the femoral condyles with the prosthesis and thus to co-align the motion axes of the device to that of the patient's knee [3]. Several studies report equal or even superior clinical outcomes compared to standard MA [4]. However, there are still critical voices. One point of criticism is about the resulting overall limb alignment and joint line obliquity in KA TKA. As the pre-arthritic situation is reconstructed, the components may be aligned in a significant varus or valgus angulation [5]. These deviations to the mechanical axis might lead to early implant failure. Further. it is questioned whether it makes sense to reconstruct pathologic situations that have led to osteoarthritis, or to better correct these with surgery. Another point of criticism is whether it is possible to properly reconstruct the individual joint surface with the use of a standard, symmetric prosthesis or if the different patient morphologies might require an individualized prosthesis [6,7]. Thus, not all patients may be suitable for KA TKA.

These concerns have led to an adaption of KA with the possibility for intraoperatively made adjustments to stay within a defined target zone of postoperative limb alignment, or to correct pathologic situations—the restricted kinematic alignment (rKA) approach [1]. Currently, there is a lack of a clear definition of when (or how often) adjustments are needed, and for what patients or phenotypes. Furthermore, there are only very limited data on the consequences for the patient—in terms of alignment, stability, and outcome [8,9]. Additional to this, there now is the need for technological support of some sort to be able to (1) identify a situation that needs to be adapted, and (2) precisely transfer this plan to the patient [10].

In this context, image-based robotics appears to be a promising tool for individualizing alignment with the concept of KA and rKA in standard TKA. Preoperative imaging enables a three-dimensional (3D) preplanning of the alignment philosophy based on the patient's knee morphotype. Intraoperative adaptions with respect to soft tissue stability are possible. The robotic assistance ensures a precise implementation of the planning. As a result, all relevant parameters are transparent and comprehensible and thus are available for further evaluation.

In our institution, we established a clear workflow for individualized alignment in robotic-assisted TKA since 09/2018. The starting point is the KA principle with certain self-defined alignment limits based on our experiences and the current literature [11]: (1) Resulting overall limb alignment of 176–181°, (2) a joint line obliquity up to 4° to the mechanical axis, and (3) a neutral rotation of the component trochlea groove to the anatomical trochlea axis. When these criteria could not be achieved with a KA-based component position, adjustments were made to a restricted KA, as described below.

Based on this, the research questions of this study were: (1) With said criteria, how often can we conduct a true KA in a standard TKA collective and how often do we have to make adaptions? (2) Are there differences in the suitability for KA (with proposed limits) between different knee morphotypes? (3) What are the differences between a true KA and an rKA in terms of alignment, resulting joint stability, and early postoperative outcome?

2. Methods

2.1. Patient Collective

The study includes a retrospective review of our institutional database on knee arthroplasties between 10/2019 and 04/2021. All patients were included who gave their informed consent to participate in the prospective data collection and received an image-based, robotic-assisted, primary unconstrained TKA for any indication in that time period. The patient demographics (age, sex, ASA score, and previous surgeries on the affected knee) and preoperative knee alignment were determined. On preoperative long leg standing X-rays (EOS System), the anatomical and the mechanical hip–knee–ankle angle (HKA) as well as the standard joint line angles (MPTA, mLDFA) were measured by an independent radiologist. Based on the determined anatomical femorotibial angle, three subgroups were defined: (1) Neutral (5–10°), (2) varus OA (<5°), and (3) valgus OA (>10°).

2.2. Application of Individualized Alignment Philosophies

All patients received an individualized alignment—true KA or rKA—based on their knee anatomy/morphotype, ligament situation, and the defined boundaries for KA following a standardized workflow.

All surgeries were conducted with the MAKO robotic arm and the Triathlon PS knee system (Stryker, Kalamazoo, MI, USA). Prior to surgery, three-dimensional preplanning of the individualized component position using the proprietary MAKO software was conducted by the operating senior surgeon following the concept of kinematic alignment (KA) (Figure 1). First, the distal and posterior resections on the femur were set symmetrically at 6 mm bone resection. This results in an individual distal femoral angulation and a 0° rotation with reference to the posterior condylar axis (PCA) (individual rotation to transepicondylar axis (TEA)). In a second step, the femoral component size was defined to best reconstruct the anterio-posterior and medio-lateral dimensions without producing an overhang. Based on this position and size, the femoral flexion was adjusted to create a smooth anterior transition without notching.

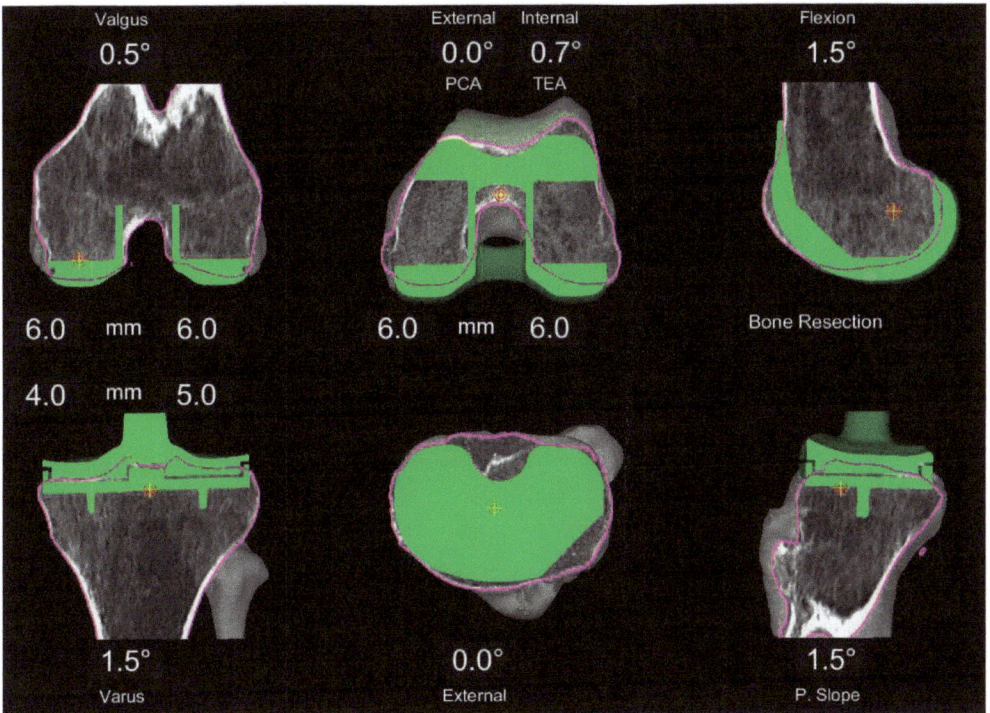

Figure 1. Example of image-based planning of the component position based on the principles of KA. Femoral resections are set to 6 mm each, resulting in 0.5° valgus position and 0.7° internal rotation with respect to the TEA. Tibia plan is preliminary at 1.5° varus, 1.5° slope and a resection level of 4 and 5 mm, respectively.

The tibia orientation was only preliminarily planned, starting with a rather conservative orientation for varus/valgus, slope, and resection level, and finally determined during surgery based on the soft tissue situation in order to achieve a symmetrically balanced extension space and an isometric gap in the medial compartment (see below).

Adaptions to this KA planning were made if the symmetric posterior resection on the femur resulted in relative malrotation of the component trochlea groove (usually internal) with respect to the native trochlea axis. In these cases, the femoral rotation was adjusted with more external rotation around a medial pivot point (constant medial posterior resection at 6 mm, less lateral post resection) (Figure 2). Adaptions to the distal femoral resection/orientation were made if the distal femoral angle deviated more than 4° from the mechanical axis or the resulting overall limb alignment was greater than 1° valgus. Again, the medial femoral resections remained at 6 mm (concept of anatomic reconstruction of the medial column), whereas the lateral resection was reduced (Figure 3). The limit for the tibia component varus and the overall varus limb alignment was 4° deviation to the mechanical axis. All these adaptions were classified as a restricted kinematic alignment (rKA) if the difference between medial and lateral resection on the femur was greater than 1 mm, or if a soft tissue release other than resection of the osteophytes and posterior capsule release was necessary to achieve balanced gaps. All other cases were defined as true KA.

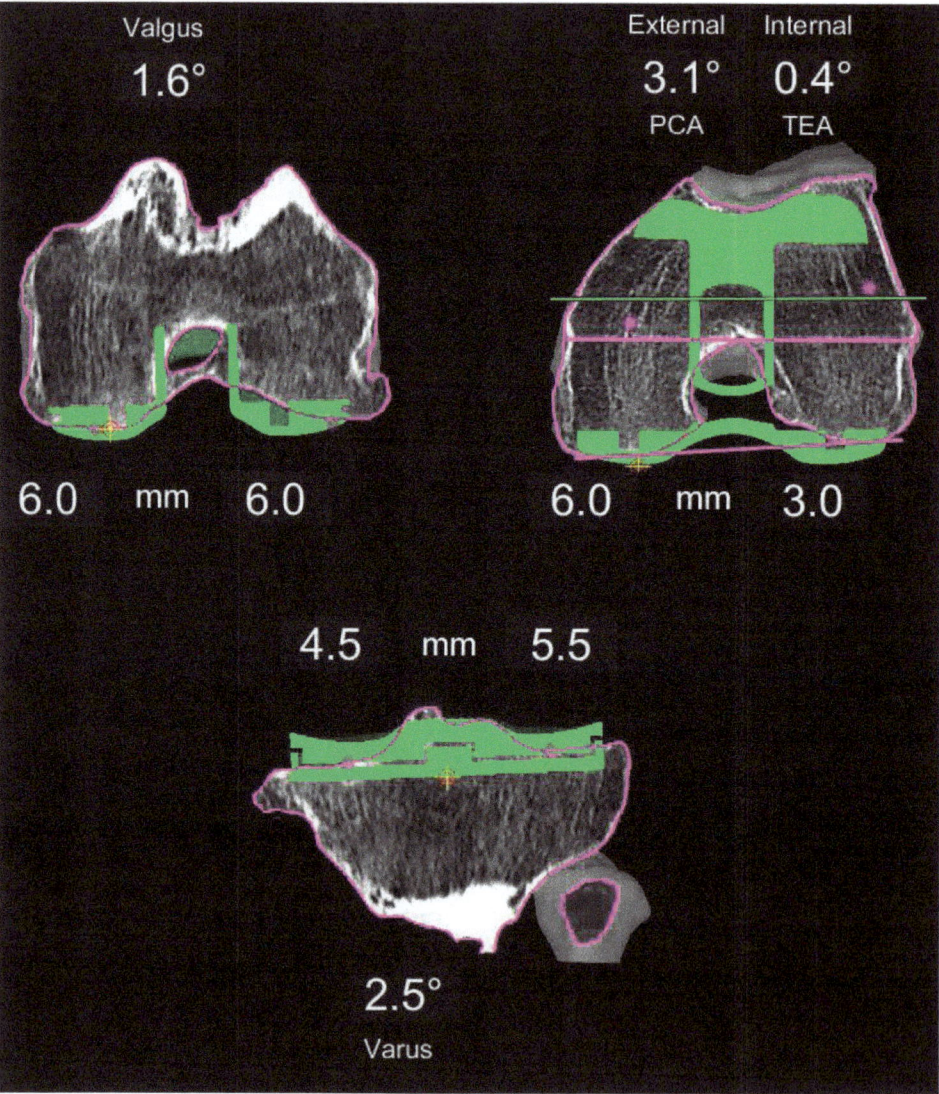

Figure 2. Example of a varus knee planned with restricted KA. The distal femoral resection is symmetric at 6 mm, whereas the posterior resection is adjusted to co-align the trochlea groove close to the native trochlea axis. This results in a 3.1° external rotation with respect to the PCA. Tibia follows the same principle as for KA (Figure 1).

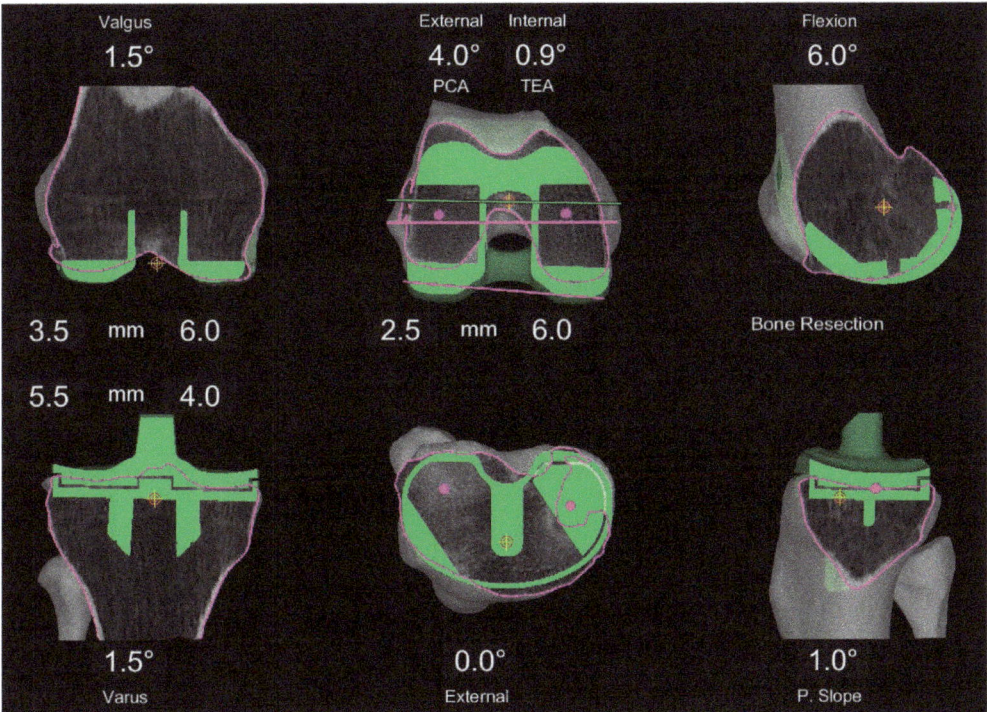

Figure 3. Example of image-based planning of the component position based on the principles of rKA in a valgus patient. Medial femoral resections are set to 6 mm each, whereas the lateral resections are adjusted. With the tibia in 1.5° varus, a 1.5° valgus on the femur is set to create a neutral overall limb alignment in the coronal plane. Femoral rotation is set to best reconstruct the trochlea axis with the component trochlea groove resulting in 4° external rotation to the PCA (0.9° internal to TEA).

The pre-planned resection level was verified intraoperatively based on the individual cartilage thickness of the knee (when available) and adjusted accordingly. Therefore, the cartilage level was added to the CT-model of the knee using the blunt probe. After that, a robotic-assisted precut of the tibia (based on the conservative preplan) was made to access and resect all relevant osteophytes affecting the soft tissue envelope. In cases of relevant extension deficit or massive posterior osteophytes, the distal and posterior femoral osteotomies were also conducted to ensure complete osteophyte removal and posterior capsule release. Additionally, both cruciate ligaments were resected prior to soft tissue analysis.

Then, a spreader was introduced in the knee to reproducibly record the extension and flexion space. Based on the predicted gap width and symmetry, the definite tibia alignment was determined to create a stable extension space at 18–19 mm medial and lateral, and the same width for the medial flexion gap ±1 mm. Mainly the varus/valgus orientation and the resection height were adjusted, and seldom the tibia slope if a flexion/extension mismatch was present. The lateral flexion gap was recorded but left as it was, unless it had been tighter than the medial. The distal femoral alignment was not adjusted, and only the femoral rotation in said rare cases. Soft tissue releases were used only if the mentioned boundaries for the overall limb alignment were reached.

This final implant position was then transposed to the knee with the help of the robotic arm. After insertion of the definite prosthesis, the final alignment (varus/valgus orientation of femur and tibia, femoral rotation, bone resection levels) and the joint stability (medial and lateral spaces) in 0° extension and 90° flexion were recorded using the robotic software.

2.3. Comparative Analysis between KA and rKA

Intraoperative robotic data on the resulting prosthesis alignment, resection levels, joint spaces, or necessary soft tissue releases were recorded as described above. The parameters of interest were analyzed in a descriptive statistical analysis using Microsoft Excel for Mac Version 15.34. The mean values as well as the range and standard deviation were calculated using the standard excel formulas. Additionally, a standardized outcome measurement using the Knee Injury and Osteoarthritis Outcome Score (KOOS), the Knee Society Score (KSS), the Oxford Knee Score (OKS), and EQ-5D was carried out preoperatively and at 2-months follow-up. Because of different preoperative mean values between the subgroups, only the improvement from preoperative to postoperative (delta between the scores) was analyzed in this study.

3. Results

3.1. Patient Collective

During the defined time period, 317 primary knee arthroplasties were performed in our institution. One hundred and forty (45%) were partial knee prosthesis (UNI), 12 (4%) were primary hinge-type prostheses, and 36 (11%) were conventional primary unconstraint TKA. The remaining 126 TKAs were performed with robotic arm assistance, out of which 111 could be included in the study (patient's consent). Patients' demographics are displayed in Table 1. The preoperative alignment parameters and distribution of the subgroups are displayed in Table 2.

Table 1. Patients' demographics of total collective.

age (range)	68 years (40–87)
sex	42 male/69 female
ASA score (I/II/III)	6%/73%/21%
previous surgeries:	
no	50 (45%)
meniscectomy	33 (30%)
ligament reconstruction	17 (15%)
patella re-alignment	15 (14%)
tibia osteotomy	8 (7%)
fracture osteosynthesis	4 (4%)
other	3 (3%)

Table 2. Preoperative alignment parameters of total collective and subgroups.

	Total (n = 111)	Neutral Group (n = 28)	Varus Group (n = 60)	Valgus Group (n = 23)
Mean HKA (range)	177° (161–196)	180° (175–184)	171° (161–178)	188° (182–196)
Mean MPTA (range)	87° (80–93)	89° (85–92)	86° (80–89)	89° (86–93)
Mean mLDFA (range)	88° (81–92)	87° (84–90)	89° (84–92)	85° (81–88)

HKA = hip-knee-ankle angle, MPTA = medial proximal tibia ankle, mLDFA = mechanical lateral distal femur ankle.

3.2. Application of Individualized Alignment Philosophies

In total, 49 patients (44%) received a true KA, whereas in 62 cases (56%), adjustments to an rKA were made. As displayed in Table 3, the suitability for KA meeting our selection criteria differed between the subgroups with 70% in varus patients, 25% in the neutral alignment group, and 0% in the valgus group.

Table 3. Distribution of alignment philosophy chosen for each subgroup.

	Neutral Group ($n = 28$)	Varus Group ($n = 60$)	Valgus Group ($n = 23$)
True KA	25% ($n = 7$)	70% ($n = 42$)	0%
Restricted KA	75% ($n = 21$)	30% ($n = 18$)	100% ($n = 23$)

3.3. Comparative Analysis between KA and rKA

In the KA group, no soft tissue releases were necessary to achieve balanced gaps. In the rKA group, releases were made in 11 cases (18%). In the rKA varus subgroup, major adjustments were made for the femoral rotation to co-align the prosthesis to the trochlea axis. In 15 of the 21 varus rKA cases, an asymmetric posterior resection was conducted. Adaptions in the coronal plane were only made in seven of the varus cases to stay within the limits of ±4° deviation to the mechanical axis. Of the 21 rKA varus cases, 2 needed additional soft tissue release (resection of medial tibia plateau and downsizing tibia, 10%).

In contrast to this, the rKA adjustments in the valgus subgroup often affected both distal and posterior asymmetric resection levels (17 of 23 cases). Seven of the valgus cases needed a soft tissue release laterally (30%).

The intraoperative alignment parameters of the components and the resulting joint spaces are displayed in Table 4. The greatest variability in the alignment was in terms of component rotation ranging from 4° internal to 3.2° external rotation with respect to the TEA. There was no difference between KA and rKA alignment parameters in the varus or neutral subgroups, except for the resection levels on the lateral condyle so they are displayed together.

Table 4. Final set component alignment intraoperatively and final gap symmetry.

	Neutral Group ($n = 28$)	Varus Group ($n = 60$)	Valgus Group ($n = 23$)
Mean tibia comp. varus (range)	1.8° (0–4°)	2.2° (1–4°)	1.2° (0–2.5°)
Mean femur comp. valgus (range)	1.4° (0–4°)	0.8° (−1–3°)	1.1° (0–2.5°)
Mean rotation to TEA (range)	−0.7° (=internal) (−3–1.5°)	−0.7° (−3.9–3.2°)	0.1° (−3–3°)
Mean diff. med. to lat. extension space (std. dev.)	0 mm (±0.46 mm)	0 mm (±0.57 mm)	0 mm (±0.52 mm)
Mean diff. med ext. to flex. space (std. dev.)	0 mm (±1.03 mm)	0 mm (±1.32 mm)	0 mm (±0.98 mm)
Mean diff. med. to lat. flexion space (std. dev.)	1 mm (±1.26 mm)	2 mm (±1.79 mm)	0 mm (±1.38 mm)

Comp. = Component, diff. = difference, med. = medial, lat. = lateral, ext. = extension, flex. = flexion, std.dev. = standard deviation.

At 2-months follow-up, the KA group showed greater improvement and faster rehabilitation in every measured outcome parameter compared to the rKA group, as displayed in Table 5.

Table 5. Improvement in outcome measurement from pre-operative to 2-months follow-up (delta) for KA and rKA group.

Score	KA Group ($n = 49$)	rKA Group ($n = 62$)
KOOS		
Symptoms	+26 pts	+17 pts
Pain	+23 pts	+20 pts
ADL	+24 pts	+20 pts
Sports	+22 pts	+16 pts
QOL	+37 pts	+30 pts
Knee Society Score	+61 pts	+55 pts
Oxford Knee Score	+10 pts	+7 pts
EQ-5D	0.25	0.13

4. Discussion

The first question was how often is KA applicable in TKA and how often are adaptations to rKA necessary? The most important finding was that in our TKA collective, "only" 44% of the patients were suitable to receive a true KA, whereas in 56%, adjustments to a symmetric resection on the distal and posterior femur were necessary to stay within our defined boundaries of overall limb alignment (HKA 176–181°) and joint line orientation ±4° or to reconstruct the anatomic trochlea groove. In the current literature, there are little comparable data to this. Almaawi et al. conducted an analysis of CT data and defined the boundaries of KA ±5° for the component position in the coronal plane and ±3° for the overall limb axis [9]. In their collective, 51% of the patients were suitable for KA without adaptions. However, it is unclear what impact possible bone defects had, that might influence measurement especially on the tibia. Only bone anatomy in the coronal plane and not the soft tissues or the axial plane were included in the analysis. Other studies aiming for true KA (with or without limits) report on necessary soft tissue releases in 7–33% of the cases [12–14]. However, it remains unclear in how many cases adjustments to KA were made. With "only" 10% soft tissue releases in the whole collective (18% in the rKA group, none in the KA group), we are at the lower end of the literature.

Nevertheless, different aspects have to be considered when evaluating the numbers presented in our study. First, our indication limits for true KA were more restrictive, especially for valgus patients compared to the mentioned literature. We did not accept more than 1° valgus deviation for the postoperative overall limb axis. This is because many valgus patients have additional pathologies at the hip and ankle joint increasing the functional valgus during gait. This has a higher risk for implant failure and secondary medial instability. In addition, the benefit of KA for valgus patients has less evidence compared to varus morphotypes. Taking a closer look at outcome data for KA versus MA, studies without indication limits for valgus patients tend to have a minor positive effect compared to those with restrictive indications [15,16]. This explains 100% of rKA in the valgus group and 75% in the neutral group—by our definition, the mild constitutional valgus patients (average LDFA 87°, MPTA 89° = 2° constitutional valgus on average). Second, our institutional proportion of uni- and bi-uni-compartmental knee arthroplasties is at 45%. Thus, our current collective for TKA probably overrepresents severe deformities, posttraumatic situations, and secondary OA after correction osteotomies. Fifty-five percent of our patients had previous surgeries on their affected knee. Lastly, all currently available studies setting limits for KA concentrate on the coronal limb alignment only as inclusion/exclusion criteria [12,17,18]. In contrast to this, we also included the axial plane and the reconstruction of the physiological trochlea axis with the prosthesis. Especially in the varus group, most of the adjustments that were conducted were made to address the rotational orientation of the femur to meet the trochlear anatomy. Riviere et al. had already raised the question of this being a critical point in KA when using standard symmetrical implants [19]. In clinical research, an equal patellofemoral complication rate is found with true KA and MA [20]. Furthermore, biomechanical research reports on a high variability on the patellofemoral kinematics in KA TKA [21]. Thus, our intension was to address this issue by optimizing the three-dimensional orientation of the component. This had a significant effect on the percentage of rKA in the varus group. On the other hand, only in seven varus patients was a correction in the coronal plane necessary.

Regarding our research question (3), we were able to display slight differences in the resulting final component alignment between the subgroups. The varus group showed an LDFA between 87° and 91° with 89.2° on average and an 87.8° MPTA (range 86°–89°). This is close to what would be expected for varus patients [22]. The valgus group differed more than what we expected. This is the result of the rKA, aiming for a neutral overall limb axis. In these classic valgus patients, the tibia joint line is much more horizontal and thus adaptions of the LDFA were necessary for the desired correction. As a result, the physiological morphotype is altered most in this valgus collective.

The overall greatest variability was seen for the component rotation (both in true KA and rKA groups) with on average 0.7° internal rotation with respect to the TEA. This completely differs from the mechanical alignment philosophy with systematic external rotation of the component by 3° in the measured resection principle. However, our findings are consistent with the current literature analyzing the native knee anatomy. Vercruysse et al. described a broad variability between the anterior trochlea line and the TEA, with internal rotation on average [23].

The last point to emphasize is the resulting joint stability created with different alignment philosophies. Whereas rKA in valgus patients on average resulted in equal and symmetric flexion and extension spaces, varus KA patients showed a symmetric extension gap, but a more trapezoidal flexion gap. The average difference between the medial and lateral flexion compartment was 2 mm and ranged 0–5 mm. Moreover, the medial flexion gap had a higher standard deviation, tending toward more laxity, compared to valgus patients. The resulting spaces are thus more physiologically reproduced compared to the native knee situation [24]. In addition, this finding is consistent with other literature analyzing the gaps in KA TKA [14,25]. Peter McEwen et al. described differences in the medial and lateral flexion gap up to 8 mm.

In the patients' outcome measurements, we found a higher improvement in all outcome scores from preoperative to 2 months follow-up in favor of the KA group. This is consistent with the literature [16]. Possibly, this is a result of the more anatomic position of the implant and more physiological soft tissue balance already improving the initial rehabilitation. However, the outcome data should not be over-interpreted as only a very short follow-up period is included and there were some differences in the preoperative scores between the subgroups.

The study has several limitations. First, it is a retrospective analysis of a preselected collective. Patients assigned for uni-compartmental prosthesis (45% in our institution), or primary hinge-type prosthesis (4%) were not included in the study. Second, the criteria to choose between KA and rKA is artificial and might differ to other institutions. Moreover, the trochlea axis, which was used to adjust the femoral component rotation, is not super precisely defined. Thus, minor deviations are possible. Third, no long-term outcome data are included in the analysis. Accordingly, no definite statement can be made as to whether the decision in favor of KA or rKA made sense and was beneficial for the patient.

5. Summary and Conclusions

In this study, we reviewed alignment parameters in TKA patients treated with an individualized alignment following the principles of KA or rKA. With a progressive indication for UNIs over TKA, and boundaries for KA in terms of overall limb axis, joint line obliquity, and rotation, only 44% of the cases were applicable for a true KA. In the KA group, a more physiological knee balance reconstructing the trapezoidal flexion gap was seen as well as a closer reconstruction of the surface anatomy and joint line in all dimensions. In the varus group, interestingly, the limiting factor for KA was less than the coronal plane and overall varus angulation than the axial plane with reconstructing the trochlea groove physiologically. Although, 70% of the varus patients were planned for KA TKA. In the valgus group, adjustments were usually made in both the coronal and axial plane and 100% were adjusted to an rKA. The initial rehabilitation phase showed a greater improvement in the KA group compared to the rKA group in all analyzed outcome scores.

Now, the interesting focus for the future is to compare the effect of adjustments on the patient´s long-term outcome; however, our data suggest that we are talking about different starting points and phenotypes that might not be perfectly comparable.

Author Contributions: K.H. was involved in the data acquisition and analysis of the data as well as in writing and revising the manuscript. B.C. was involved in the data acquisition, conception and supervision of the study design and the preparation of the manuscript. S.C. was involved in data acquisition and data analysis and interpretation. T.C. designed the study concept, supervised the data evaluation, wrote and revised the manuscript and took care of resources and financing. All authors have read and agreed to the published version of the manuscript.

Funding: This research received no external funding.

Institutional Review Board Statement: The data acquisition was conducted according to the guidelines of the Declaration of Helsinki. All subjects gave their informed consent for data collection before their inclusion into the data base. The study includes a retrospective analysis of an existing, anonymized data-base on robotic assisted TKA routine data. Thus, no specific approval of the local ethics committee or institutional review board was required for the evaluation.

Informed Consent Statement: Informed consent was obtained from all subjects involved in the data collection for this study.

Conflicts of Interest: B.C. and T.C. are paid consultants for Stryker.

Ethical Statement: All subjects gave their informed consent for data collection before their inclusion. The study was conducted in accordance with the Declaration of Helsinki. As this is a retrospective analysis of fully anonymized and patient independent data, no approval by the Ethics Committee was required.

References

1. Rivière, C.; Lazic, S.; Boughton, O.; Wiart, Y.; Villet, L.; Cobb, J. Current concepts for aligning knee implants: Patient-specific or systematic? *EFORT Open Rev.* **2018**, *3*, 1–6. [CrossRef]
2. Nisar, S.; Palan, J.; Rivière, C.; Emerton, M.; Pandit, H. Kinematic alignment in total knee arthroplasty. *EFORT Open Rev.* **2020**, *5*, 380–390. [CrossRef] [PubMed]
3. Howell, S.M.; Hull, M.L. Kinematic Alignment in Total Knee Arthroplasty. In *Surgery of the Knee*; Insall, J.N., Scott, W.N., Eds.; Elsevier, Churchill Livingstone: London, UK, 2011; pp. 1255–1268.
4. Woon, J.T.K.; Zeng, I.S.; Calliess, T.; Windhagen, H.; Ettinger, M.; Waterson, H.B.; Toms, A.D.; Young, S.W. Outcome of kinematic alignment using patient-specific instrumentation versus mechanical alignment in TKA: A meta-analysis and subgroup analysis of randomised trials. *Arch. Orthop. Trauma Surg.* **2018**, *138*, 1293–1303. [CrossRef] [PubMed]
5. Vandekerckhove, P.-J.; Lanting, B.; Bellemans, J.; Victor, J.; Macdonald, S. The current role of coronal plane alignment in Total Knee Arthroplasty in a preoperative varus aligned population: An evidence based review. *Acta Orthop. Belg.* **2016**, *82*, 129–142. [PubMed]
6. Maillot, C.; Leong, A.; Harman, C.; Morelli, A.; Mospan, R.; Cobb, J.; Rivière, C. Poor relationship between frontal tibiofemoral and trochlear anatomic parameters: Implications for designing a trochlea for kinematic alignment. *Knee* **2019**, *26*, 106–114. [CrossRef] [PubMed]
7. Meier, M.; Zingde, S.; Steinert, A.; Kurtz, W.; Koeck, F.; Beckmann, J. What Is the Possible Impact of High Variability of Distal Femoral Geometry on TKA? A CT Data Analysis of 24,042 Knees. *Clin. Orthop. Relat. Res.* **2019**, *477*, 561–570. [CrossRef] [PubMed]
8. Blakeney, W.; Beaulieu, Y.; Kiss, M.-O.; Rivière, C.; Vendittoli, P.-A. Less gap imbalance with restricted kinematic alignment than with mechanically aligned total knee arthroplasty: Simulations on 3-D bone models created from CT-scans. *Acta Orthop.* **2019**, *90*, 602–609. [CrossRef]
9. Almaawi, A.M.; Hutt, J.R.; Masse, V.; Lavigne, M.; Vendittoli, P.-A. The Impact of Mechanical and Restricted Kinematic Alignment on Knee Anatomy in Total Knee Arthroplasty. *J. Arthroplast.* **2017**, *32*, 2133–2140. [CrossRef]
10. Vendittoli, P.-A.; Rivière, C.; Macdessi, S. The rebirth of computer-assisted surgery. Precise prosthetic implantation should be considered when targeting individualized alignment goals in total knee arthroplasty. *Knee Surg. Sports Traumatol. Arthrosc.* **2020**, 1–4. [CrossRef] [PubMed]
11. Calliess, T.; Ettinger, M. Limits of kinematic alignment and recommendations for its safe application. *Orthopäde* **2020**, *49*, 617–624. [CrossRef]
12. Hutt, J.; LeBlanc, M.-A.; Massé, V.; Lavigne, M.; Vendittoli, P.-A. Kinematic TKA using navigation: Surgical technique and initial results. *Orthop. Traumatol. Surg. Res.* **2016**, *102*, 99–104. [CrossRef] [PubMed]
13. Howell, S.M.; Papadopoulos, S.; Kuznik, K.T.; Hull, M.L. Accurate alignment and high function after kinematically aligned TKA performed with generic instruments. *Knee Surg. Sports Traumatol. Arthrosc.* **2013**, *21*, 2271–2280. [CrossRef] [PubMed]
14. McEwen, P.; Balendra, G.; Doma, K. Medial and lateral gap laxity differential in computer-assisted kinematic total knee arthroplasty. *Bone Jt. J.* **2019**, *101-B*, 331–339. [CrossRef]

15. Waterson, H.B.; Clement, N.D.; Eyres, K.S.; Mandalia, V.I.; Toms, A. The early outcome of kinematic versus mechanical alignment in total knee arthroplasty: A prospective randomised control trial. *Bone Jt. J.* **2016**, *98-B*, 1360–1368. [CrossRef]
16. Calliess, T.; Bauer, K.; Stukenborg-Colsman, C.; Windhagen, H.; Budde, S.; Ettinger, M. PSI kinematic versus non-PSI mechanical alignment in total knee arthroplasty: A prospective, randomized study. *Knee Surg. Sports Traumatol. Arthrosc.* **2017**, *25*, 1743–1748. [CrossRef]
17. Laforest, G.; Kostretzis, L.; Kiss, M.-O.; Vendittoli, P.-A. Restricted kinematic alignment leads to uncompromised osseointegration of cementless total knee arthroplasty. *Knee Surg. Sports Traumatol. Arthrosc.* **2021**, 1–8. [CrossRef]
18. Macdessi, S.J.; Griffiths-Jones, W.; Chen, D.B.; Griffiths-Jones, S.; Wood, J.A.; Diwan, A.D.; Harris, I.A. Restoring the constitutional alignment with a restrictive kinematic protocol improves quantitative soft-tissue balance in total knee arthroplasty: A randomized controlled trial. *Bone Jt. J.* **2020**, *102-B*, 117–124. [CrossRef]
19. Rivière, C.; Dhaif, F.; Shah, H.; Ali, A.; Auvinet, E.; Aframian, A.; Cobb, J.; Howell, S.; Harris, S. Kinematic alignment of current TKA implants does not restore the native trochlear anatomy. *Orthop. Traumatol. Surg. Res.* **2018**, *104*, 983–995. [CrossRef] [PubMed]
20. Dossett, H.G.; Estrada, N.A.; Swartz, G.J.; Lefevre, G.W.; Kwasman, B.G. A randomised controlled trial of kinematically and mechanically aligned total knee replacements. *Bone Jt. J.* **2014**, *96-B*, 907–913. [CrossRef]
21. Theodore, W.; Twiggs, J.; Kolos, E.; Roe, J.; Fritsch, B.; Dickison, D.; Liu, D.; Salmon, L.; Miles, B.; Howell, S. Variability in static alignment and kinematics for kinematically aligned TKA. *Knee* **2017**, *24*, 733–744. [CrossRef]
22. Hirschmann, M.T.; Moser, L.B.; Amsler, F.; Behrend, H.; Leclercq, V.; Hess, S. Phenotyping the knee in young non-osteoarthritic knees shows a wide distribution of femoral and tibial coronal alignment. *Knee Surg. Sports Traumatol. Arthrosc.* **2019**, *27*, 1385–1393. [CrossRef] [PubMed]
23. Vercruysse, C.; Vandenneucker, H.; Bellemans, J.; Scheys, L.; Luyckx, T. The shape and orientation of the trochlea run more parallel to the posterior condylar line than generally believed. *Knee Surg. Sports Traumatol. Arthrosc.* **2018**, *26*, 2685–2691. [CrossRef] [PubMed]
24. Roth, J.D.; Howell, S.; Hull, M.L. Native Knee Laxities at 0°, 45°, and 90° of Flexion and Their Relationship to the Goal of the Gap-Balancing Alignment Method of Total Knee Arthroplasty. *J. Bone Jt. Surg. Am. Vol.* **2015**, *97*, 1678–1684. [CrossRef]
25. Roth, J.D.; Howell, S.M.; Hull, M.L. Analysis of differences in laxities and neutral positions from native after kinematically aligned TKA using cruciate retaining implants. *J. Orthop. Res.* **2019**, *37*, 358–369. [CrossRef] [PubMed]

Article

Variation of the Three-Dimensional Femoral J-Curve in the Native Knee

Sonja A. G. A. Grothues *[ ] and Klaus Radermacher

Chair of Medical Engineering, Helmholtz Institute for Biomedical Engineering, RWTH Aachen University, 52074 Aachen, Germany; radermacher@hia.rwth-aachen.de
* Correspondence: grothues@hia.rwth-aachen.de

Citation: Grothues, S.A.G.A.; Radermacher, K. Variation of the Three-Dimensional Femoral J-Curve in the Native Knee. *J. Pers. Med.* **2021**, *11*, 592. https://doi.org/10.3390/jpm11070592

Academic Editor: Maximilian Rudert

Received: 18 May 2021
Accepted: 16 June 2021
Published: 23 June 2021

Publisher's Note: MDPI stays neutral with regard to jurisdictional claims in published maps and institutional affiliations.

Copyright: © 2021 by the authors. Licensee MDPI, Basel, Switzerland. This article is an open access article distributed under the terms and conditions of the Creative Commons Attribution (CC BY) license (https://creativecommons.org/licenses/by/4.0/).

Abstract: The native femoral J-Curve is known to be a relevant determinant of knee biomechanics. Similarly, after total knee arthroplasty, the J-Curve of the femoral implant component is reported to have a high impact on knee kinematics. The shape of the native femoral J-Curve has previously been analyzed in 2D, however, the knee motion is not planar. In this study, we investigated the J-Curve in 3D by principal component analysis (PCA) and the resulting mean shapes and modes by geometric parameter analysis. Surface models of 90 cadaveric femora were available, 56 male, 32 female and two without respective information. After the translation to a bone-specific coordinate system, relevant contours of the femoral condyles were derived using virtual rotating cutting planes. For each derived contour, an extremum search was performed. The extremum points were used to define the 3D J-Curve of each condyle. Afterwards a PCA and a geometric parameter analysis were performed on the medial and lateral 3D J-Curves. The normalized measures of the mean shapes and the aspects of shape variation of the male and female 3D J-Curves were found to be similar. When considering both female and male J-Curves in a combined analysis, the first mode of the PCA primarily consisted of changes in size, highlighting size differences between female and male femora. Apart from changes in size, variation regarding aspect ratio, arc lengths, orientation, circularity, as well as regarding relative location of the 3D J-Curves was found. The results of this study are in agreement with those of previous 2D analyses on shape and shape variation of the femoral J-Curves. The presented 3D analysis highlights new aspects of shape variability, e.g., regarding curvature and relative location in the transversal plane. Finally, the analysis presented may support the design of (patient-specific) femoral implant components for TKA.

Keywords: native knee morphology; femoral J-Curve; principal component analysis; geometric parameter analysis

1. Introduction

The sagittal shape of the femoral condyles, which is often referred to as J-Curve, is known to be a significant determinant of knee biomechanics [1]. Similarly, in total knee arthroplasty (TKA), the J-Curve of the femoral component is reported to have a high impact on knee kinematics [2] and its relevance is reflected in various implant design philosophies, including single-, dual-, and multi-radius designs. The medial and lateral J-Curve approximate the contours being in contact with the tibial plateaus and thereby they are highly relevant for tibiofemoral articulation. Therefore, the J-Curve is related to relevant motion phenomena of the native knee, such as femoral rollback and medial pivot [1,3]. Those are linked to flexion range of motion [4] and patient satisfaction in general [5]. In addition, the J-Curve or rather its alteration is highly relevant for ligament strain and tension as well as for the resulting tibiofemoral contact forces. With a ligament stiffness of 60–80 N/mm of medial and lateral collateral ligaments (MCL/LCL) [6,7], a local condylar offset compared to the native J-Curve of only 1 mm will result either in 60–80 N additional lateral and medial tibiofemoral contact force and increased ligament strain; or in ligament relaxation and potential (mid-flexion) instability. In addition, first structural damage is occurring in ligaments from about 5% strain [8]. With an assumed average length of the MCL(LCL) of 100(60) mm, a medial (lateral) offset limit would be 5(3) mm (corresponding to 5% maximum strain) which would result in additional medial (lateral) forces of ~300–400(180–240)N for an average knee. Taking into account, that knee arthroplasty should not extend ligament strain up to the limits of structural damage, and that loads of 10 N (corresponding to less than 1 mm offset) already activate afferent nerves from receptors in the ligaments triggering the knee joint stabilizing muscles (Sojka et al., 1991), we assume, that local J-Curve offset limits would have to be reduced to the range of 1–2 mm maximum. This is in agreement with literature regarding recommendations for varus-valgus laxity between 0.5 and 1 mm for extension and 0.7–1.2 mm for flexion [9].

Consequently, the analysis of the native femoral J-Curve is essential for a better understanding of native knee biomechanics and for optimizing the femoral implant component design in TKA. Previous analyses of the femoral J-Curve have focused on its 2D shape in one specific cutting plane or through projection. Most studies used geometrical primitives such as ellipses and circles and fitted them to the respective 2D J-Curve contours for investigation [10–15]. In a previous study, we evaluated the variation in the native femoral J-Curve by principal component analysis (PCA), enabling a more comprehensive investigation of the shape variation [16]. However, due to the 3D nature of knee motion, the restriction to a 2D evaluation remained a limitation of this study. Hiss and Schwerbrock [17] analyzed the condylar extremum points of a cadaveric knees in 3D, by a comprehensive manual analysis. A limitation of their labor-intensive method is that it is not applicable to large sample sizes. A limitation of their analysis was that they neglected the J-Curve's orientation with regard to the mechanical axis, whereby a relevant amount of variation was neglected. Other authors analyzed the tibiofemoral process of contacts e.g., by finite element simulations [18], but did not evaluate the derived points regarding shape variation.

The aim of this study was to investigate the 3D femoral J-Curve of the native knee by principal component and geometric parameter analysis.

2. Materials and Methods

2.1. Patient Datasets

Bone surface models of 90 cadaveric femora, which have been segmented semiautomatically (control by experts) from CT data (voxel size: 0.49/0.53 mm), were provided by ConforMIS (ConforMIS Inc., Billerica, MA, USA). Of the 90 cadavers, 56 were male, 32 female, and for two no gender information was available. The bone models showed no osteophytes or other signs of osteoarthritis. All further processing was performed in semiautomatic self-written MATLAB scripts (Version R2018b, The MathWorks, Inc., Natick, MA, USA).

2.2. Contour Derivation

First, the bone models were transferred to a bone-specific coordinate system [19]. Left femora were mirrored. In order to determine relevant bony contours, the concept of rotating cutting planes was used, which has been previously applied in the context of surface parametrization [19,20]. The concept is depicted in Figure 1A. The transepicondylar axis was used as origin of the cutting planes. Overall 300 cutting planes between extremum points of the articulating areas on the condyles and the trochlea were used (note Figure 1A shows only 18 cutting planes for better visibility of the individual cutting planes). For each cutting plane a cutting contour was derived. Subsequently, for each contour an extremum search was performed, as it can be seen in Figure 1B. Therefore, the contours were transformed to the x-y plane, and extrema (maxima) regarding the y-axis were identified. For the contours defined by the extrema, a curvature analysis was performed, in order to determine the boundaries of the articulating area, according to Li et al. [13]. The contours were then cut accordingly and interpolated by 300 equidistant points.

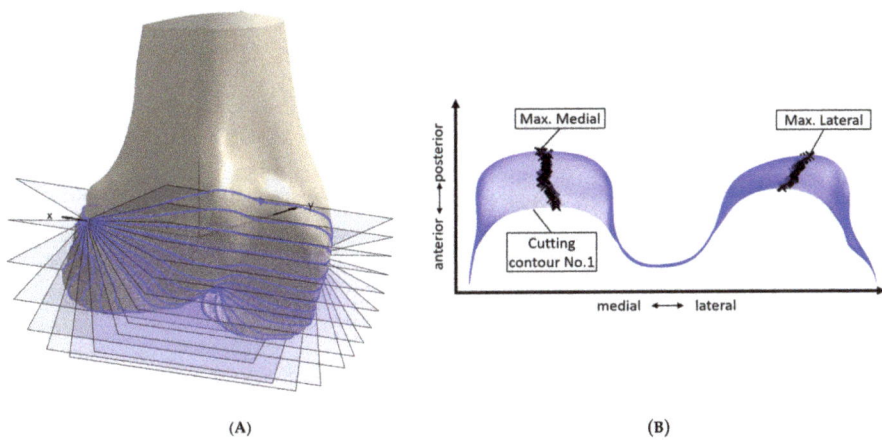

Figure 1. Elements of the process of contour derivation. (**A**) Example femur with rotating cutting planes for the derivation of cutting contour (note: only 18 cutting planes displayed here, to enable better visualization of the individual planes). (**B**) Cutting contours (blue) and extrema (black) for cutting planes 1 to 63.

2.3. Principal Component Analysis

Principal component analysis (PCA) is a mathematical method, which is used for reducing dimensionality of multivariate datasets. In PCA, the principal components are calculated, which represent the directions along which the data varies the most. The principal components can be derived by calculating the eigenvectors of the covariance matrix, and they are ordered according to the amount of variance they account for [21].

In the present study, PCA was used to identify dominant patterns of contour variation. PCA requires corresponding data points (landmarks) between the subjects. This is enabled by the use of a consistent bone-specific coordinate system for the contour derivation, and the standardized definition of boundary points. The PCA was performed combined on both the medial and lateral femoral 3D J-Curves. The analysis was performed according to Shlens [22]. The principal modes were defined according to Stegmann and Gomez [23]. The female and male cadavers were analyzed separately as well as combined, in order to evaluate differences in gender.

2.4. Geometric Parameter Analysis

A geometric parameter analysis was applied to the mean shape as well as to the first five modes. General size parameters, arc lengths, radii describing the curvature, and the mean and maximum local condylar offsets were considered. The parameters are listed and described in detail in Table 1. In addition, the parameters are displayed in Figure 2. Changes in parameter measures originating from the modes were quantified in absolute deviations and in percent.

Table 1. Description of the parameters considered in the geometric parameter analysis. Parameters are either defined for the combined overall shape of both J-Curves or individually for the medial and lateral side (column: overall/medial and lateral).

Parameter Name	Overall/Medial and Lateral	Unit	Description
Mean distal ML spacing	Overall	mm	Mean mediolateral distance of the distal points of the lateral/medial 3D J-Curve (15° of extension to 20° of flexion, reference: radius of the circle fitted to the distal portion of the condyles). Inspired by Walker [24].
Mean posterior ML width	Overall	mm	Mean mediolateral distance of the posterior points of the lateral/medial 3D J-Curve (20°–120° of flexion, reference: radius of the circle fitted to the posterior portion of the condyles). Inspired by Mahfouz [25].
AP length	Medial and lateral	mm	Anteroposterior length of the medial/lateral 3D J-Curve.
Distal radius	Medial and lateral	mm	Radius of the circle fitted to the distal portion of the medial/lateral 3D J-Curve. The calculation was performed according to Nuno and Ahmed [15] and is described in more detail in Asseln et al. [26].
Posterior radius	Medial and lateral	mm	Radius of the circle fitted to the posterior portion of the medial/lateral 3D J-Curve. The calculation was performed according to Nuno and Ahmed [15] and is described in more detail in Asseln et al. [26].
Functional arc length	Medial and lateral	mm	Arc length of the medial/lateral 3D J-Curve between 15° of extension until 120° of flexion (reference: center of the circle fitted to the distal/posterior portion of the condyles).
Arc length 15° Ext.–20° Flex.	Medial and lateral	mm	Arc length of the medial/lateral 3D J-Curve between 15° of extension until 20° of flexion (reference: center of the circle fitted to the distal portion of the condyles).
Arc length 20°–120° Flex.	Medial and lateral	mm	Arc length of the medial/lateral 3D J-Curve between 20° until 120° of flexion (reference: center of the circle fitted to the distal/ posterior portion of the condyles).
Mean abs. deviation	Medial and lateral	mm	Mean absolute deviation (mean condylar offset) regarding anteroposterior and proximodistal direction.
Max abs. deviation	Medial and lateral	mm	Maximum absolute deviation (maximum condylar offset) regarding anteroposterior and proximodistal direction.

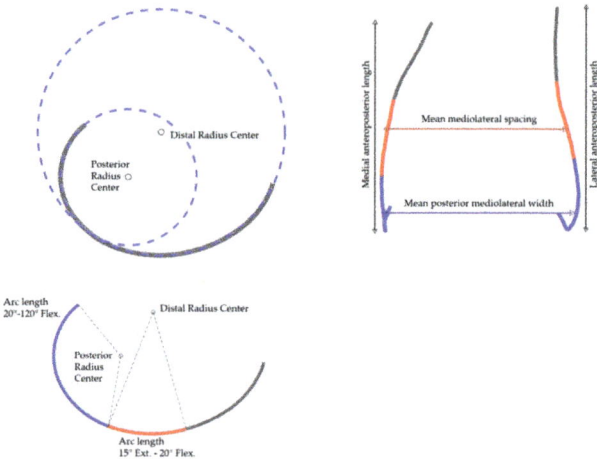

Figure 2. Visualization of the geometric parameter analysis on the example of the mean shape (combined population).

3. Results

In total, 85 of the 90 cadaver cases could be processed without errors (54 male, 29 females, 2 without gender information). Figure 3 shows an example of the derived contours of one femur, together with the respective bone model. An overview of all derived 3D J-Curves is given in Figure 4.

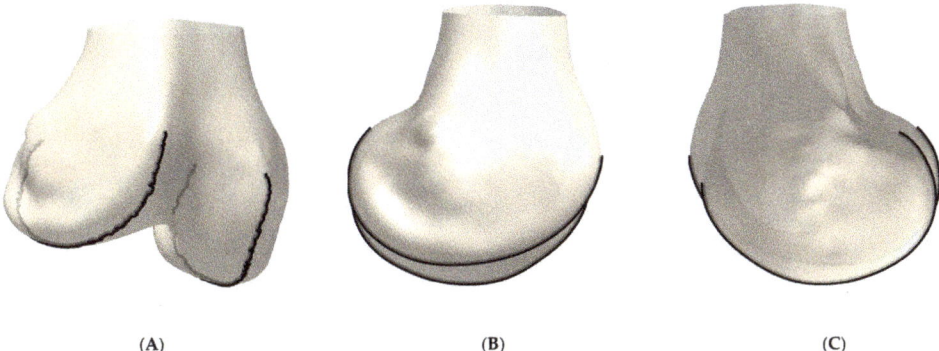

Figure 3. Example of the derived 3D J-Curve contours. (**A**) Anterior/lateral-posterior/medial view. (**B**) Lateral-medial view. (**C**) Medial-lateral view.

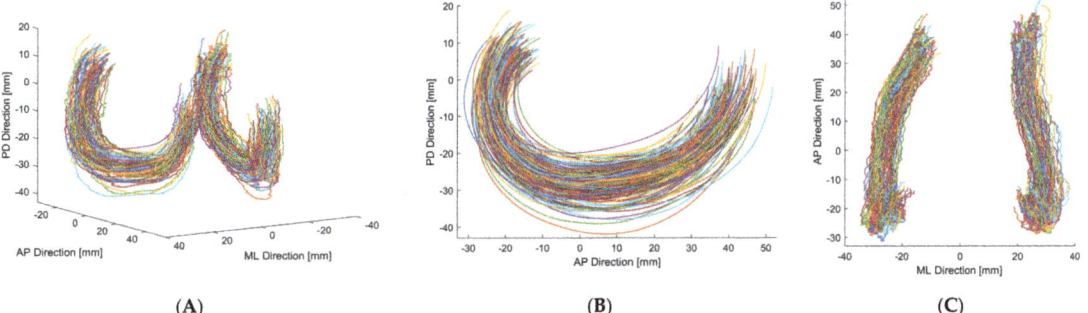

Figure 4. 3D J-Curve contours of both genders. (**A**) Anterior/lateral-posterior/medial view. (**B**) Lateral-medial view. (**C**) Superior-inferior view.

The mean shapes of the male, female and combined population differed regarding the morphological measures considered (Table 2). However, after normalization of the measures according to their direction of measurement (mediolateral measures by the posterior mediolateral width, anteroposterior measures by the anteroposterior size) as suggested by Asseln et al. [27], those normalized measures were comparable for the male, female and combined population, as it can be seen in Table 2.

The results of the separate PCA of female and male 3D J-Curves showed similarities regarding the aspects of shape variations (e.g., arc lengths, orientation, aspect ratio). For the combined analysis (Figure 5), the first mode consisted almost solely of changes in size, highlighting size differences between female and male femora. Apart from this first mode, the aspects of shape variation were similar for all analyses. Due to similarities in normalized measures of the mean shapes and in the aspects of shape variation, in the following only the detailed results of the combined analysis of both genders are presented.

Figure 5 shows the PCA results regarding the first five modes. The percentage of variation explained by modes 1–5 were 31.5, 23.4, 20.1, 7.4, and 5.5%, respectively (sum: 87.8%). In Table 3 the results of the respective geometric parameter analysis are presented.

The first mode involved changes in size, which lead to an increase of all parameters in the geometric parameter analysis, when adding 3 standard deviations to the mean shape (Table 3). Furthermore, for the medial side, also slight changes in 3D J-Curve orientation were associated. With the second mode, the most prominent changes were seen regarding the anterior region of the lateral J-Curve. For the medial side, only slight changes in curvature and size were observed. The third mode consisted of changes in medial J-Curve orientation, in lateral J-Curve size and in mediolateral width. The fourth mode primarily represented changes in aspect ratio. The fifth mode mostly consisted of changes in relative location of the medial vs. the lateral 3D J-Curve.

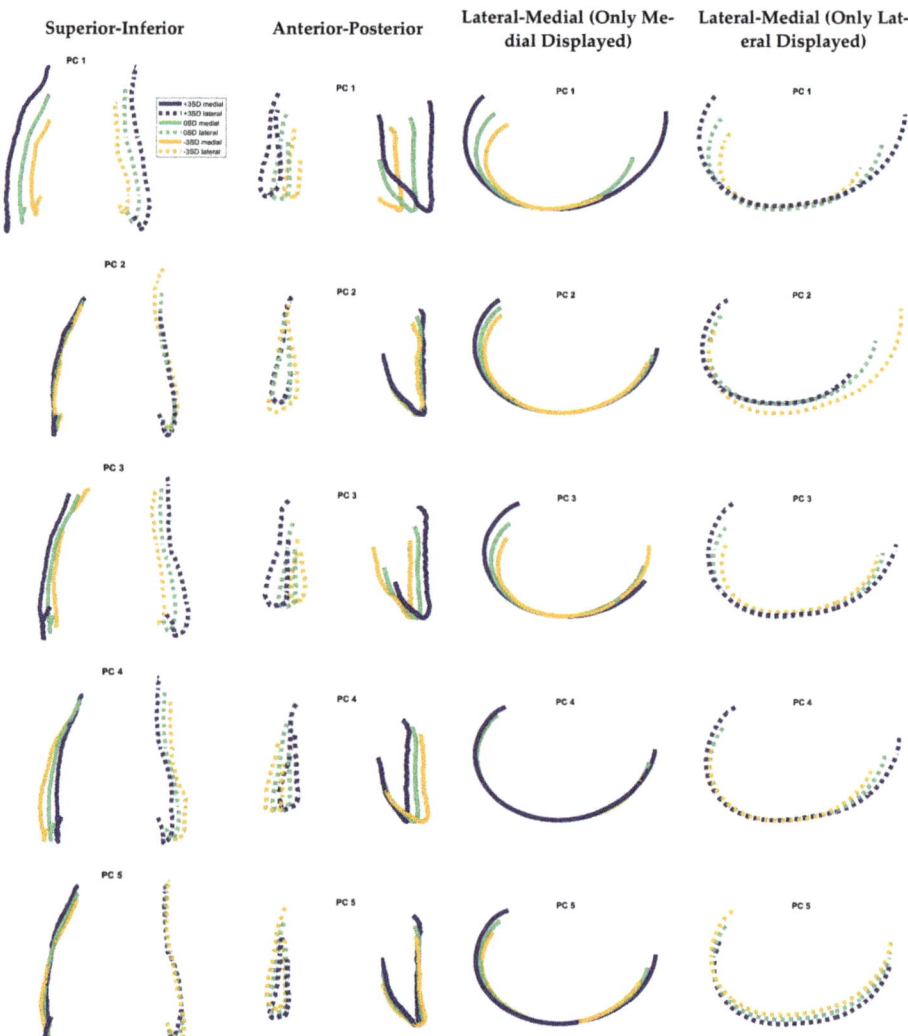

Figure 5. Modes 1–5 of the cadavers' 3D J-Curves in different views. Solid line: medial, dashed line: lateral. 3SD = 3 standard deviations. All contours were oriented to their most distal point in proximodistal direction, for better comparison of the respective variance. Variation explained by the modes 1–5: 31.5, 23.4, 20.1, 7.4, and 5.5%, respectively.

Table 2. Results of the geometric parameter analysis: measures of the mean shapes of the male, female, and combined population are listed. In addition, normalized measures are given in brackets.

Parameter (Normalized by ML/AP)	Mean ML Spacing	Mean Posterior ML Width		AP Length	Distal Radius	Posterior Radius	Funct. Arc Length	Arc Length 15° Ext.–20° Flex.	Arc Length 20°–120° Flex.
Mean shape (combined)	51.2 mm (0.95)	53.7 mm	Lateral	64.2 mm (0.99)	48.8 mm (0.75)	20.3 mm (0.31)	67.4 mm (1.04)	32.5 mm (0.50)	34.9 mm (0.54)
			Medial	60.1 mm (0.93)	35.1 mm (0.54)	19.3 mm (0.30)	67.5 mm (1.04)	22.8 mm (0.35)	44.7 mm (0.69)
Mean shape (Male)	53.7 mm (0.96)	56.1 mm	Lateral	66.9 mm (0.99)	50.5 mm (0.75)	21.4 mm (0.32)	69.7 mm (1.03)	33.7 mm (0.50)	35.9 mm (0.53)
			Medial	62.8 mm (0.93)	36.9 mm (0.55)	20.2 mm (0.30)	70.1 mm (1.04)	23.9 mm (0.36)	46.2 mm (0.69)
Mean shape (Female)	46.2 mm (0.94)	49.1 mm	Lateral	60.5 mm (0.99)	46.9 mm (0.77)	18.6 mm (0.31)	64.0 mm (1.05)	30.9 mm (0.51)	33.2 mm (0.54)
			Medial	55.2 mm (0.91)	31.5 mm (0.52)	17.7 mm (0.29)	62.9 mm (1.03)	20.4 mm (0.33)	42.5 mm (0.70)

Table 3. Results of the geometric parameter analysis: Effect sizes for the first five modes are listed (+3SD). Deviations with regard to the mean shape are quantified in millimeter and in percent. Changes exceeding predefined limits are highlighted (color code below). Abbreviations: AP = anteroposterior, ML = mediolateral.

Parameter		Mean ML Spacing	Mean Posterior ML Width		AP Length	Distal Radius	Posterior Radius	Funct. Arc Length	Arc Length 15° Ext.–20° Flex.	Arc Length 20°–120° Flex.	Mean Abs. Deviation
Mode	1	11.79 mm (23.0%)	10.96 mm (20.4%)	Lateral	12.15 mm (18.9%)	7.31 mm (15%)	4.85 mm (23.9%)	12.3 mm (18.3%)	5.42 mm (16.7%)	6.88 mm (19.7%)	5.34 mm
				Medial	16.84 mm (28%)	8.31 mm (23.7%)	5.26 mm (27.2%)	13.35 mm (19.8%)	6.01 mm (26.4%)	7.35 mm (16.4%)	8.81 mm
	2	3.71 mm (7.2%)	−0.3 mm (−0.6%)	Lateral	−7.11 mm (−11.1%)	2.33 mm (4.8%)	0.54 mm (2.7%)	10.85 mm (16.1%)	1.56 mm (4.8%)	9.29 mm (26.6%)	9.36 mm
				Medial	3.4 mm (5.7%)	1.99 mm (5.7%)	0.87 mm (4.5%)	6.84 mm (10.1%)	1.72 mm (7.6%)	5.12 mm (11.4%)	4.56 mm
	3	4.72 mm (9.2%)	7.7 mm (14.3%)	Lateral	6.59 mm (10.3%)	9 mm (18.4%)	3.44 mm (16.9%)	16.2 mm (24%)	7.76 mm (23.9%)	8.44 mm (24.2%)	4.37 mm
				Medial	3.32 mm (5.5%)	4.08 mm (11.6%)	2.53 mm (13.1%)	11.75 mm (17.4%)	2.82 mm (12.4%)	8.93 mm (20%)	7.08 mm
	4	−4.72 mm (−9.2%)	−6.31 mm (−11.7%)	Lateral	6.49 mm (10.1%)	7.97 mm (16.3%)	1.75 mm (8.6%)	12.93 mm (19.2%)	6.17 mm (19%)	6.76 mm (19.4%)	3.86 mm
				Medial	2.63 mm (4.4%)	−0.24 mm (−0.7%)	0.29 mm (1.5%)	3.45 mm (5.1%)	−0.07 mm (−0.3%)	3.52 mm (7.9%)	2.09 mm
	5	−0.56 mm (−1.1%)	−0.72 mm (−1.3%)	Lateral	−0.49 mm (−0.8%)	−3.33 mm (−6.8%)	−0.17 mm (−0.8%)	−4.02 mm (−6%)	−1.61 mm (−4.9%)	−2.4 mm (−6.9%)	2.97 mm
				Medial	4.48 mm (7.4%)	3.28 mm (9.3%)	0.76 mm (3.9%)	6.22 mm (9.2%)	2.39 mm (10.5%)	3.83 mm (8.6%)	3.66 mm

Color code: Deviations: ≥ ±10%: ▨ | ≥ ±20%: ■ Mean abs. deviation: ≥2 mm: ▨ | ≥5 mm: ■.

4. Discussion

In contrast to previous analyses on the 2D J-Curve shape, the analysis presented enabled the consideration of shape and shape variation in the transversal plane. Compared to a previous study by Hiss and Schwerbrock [17] on femoral J-Curves in 3D, the presented analysis was performed semiautomatically, which enabled the processing of a higher number of femora.

Similar aspects of shape variation of the femoral 3D J-Curves were found in men and in women. The amount of variation explained by changes in size was higher for the combined than for the gender-specific analyses. This is reasonable, as men in general have larger knees compared to women [27]. Hence, the combination of both genders probably is the reason for the increased variability in size.

For the combined analyses, the identified radii of the 3D J-Curve's mean shape are comparable to those of previous studies on the 2D J-Curve [11,12,15,27]. Most of the parameter values derived in this study are also comparable to a previous study on the 2D J-Curve by our group [16]. However, a relevant difference regarding the AP length of the medial J-Curve can be seen. The medial 3D J-Curve shows a higher AP length compared to the medial 2D J-Curve. This may be explained by the distribution of the medial condyle's extremum points in the transversal plane (Figure 4C). The extrema of both condyles do not lie in a single sagittal plane. Especially the medial extrema rather form a curve. As for the 2D J-Curve derivation a single sagittal cutting plane was used, parts of the medial J-Curve may have been neglected. This effect may also be present to a lower extent for the lateral side, as the lateral 2D J-Curve is also slightly smaller in AP direction compared to the lateral 3D J-Curve.

The general relevance of morphological parameters for knee kinematics has been shown in a previous study by our group [28]. In the first degrees of flexion, the share of rolling vs. gliding of the femur on the tibia is estimated to be 1:2 [29]. Afterwards, the motion can be characterized as primarily gliding (in late flexion: rolling/gliding 1:4) [29]. Therefore, the arc length in the beginning of flexion is of higher functional relevance, as it represents the primary running surface of the respective condyle and thereby influences the range of tibiofemoral anterior-posterior translation and internal-external rotation. In the PCA results, changes in the distal arc length differed between the medial and lateral side and were even counteracting for modes 4 and 5 (Table 3).

In our study, mean absolute condylar offsets in the range of 2.09–9.36 mm and local maximum offsets in the range of 2.61–16.0 mm were found. Those exceed the derived offset limits of 1–2 mm. It has to be noted that with ± 3 standard deviations, a wide range of variation was considered. However, every patient needs to be provided with an adequate implant. In addition, all mean offsets were larger than 2 mm, suggesting that a relevant share of the patient population may receive an implant with local condylar offsets exceeding those limits. Some of the variation regarding size and aspect ratio is accounted for by different implant sizes and narrow/standard implant versions. Remaining variation, however, is not accounted for with standard implants.

Limitations

The study presented involved limitations. First, the start and end points of the J-Curves were determined automatically by curvature analysis and not by a visual inspection of the clinical images. However, this automation was necessary in order to enable the processing of a large number of cases.

Second, the use of an extremum search still is an approximation of an actual course of tibiofemoral contact points on the femur. However, the extremum search used in this study identified relevant points on the contours, which correspond to contact points of femoral and tibial implant components in TKA. Therefore, we believe the contours to be of relevance for implant design.

Third, the database is limited to 90 cases of unknown ethnicity. Further analyses are necessary to investigate more cases and evaluate differences between ethnicities. In addition, this study is restricted to the analysis of the femur. Future analyses should also investigate the tibial sagittal contours and the patellofemoral contact (native vs. alloplastic).

Lastly, this study only addresses implant design as one factor with influence on clinical outcome and patient satisfaction in TKA. There are many other potentially relevant influencing factors, such as surgical technique, muscular and ligamentous situation, patient's expectations, etc. However, by optimizing the J-Curve "fit", the potential for superior outcomes may be enabled.

5. Conclusions

The results of this study suggest that variation in the native femoral 3D J-Curves does not only involve scaling and aspect ratio changes, but other aspects such as changes in curvature or circularity, arc lengths, and relative location. Current OTS implant manufacturers offer various implant sizes (i.e., scaling only) as well as narrow and wide implants, accounting for differences in size and in aspect ratio. Differences in other aspects such as in curvature are not accounted for so far. The industry aims at a better restoration of knee morphology, e.g., by introducing more sizes or gender-specific implants. Hence, for future implant systems it might be valuable not only to consider narrow and standard versions but, e.g., high and low curvature implants as well as versions with different offsets. Taking into account the importance of shape mismatches along the articulating surfaces [9,30] as well as the discrepancy between actual implant designs and patient specific J-Curves [16], the number of additional sizes needed potentially will be very high. Against this background, we agree to the conclusion of Delport et al., that another way could be to customize the implant design to each patient individually [9]. In such cases, however, additional attention to force distribution and contact areas between implant surfaces may be needed, depending upon factors such as the nature and degree of the customization of the implant design.

Due to the relevance of bone morphology for active kinematics, related soft tissue strains and for the overall clinical outcome [1,3–5], patient specific 3D J Curves derived from individual image data could be used to evaluate therapeutic options (OTS implants vs. patient specific implants (intrinsically reflecting patient specific J-Curve shape)) and to decide for an adequate match for each patient individually.

Author Contributions: Conceptualization, S.A.G.A.G. and K.R.; formal analysis, S.A.G.A.G.; writing—original draft, S.A.G.A.G.; writing—review and editing, K.R. All authors have read and agreed to the published version of the manuscript.

Funding: This work was partially supported by ConforMIS, Inc., Billerica, USA (RWTH 419410.0013).

Institutional Review Board Statement: Ethical approval was not required for this study since the surface bone models and associated data used in this investigation were from cadaveric specimens. No donor identifying information was accessed for the conduct of the study.

Informed Consent Statement: Not applicable.

Conflicts of Interest: The funding did not affect the outcome of the study in any respect. The cadaveric specimens were chosen solely based on osteophyte volume. The principal components were ranked and chosen for closer analysis based on the amount of variance explained. ConforMIS had no role in the study design, the collection, analysis and interpretation of data, in the writing of the manuscript or in the decision to submit the manuscript for publication.

References

1. Klein, P.; Sommerfeld, P. *Biomechanik der Menschlichen Gelenke—Biomechanik der Wirbelsäule*; Nachdr. d. Aufl von 2004 in 1 Bd; Urban & Fischer in Elsevier: München, Germany, 2012; ISBN 3437552031.
2. Kessler, O.; Dürselen, L.; Banks, S.; Mannel, H.; Marin, F. Sagittal curvature of total knee replacements predicts in vivo kinematics. *Clin. Biomech. (Bristol Avon)* **2007**, *22*, 52–58. [CrossRef] [PubMed]
3. Freeman, M.A.R.; Pinskerova, V. The movement of the normal tibio-femoral joint. *J. Biomech.* **2005**, *38*, 197–208. [CrossRef] [PubMed]
4. Pfitzner, T.; Moewis, P.; Stein, P.; Boeth, H.; Trepczynski, A.; von Roth, P.; Duda, G.N. Modifications of femoral component design in multi-radius total knee arthroplasty lead to higher lateral posterior femoro-tibial translation. *Knee Surg. Sports Traumatol. Arthrosc.* **2018**, *26*, 1645–1655. [CrossRef] [PubMed]
5. Fantozzi, S.; Catani, F.; Ensini, A.; Leardini, A.; Giannini, S. Femoral rollback of cruciate-retaining and posterior-stabilized total knee replacements: In vivo fluoroscopic analysis during activities of daily living. *J. Orthop. Res.* **2006**, *24*, 2222–2229. [CrossRef]
6. Völlner, F.; Weber, T.; Weber, M.; Renkawitz, T.; Dendorfer, S.; Grifka, J.; Craiovan, B. A simple method for determining ligament stiffness during total knee arthroplasty in vivo. *Sci. Rep.* **2019**, *9*, 5261. [CrossRef]
7. Wilson, W.T.; Deakin, A.H.; Payne, A.P.; Picard, F.; Wearing, S.C. Comparative analysis of the structural properties of the collateral ligaments of the human knee. *J. Orthop. Sports Phys. Ther.* **2012**, *42*, 345–351. [CrossRef]
8. Provenzano, P.P.; Heisey, D.; Hayashi, K.; Lakes, R.; Vanderby, R. Subfailure damage in ligament: A structural and cellular evaluation. *J. Appl. Physiol. (1985)* **2002**, *92*, 362–371. [CrossRef]
9. Delport, H.; Labey, L.; de Corte, R.; Innocenti, B.; Vander Sloten, J.; Bellemans, J. Collateral ligament strains during knee joint laxity evaluation before and after TKA. *Clin. Biomech. (Bristol Avon)* **2013**, *28*, 777–782. [CrossRef]
10. Biscević, M.; Hebibović, M.; Smrke, D. Variations of femoral condyle shape. *Coll. Antropol.* **2005**, *29*, 409–414.

11. Howell, S.M.; Howell, S.J.; Hull, M.L. Assessment of the radii of the medial and lateral femoral condyles in varus and valgus knees with osteoarthritis. *J. Bone Jt. Surg. Am.* **2010**, *92*, 98–104. [CrossRef]
12. Li, K.; Langdale, E.; Tashman, S.; Harner, C.; Zhang, X. Gender and condylar differences in distal femur morphometry clarified by automated computer analyses. *J. Orthop. Res.* **2012**, *30*, 686–692. [CrossRef]
13. Li, K.; Tashman, S.; Fu, F.; Harner, C.; Zhang, X. Automating analyses of the distal femur articular geometry based on three-dimensional surface data. *Ann. Biomed. Eng.* **2010**, *38*, 2928–2936. [CrossRef]
14. Martelli, S.; Pinskerova, V. The shapes of the tibial and femoral articular surfaces in relation to tibiofemoral movement. *J. Bone Jt. Surg. Br.* **2002**, *84*, 607–613. [CrossRef]
15. Nuño, N.; Ahmed, A.M. Sagittal profile of the femoral condyles and its application to femorotibial contact analysis. *J. Biomech. Eng.* **2001**, *123*, 18–26. [CrossRef]
16. Grothues, S.A.G.A.; Asseln, M.; Radermacher, K. Variation of the femoral J-Curve in the native knee. In Proceedings of the 20th Annual Meeting of the International Society for Computer Assisted Orthopaedic Surgery (CAOS 2020), Brest, France, 10–13 June 2020; pp. 86–91.
17. Hiss, E.; Schwerbrock, B. Untersuchungen zur räumlichen Form der Femurkondylen. *Z. Orthop. Ihre Grenzgeb.* **1980**, *118*, 396–404. [CrossRef]
18. Gu, W.; Pandy, M. Direct Validation of Human Knee-Joint Contact Mechanics Derived from Subject-Specific Finite-Element Models of the Tibiofemoral and Patellofemoral Joints. *J. Biomech. Eng.* **2019**. [CrossRef]
19. Asseln, M. *Morphological and Functional Analysis of the Knee Joint for Implant Design Optimization*; [1. Auflage]; Shaker Verlag: Düren, Germany, 2019; ISBN 978-3-8440-7047-7.
20. Asseln, M.; Hänisch, C.; Alhares, G.; Eschweiler, J.; Radermacher, K. Automatic Parameterisation of the Distal Femur Based on 3D Surface Data: A Novel Approach for Systematic Morphological Analysis and Optimisation. In Proceedings of the 15th Annual Meeting of the International Society for Computer Assisted Orthopaedic Surgery (CAOS 2015), Vancouver, BC, Canada, 17–20 June 2015; p. 68.
21. Ringnér, M. What is principal component analysis? *Nat. Biotechnol.* **2008**, *26*, 303–304. [CrossRef]
22. Shlens, J. *A Tutorial on Principal Component Analysis*. 2005. Available online: https://www.cs.cmu.edu/~{}elaw/papers/pca.pdf (accessed on 14 January 2020).
23. Stegmann, M.B.; Gomez, D.D. *A Brief Introduction to Statistical Shape Analysis*. 2002. Available online: http://www2.imm.dtu.dk/pubdb/edoc/imm403.pdf (accessed on 31 May 2021).
24. Walker, P.S. Bearing Surfaces for Motion Control in Total Knee Arthroplasty. In *Total Knee Arthroplasty*; Bellemans, J., Ries, M.D., Victor, J.M.K., Eds.; Springer: Berlin/Heidelberg, Germany, 2005; pp. 295–302. ISBN 3-540-20242-0.
25. Mahfouz, M.; Abdel Fatah, E.E.; Bowers, L.S.; Scuderi, G. Three-dimensional morphology of the knee reveals ethnic differences. *Clin. Orthop. Relat. Res.* **2012**, *470*, 172–185. [CrossRef]
26. Asseln, M.; Fischer, M.C.M.; Chan, H.Y.; Meere, P.; Walker, P.; Radermacher, K. Automatic standardized shape analysis of the sagittal profiles (J-Curves) of the femoral condyles based on three-dimensional (3D) surface data. In Proceedings of the 19th Annual Meeting of the International Society for Computer Assisted Orthopaedic Surgery (CAOS 2019), New York, NY, USA, 19–22 June 2019; pp. 21–25.
27. Asseln, M.; Hänisch, C.; Schick, F.; Radermacher, K. Gender differences in knee morphology and the prospects for implant design in total knee replacement. *Knee* **2018**, *25*, 545–558. [CrossRef]
28. Asseln, M.; Grothues, S.A.G.A.; Radermacher, K. Relationship between the form and function of implant design in total knee replacement. *J. Biomech.* **2021**, *119*, 110296. [CrossRef] [PubMed]
29. Menschik, A. *Biometrie: Das Konstruktionsprinzip des Kniegelenks, des Hüftgelenks, der Beinlänge und der Körpergröße*; Springer: Berlin/Heisenberg, Germany, 1987; ISBN 3-540-17737-X.
30. Mihalko, W.M.; Saleh, K.J.; Krackow, K.A.; Whiteside, L.A. Soft-tissue balancing during total knee arthroplasty in the varus knee. *J. Am. Acad. Orthop. Surg.* **2009**, *17*, 766–774. [CrossRef] [PubMed]

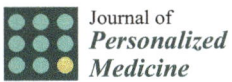

Review

Clinical and Radiological Outcomes after Knee Arthroplasty with Patient-Specific versus Off-the-Shelf Knee Implants: A Systematic Review

Céline Saphena Moret [1,2,†], Benjamin Luca Schelker [1,2,†] and Michael Tobias Hirschmann [1,2,*]

1. Department of Orthopaedic Surgery and Traumatology, Kantonsspital Baselland (Bruderholz, Liestal, Laufen), CH-4101 Bruderholz, Switzerland; celinesaphena.moret@unibas.ch (C.S.M.); benjamin.schelker@unibas.ch (B.L.S.)
2. Department of Clinical Research, Research Group Michael T. Hirschmann, Regenerative Medicine & Biomechanics, University of Basel, CH-4001 Basel, Switzerland
* Correspondence: michael.hirschmann@unibas.ch; Tel.: +41-765105865
† These authors contributed equally to the work.

Abstract: Customised, patient-specific implants (PSI) manufactured based on computed tomography data are intended to improve the clinical outcome by restoring more natural knee kinematics as well as providing a better fit and a more precise positioning. The aim of this systematic review is to investigate the effect of these PSI on the clinical and radiological outcome compared to standard, off-the-shelf (OTS) implants. Thirteen comparative studies including a total of 2127 knee implants were identified. No significant differences in clinical outcome assessed with the range of motion, the Knee Society Score (KSS), and the Forgotten Joint Score (FJS-12) were found between PSI and OTS implants. PSI showed fewer outliers from the neutral limb axis and a better implant fit and positioning. Whether these radiological differences lead to long-term advantages in terms of implant survival cannot be answered based on the current data. Patients receiving PSI could be discharged home earlier at the same or at an even lower total cost. The effective overall superiority of PSI has yet to be proven in long-term studies.

Keywords: total knee arthroplasty; customised; patient specific; personalised; knee replacement

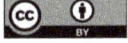

1. Introduction

Total knee arthroplasty (TKA) is a successful and effective treatment for end-stage knee osteoarthritis (OA) [1,2]. With the increase in life expectancy and in the prevalence of obesity, OA has become a relevant cause of disability worldwide, thus leading to a rise in the number of TKA performed [3,4]. However, up to 20% of patients are dissatisfied with the clinical outcome of the surgery as they suffer from persistent pain, instability, persistent or recurrent effusion, and limited knee function [5–9]. The possible reasons for these unsatisfactory outcomes are manifold and often lead to revision arthroplasty. In particular, aseptic loosening, instability, and patellofemoral disorders, which are responsible for about 40% of all revision causes, are known to be affected by the size or positioning of the implant [10–12]. A potentially relevant approach to improve the outcome after knee arthroplasty, which besides enhancing surgical precision and defining an optimal alignment strategy, consists of developing new implant designs. Conventional, off-the-shelf (OTS) implants were developed on the basis of anthropometric measurements of a defined standard population [13]. Although different models and sizes of OTS implants exist, it can be challenging to find the best fitting implant design and size for the individual patient's knee morphology. In addition, the choice of implant is also limited by the surgeon's preferences and experience with different models or the availability in a particular hospital. Modern imaging and implant fabrication techniques make it possible to produce patient-specific instrumentation and implants in order to better fit the individual anthropometric knee joint morphology. The crucial question is whether patients benefit from a more individualised approach using patient-specific implants (PSI). Hence, the aim of this systematic review is to (1) compare clinical outcomes of patient-specific unicompartmental knee arthroplasty (UKA) and TKA implants (PSI) with OTS implants, (2) investigate the radiological outcome such as the implant and limb alignment, and (3) examine the impact of individualised implants on procedure-related factors such as cost, length of hospital stay, discharge destination, and blood loss.

2. Materials and Methods

2.1. Search Strategy

A systematic literature search was conducted on PubMed, Medline, Embase, Cochrane, Scopus, and World of Science from their inception until 5 March 2021 to identify potentially relevant articles for this review. Terms including "unicondylar knee replacement", "unicondylar knee arthroplasty", "unicondylar knee prosthesis", "partial knee replacement", "partial knee arthroplasty", "unicompartmental knee replacement", "unicompartmental knee arthroplasty", "unicompartmental knee prosthesis", "UKA", "total knee replacement", "total knee arthroplasty", "total knee prosthesis", "TKA", "patient-specific", custom*, "individually made", "off-the-shelf", commercial*, and convention* were searched for in both the title and abstract.

Inclusion criteria comprised publications in English or German in peer-reviewed journals comparing patient-specific with standard implants. Only full-text articles were included. Following the compilation of all identified articles and removal of duplicates, two investigators (BLS, CSM) independently screened the studies for inclusion criteria by title and abstract. Then, selected articles were scanned by full text on their eligibility. In case of discrepancies, a third author was consulted (MTH). In addition, manual screening of the reference lists of articles that met the above-mentioned criteria was conducted for additional studies that were not covered by the original search terms.

For this systematic review, only studies comparing clinical outcomes with validated assessment methods or clear endpoints between PSI and OTS implants for UKA and TKA were included. These outcomes contained the Knee Society Score (KSS) [14], specific patient-reported outcome measures (PROMs), the range of motion (ROM), and radiological measurements as well as manipulation under anaesthesia (MUA) and revision rates. Further studies assessing procedure-related factors such as costs, length of hospital stay, discharge destination, and blood loss were also included. All prospective trials and retrospective studies were considered.

Articles regarding patient-specific knee implants for complex bony reconstructions or tumour surgery and patient-specific instrumentation solely (without patient-specific implants) as well as simulation studies, review articles, case reports and editorial comments were excluded.

2.2. Quality Assessment

The methodological quality of the included studies and the risk of bias were assessed using the Methodological Index for Non-Randomised Studies (MINORS) for non-randomised comparative and non-comparative clinical intervention studies [15]. MINORS proposes a global ideal score of 16 for non-comparative studies and of 24 for comparative studies.

2.3. Data Extraction

One of the authors (BLS) extracted the data from the selected publications into a Microsoft Excel spreadsheet. Then, the other author (CSM) checked the input for errors. The following information was extracted from the studies: title, author, year of publication, study design, level of evidence, number of knees in each study group, implant types, follow-up time, patient demographics, clinical outcome scores, revision rates, MUA rates, ROM, costs, hospitalisation time, discharge destination, blood loss, and radiological outcome measures.

2.4. Statistical Analysis

Continuous variables were described with means and standard deviations or medians and ranges. Categorical variables were given with absolute and relative frequencies. Some of the results were only available as ranges and not as standard deviations (SD), limiting the comparability of the individual studies. Due to the great heterogeneity of the available studies, it was not possible to conduct a meta-analysis. For data interpretation, a $p < 0.05$ was considered statistically significant.

3. Results

3.1. Search Results and Characteristics of Included Studies

The literature search yielded a total of 1430 publications and, after allocation processes shown in Figure 1, 13 articles met the criteria for this systematic review. Of these articles, 11 investigated the outcomes after TKA [16–26] and two investigated the outcomes after UKA [27,28] with PSI versus OTS implants. There were four prospective cohort studies and nine retrospective cohort studies. According to MINORS for comparative studies, the mean global score was 17.7 (SD ± 2). Further characteristics of the included studies are listed in Table 1.

Table 1. Overview selected studies.

Author (Year)	Implant Type	Outcome Measurements	Study Design	Studied Implants OTS	Studied Implants PSI	Level of Evidence	Minors Score
Demange (2015) [27]	UKA	Clinical and radiological (coverage, alignment)	Retrospective cohort study	Miller-Galante (Zimmer Biomet)	iUni® G1 (ConforMIS)	III	16
Mayer (2020) [28]	UKA	Procedure-associated parameters, radiological (alignment), and revision rate	Retrospective cohort study	Oxford® MB (Zimmer Biomet)	iUni® FB (ConforMIS)	III	20
Arbab (2018) [16]	TKA	Radiological (alignment)	Retrospective cohort study	Triathlon® (Stryker)	iTotal® G2 CR (ConforMIS)	III	19
Buch (2019) [17]	TKA	Procedure-associated parameters, clinical, MUA, revision rate	Prospective cohort study	Columbus® (B. Braun) or Vanguard® (Zimmer Biomet)	iTotal® G2 CR (ConforMIS)	II	20
Culler (2017) [18]	TKA	Procedure-related parameters, costs	Prospective cohort study	N/A	N/A	II	18
Ivie (2014) [19]	TKA	Radiological (alignment)	Retrospective cohort study	NK II® PS (Zimmer Biomet)	iTotal® G2 CR (ConforMIS)	III	18
Meheux (2019) [20]	TKA	Clinical, revision rate, radiological, procedure-associated parameters	Retrospective cohort study	GENESIS II PS (Smith&Nephew)	iTotal® G2 CR (ConforMIS) and iTotal® G2 plus CR (ConforMIS)	III	17
O'Connor (2019) [21]	TKA	Procedure parameters	Retrospective cohort study	N/A	iTotal® (ConforMIS)	III	20
Reimann (2019) [22]	TKA	Clinical	Retrospective cohort study	Triathlon® CR (Stryker)	iTotal® G2 CR (ConforMIS)	III	16
Schroeder (2019) [23]	TKA	Radiological	Prospective cohort study	NexGen® (Zimmer Biomet) or Vanguard® (Zimmer Biomet) or SIGMA® (DePuy Synthes)	iTotal® CR (ConforMIS)	II	14
Schwarzkopf (2015) [24]	TKA	Clinical, procedure parameters	Retrospective cohort study	GENESIS II PS (Smith&Nephew) or SIGMA® (DePuy Synthes) or P.F.C.™ SIGMA® (DePuy Synthes)	iTotal® G2 CR (ConforMIS)	III	15
Wheatley (2019) [25]	TKA	Clinical	Retrospective cohort study	Persona® PS (Zimmer Biomet)	iTotal® PS (ConforMIS)	III	18
White and Ranawat (2016) [26]	TKA	Clinical radiological	Retrospective cohort study	P.F.C.™ SIGMA® PS FB cem (DePuy Synthes) or P.F.C.™ SIGMA® CR RP non-cem (DePuy Synthes)	iTotal® CR (ConforMIS)	III	19

Abbreviation: OTS: off-the-shelf implant, PSI: patient-specific implant, UKA: unicompartmental knee arthroplasty, TKA: total knee arthroplasty, MB: mobile bearing, FB: fixed bearing, CR: cruciate retaining, PS: posterior-stabilised, RT: rotating platform, cem: cemented, non-cem: non-cemented, N/A: not available.

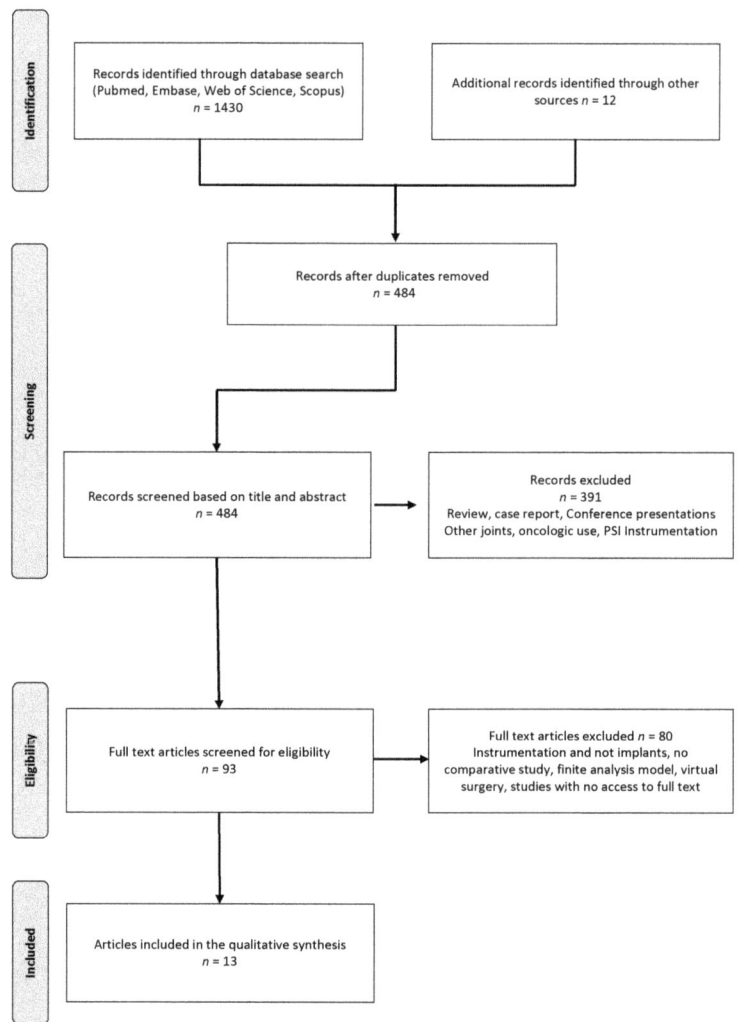

Figure 1. Flowchart of the study selection process according to the PRISMA Statement for the Conduct of Systematic Reviews.

3.2. Patient Characteristics

In this review, a total of 2127 knee implants were assessed. Of the these, 2034 and 93 underwent TKA and UKA, respectively. TKA patients received 1028 PSI systems and UKA patients received 53 PSI systems. In addition, O'Conner et al. [21] examined 4434 knees for the resulting costs only. Patient demographics of the included studies can be found in Table 2.

3.3. Implant Types

For TKA, ConforMIS' first and second generation iTotal® implants were used as PSI and compared to one or two different OTS implants (Table 2). In patients requiring a UKA, ConforMIS' iUni® implants were compared to OTS implants (Table 2).

Table 2. Patient demographics at surgery.

Author (Year)	Implant System	Number of Knees	Mean Age, Years (Range) or (SD)		Gender, Female (%)		Mean BMI, kg/m² (Range) or (SD)		Mean Follow-Up Time, Months (SD)	
Demange (2015) [27]	OTS	20	56 (6.9)	ns	52.6		32.7 (7.2)		75 (20)	
	PSI	33	59 (10.9)		65.6		28.7 (5.3)		37 (8.6)	
Mayer (2020) [28]	OTS	20	61.4 (8.4)		45		31.3 (5.5)		18	
	PSI	20	62.9 (9.2)		45		29.7 (5.6)		18	
Arbab (2018) [16]	OTS	88								
	PSI	113								
Buch (2019) [17]	OTS	30	57.2 (34–67)	ns	53	ns	31 (22–38)	ns	28	
	PSI	32	57.3 (42–72)		41		33.4 (24–53)		28	
Culler (2017) [18]	OTS	122	68.3 (9.5)	ns	43.9	ns	32.3 (7.8)	ns		
	PSI	126	69.7 (8.4)		41.9		30.8 (6.5)			
Ivie (2014) [19]	OTS	100								
	PSI	100								
Meheux (2019) [20]	OTS	41	63 (10.1)				34.4 (7.1)	**	37.2 (18)	
	PSI 1	77	62.7 (8.3)				30.3 (4.5)		37.2 (18)	
	PSI 1	36	62.8 (6.7)				28.9 (5.2)		37.2 (18)	
O'Connor (2019) [21]	OTS	3695								
	PSI	739								
Reimann (2019) [22]	OTS	103	70.9 (7.1)	***	68.4	ns	31.4 (5.5)	ns	33 (7.6)	***
	PSI	125	65.5 (9.3)		63.1		30.5 (5.2)		27.5 (5.7)	
Schroeder (2019) [23]	PSI	44	70.5 (57–87)		40.9		30.7 (22–49.1)			
Schwarzkopf (2015) [24]	OTS	314	65	ns	65		32.11	ns		
	PSI	307	61.4		60.2		30.85			
Wheatley (2019) [25]	OTS	124	70 (8.5)	*	64.6	ns	30.3 (8.5)	ns	3	
	PSI	47	66.9 (7.7)		61.7		30.3 (8.5)		3	
White and Ranawat (2016) [26]	OTS, CR	42	59.8 (6.7)	ns	66.7	ns	31.8 (5.5)	ns	31.2 (8.4)	ns
	OTS, PS	11	53.9 (6.0)	*	9.1	**	34.4 (6.5)	**	27.6 (4.8)	
	PSI, CR	21	59.1 (7.4)		66.7		28.7 (4.8)		28.8 (4.8)	

Abbreviations: BMI: body mass index, kg: kilogram, m: meter, SD: standard deviation, OTS: off-the-shelf implants, PSI: patient-specific implants, CR: cruciate retaining, PS: posterior-stabilised, ns: no statistically significant difference * $p < 0.05$, ** $p < 0.01$, *** $p < 0.001$.

3.4. Clinical Outcome

White and Ranawat [26] asked patients to rate their satisfaction regarding their knee implant on a scale from 1 (unsatisfied) to 10 (fully satisfied). The OTS CR (mean 8.3, SD ± 2.2, $p = 0.04$) and OTS PS (mean 8.9, SD ± 1.0, $p = 0.01$) implant group reported significantly higher satisfaction than PSI (mean 7.0, SD ± 2.1).

Buch et al. [17] found a significantly greater mean postoperative ROM in the PSI group compared to the OTS implant group (122° versus 114°, $p < 0.001$). In contrast, Schwarzkopf et al. [24] reported a decrease of 3.44° (range, −83° to 55°) in ROM after TKA with PSI, whereas patients receiving OTS implants showed an increase of 1.54° (range, −80° to 90°, $p < 0.1$). The remaining authors did not observe statistically significant differences in ROM between both groups [20,22,25–27].

With regard to the KSS, Wheatley et al. [25] only found a non-significant difference in both the knee score and the function score. Reimann et al. [22], on the other hand, found a significantly better function score in the PSI compared to the OTS implant group. White and Ranawat [26] determined a significantly lower the knee score in the PSI group (85.4 points) compared to both OTS implant groups (95.5 and 97.3 points), whereas Meheux et al. [20] found no significant differences.

Wheatley et al. [25] also assessed the Forgotten Joint Score (FJS-12), which showed no significant difference between PSI and OTS implant groups. Furthermore, the Western Ontario and McMaster Universities Arthritis (WOMAC) questionnaire was conducted by White and Ranawat [26]. The OTS CR implant group showed a significantly better total score than the PSI group ($p = 0.04$). Further results regarding the clinical outcome are provided in Table 3.

Table 3. Revisions, ROM, clinical outcomes.

Author (Year)	Implant System	Revision n (%)	Mean ROM (SD)	MUA n (%)	Mean KSS (SD) [1] Preoperative	Mean KSS (SD) [1] Postoperative	FJS [1]	WOMAC [1] Preoperative	WOMAC [1] Postoperative
Demange (2015) [27]	OTS	3 (15)	pre: 122° (±9.5°) post: 127° (±7.5°)		KS: 48 (16.2)	KS: 94 (7.6)			
Mayer (2020) [28]	PSI	2 (6.1)	pre: 125° (±8.5°) post: 125° (±6.2°)		*				
Buch (2019) [17]	OTS PSI OTS PSI	2 (10) 1 (5) 2 (6.7) 1 (3.1)	post: 144° post: 122° post: 122.7° (±8.2°)	1 (3.3) 2 (6.3) ns					
Meheux (2019) [20]	OTS PSI 1 PSI 2	1 (2.4) 18 (23) 0 (0)	post: 124.2° (±6.0°) post: 123.8° (±7.4°) ns		KS: 53.7 (10.1) KS: 55.5 (8.3) KS: 54.2 (6.7) ns	KS: 91.9 (11.9) KS: 94.6 (7.6) KS: 95.3 (13.3) ns			
Reimann (2019) [22]	OTS PSI	1 (1.8) 1 (1.2)	pre: 110° (±13.8°) ns post: 105° (±9.2°) pre: 110° (±15°) ns post: 105° (±9.9°)			KS: 78.3 (13.8) FS: 68.0 (18.7) KS: 82.4 (13.1) FS: 82.4 (13.1) ns **			
Schwarzkopf (2015) [24]	OTS PSI OTS	1 (0.8)	pre: 109.4° (±9.6°) post: 119.3° (±6.1°)	2 (1.6) ns	KS: 52.7 (10.8) FS: 56.3 (16.3) ns	KS: 91.7 (10.2) FS: 77.6 (19.4) ns	62.1 (25.7)		
Wheatley (2019) [25]	PSI	1 (2.1)	pre: 109.3° (±9.1°) post: 118.8° (±11.0°) ns	1 (2.1)	KS: 55.1 (12.5) FS: 51.8 (16)	KS: 91.1 (9.6) FS: 81.4 (15.3)	56.0 (26.9) ns		

Table 3. Cont.

Author (Year)	Implant System	Revision n (%)	Mean ROM (SD)		MUA n (%)	Mean KSS (SD) Preoperative		Mean KSS (SD) [1] Postoperative		FJS [1]	WOMAC Preoperative	WOMAC [1] Postoperative
White and Ranawat (2016) [26]	OTS, CR	0 (0)	pre: 111° (12°) post: 118° (8°)	**	0	KS: 45.7 (9) FS: 51.1 (10.4)		KS: 95.5 (7.1) FS: 88.9 (13.8)	ns		TS: 52.4 (12.8) PS: 11.1 (2.8) SS: 5.1 (1.4) FS: 36.2 (9.7)	TS: 7.8 (8.4) * PS: 1.2 (2.5) SS: 1.3 (2.1) FS: 5.2 (5.8)
	OTS, PS	0 (0)	pre: 114° (10°) post: 120° (4°)		0	KS: 45.2 (9) FS: 54.1 (13.2)		KS: 97.3 (3.9) FS: 96.4 (5)	*		TS: 41.3 (9.6) PS: 7.8 (1.9) SS: 3.4 (1.6) FS: 30.1 (7.36)	TS:15.4 (18.3) PS:2.8 (4) SS: 2.2 (2.3) FS: 10.4 (12.9)
	PSI, CR	1 (4.8)	pre: 120° (12°) post: 115° (10°)	ns	6 (28.6)	KS: 53.6 (8.3) FS: 54 (12.2)	**	KS: 85.4 (15.5) FS: 86 (14.8)	**		TS: 51.4 (17) PS: 11.5 (3.9) SS: 4.6 (2.5) FS: 35.3 (12.3)	TS: 23.4 (23.1) * PS: 4.8 (5.3) SS: 3 (2.4) FS: 15.2 (16.3)

Abbreviations: ROM: range of motion, MUA: manipulation under anaesthesia, KSS: Knee Society Score, KS: knee score, FS: function score, FJS: Forgotten Joint Score, WOMAC: Western Ontario and McMaster Universities Arthritis Index, TS: total score, PS: pain score, SS: stiffness score, FS: function score, SD: standard deviation, OTS: off-the-shelf implants, PSI: patient-specific implants, CR: cruciate-retaining, PS: posterior-stabilised, pre: preoperative, post: postoperative, ns: no statistically significant difference * $p < 0.05$, ** $p < 0.01$, *** $p < 0.001$. [1] clinical outcome scores at last follow up.

3.5. Revisions and Reoperations

Looking at the rate of MUA, White and Ranawat [26] observed that six of the 21 (28.6%) patients in the PSI group required manipulation compared to none in the OTS implant group. However, these results were not replicated in the other studies, where the rate of MUA did not differ between both PSI and OTS implant groups [17,25]. In the study by Meheux et al. [20], the iTotal® G2 (ConforMIS) system showed a revision rate of 23% (18/77) compared to 2.4% (1/41) for the OTS implant. This led the PSI system to be discontinued during the study period and exchanged for the iTotal® G2 plus (ConforMIS) system. None of the patients subsequently operated on with the new system required revision within the two-year follow-up period. Wheatley et al. [25] reported four patients needing arthroscopic debridement due to retropatellar crepitations in the PSI group compared to one arthroscopic debridement in the OTS group. However, all but one of the included studies assessing revisions after TKA found higher revision rates in the OTS groups [17,22,27,28].

3.6. Radiological Outcomes

Comparing the frontal tibial component angle (FTC) of the implants to the target values of 90°, Meheux et al. [20] demonstrated that the PSI-1 and OTS implant groups deviated significantly from the target in contrast to the PSI-2 group. The study by Ivie et al. [19] could not confirm these results. However, the same authors [19] found a significant difference in the frontal femoral component angle (FFC) angle between OTS implants and PSI. Although the mean FFC was within the desired +3° of deviation from the neutral axis (90°) for both groups, the femoral component of the PSI was 1.5 times more likely to be within this desired range than that of the OTS implants. No further studies included in the review reported on the FFC (Table 4).

Ivie et al. [19] found a mean postoperative hip–knee–ankle angle (HKA) significantly closer to the neutral limb alignment in the PSI group (PSI, 0.47° of varus ± 3.15° versus OTS implants, 1.68° of valgus ± 3.65°; $p \leq 0.01$). In contrast, Arbab et al. [16] and Meheux et al. [20] found no significant difference in the HKA between PSI and OTS implant cohorts. However, Arbab et al. [16] and Ivie et al. [19] reported fewer outliers from neutral alignment (±3°) in the PSI group compared to the OTS implant group.

Schroeder et al. [23] investigated the fit of different types of tibial components intraoperatively. PSI achieved an optimal fit (i.e., ≤1 mm of overhang or undercoverage) or relative undercoverage of 1–3 mm in 80% of case in contrast to 27% for OTS implants ($p < 0.001$). Demange et al. [27], who investigated the optimal fit of UKA implants, found that 75.8% of PSI and 21.1% of OTS implants achieved of an optimal fit.

The rotational alignment of the tibial component was also analysed by Schroeder et al. [23] using a computer-aided design (CAD) during a virtual surgery. When a maximal tibial bone coverage was opted for, the rotational alignment did not have to be compromised in the PSI group in contrary to OTS implant group, which showed a greater mean deviation from the adequate alignment.

3.7. Procedure-Related Factors

O'Connor et al. [21] attributed a statistically significant average savings of 1695 USD ($18,585 versus $20,280; <0.0001) in total costs to PSI. However, another author only found a non-significant differences in costs in favour of PSI (PSI $21,591 ± 4439 versus OTS $22,092 ± 5940) [18]. Significantly lower were also the costs for follow-up care in the PSI group ($5048 ± $2929 versus $6361 ± $4482; $p = 0.007$).

In terms of length of hospital stay, patients undergoing UKA with a PSI spent an average of 8.4 days (SD ± 1.5, $p < 0.003$) in hospital compared to 10.9 days (SD ± 2.9) with an OTS implant [28]. Similarly, a significantly shorter length of stay was calculated for TKA using PSI by Schwarzkopf et al. [24] (2.44 vs. 3.18, $p < 0.01$), Meheux et al. [20] (OTS vs. PSI 1 vs. PSI 2, 3.3 ± 1.2 vs. 2.88 ± 1.1 vs. 2.08 ± 0.6, $p < 0.01$) and Buch et al. [17] (OTS vs. PSI, 2.7 vs. 1.6, $p = 0.004$).

Table 4. Radiological outcome.

Author (Year)	Implant System	Mean FFC (SD)	Mean FTC (SD)	Mean Tibial Slope (SD)	Mean HKA [1] (SD) or (Range) Pre-Op	Mean HKA [1] (SD) or (Range) Post-Op	>±3° HKA Outliers	Femorotibial Angle [1] Pre-Op	Femorotibial Angle [1] Post-Op	Optimal Tibial Fit [a] Resp. Relative Undercoverage [b]
Demange (2015) [27]	OTS				3.3° (4.9°) (−5.4°–+8.5°) 8.2°	−0.9° (3.8°) (−8.0°–−3.4°) 2.3°				21.1% [a]
	PSI									75.8% [a]
Arbab (2018) [16]	OTS, CR				(−18.2°–+15.7°) median 5.6° 9.0°	(−10.1°–+12.5°) median 11.7° 3.2°	26%			
	PSI, CR				(−27.3°–−18.9) median 5.7°	(−7.6°–−8.4°) median 0.7°	16%			
Ivie (2014) [19]	OTS	88.32° (1.51°) *	87.81 (1.54°) ns	87.12° (1.73°) ns		1.68° (3.65°) **	43.1%			
	PSI	87.37° (3.87°)	87.71° (1.44°)	86.42° (2.61°)		−0.47° (3.15°)	29.6%			
Meheux (2019) [20]	OTS		88.54° (1.5°)	4.00° (2.5°)	−3.32° (5.2°)	−3.32° (5.2°)			2.29° (3.8°)	
	PSI 1		91.08° (1.9°)	6.40° (2.9°)	−3.97° (3.5°) ns	−1.34° (4.6°) ns			4.09° (2.7°)	
	PSI 2		89.89° (1.0°)	5.53° (3.9°)	−3.89° (3.46°)	−0.35° (1.8°)			4.1° (3°)	
Schroeder (2019) [23]	OTS 1									23% a+b
	OTS 2									25% a+b ***
	OTS 3									34% a+b
	PSI									80% a+b
White and Ranawat (2016) [26]	OTS, CR			5° (1°)				−4° (3°)	2°	
	OTS, PS			4° (1°)				−1° (7°) ns	2° ns	
	PSI, CR			5° (1°)				−3° (4°)	2°	

Abbreviations: FFC: frontal femoral component angle, FTC: frontal tibial component angle, pre-op: preoperative, post-op: postoperative, HKA: hip–knee–ankle, SD: standard deviation, OTS: off-the-shelf implants, PSI: patient-specific implants, CR: cruciate retaining, PS: posterior-stabilised, ns: no statistically significant difference. * $p < 0.05$, ** $p < 0.01$, *** $p < 0.001$. [1] varus knees were recorded as negative values and valgus as positive [a] 1 mm implant overhang to 1 mm tibial bone undercoverage [b] 1–3 mm tibial undercoverage.

No significant differences were seen in the duration of surgery in both groups for UKA and TKA [24,28]. Buch et al. [17] found the proportion of patients discharged home to be significantly higher in the PSI group (97% versus 80%, $p = 0.05$), whereas Culler et al. [18] found no significant difference between groups. In addition, Meheux et al. [20] also recorded a lower postoperative haemoglobin (Hg) drop in the PSI 2 group compared to the OTS implant group (0.61 ± 0.3 vs. 1.20 ± 1.3, $p < 0.05$).

4. Discussion

The key question to be answered by this review is whether patients undergoing TKA or UKA with a PSI present a better clinical outcome than with OTS implants. Based on the results of the included studies, no clear advantage of PSI over OTS implants were identified. Nonetheless, the results of the included studies have proven the non-inferiority of PSI in terms of clinical outcomes compared to OTS implants.

Implications for decisive improvements in clinical outcome favouring PSI are drawn from promising results of kinematic and biomechanical studies as well as PROMs data from various case series [29–32]. For instance, Zeller et al. [33] howed that PSI have more normal and physiological kinematics corresponding to the native knee than OTS implants. Patil et al. [34] came to a similar conclusion based on the results of their cadaver study. Due to the lack of an OTS implant control group, case series regarding the clinical and radiological outcome of PSI were excluded from the present study [29–32].

In this study, only one publication addressed patient satisfaction [26]. However, the determined inferiority of PSI compared to OTS implants is inconsistent with the data presented by Katthagen et al. [35], which was not included in the present study due to the unavailability of the full text manuscript. In contrary to White and Ranawat [26], reporting an increased rate of MUA in the PSI group, more recent studies did not support those findings [25,36]. Hence, future studies should potentially take this aspect into account.

Considering the revision rate, most of the included studies reported lower revision rates in the PSI group [17,27,28]. However, no explanation could be found for the increased incidence of patellar crepitations, requiring arthroscopic debridement, in said group in the study by Wheatley et al. [25]. This complication was not described by the other authors.

The mechanical alignment most surgeons aim for still remains the standard alignment target. A postoperative limb alignment within $\pm 3°$ from the neutral axis is generally considered a "safe zone", as studies by Ritter et al. [37] and Fang et al. [38] have shown that deviation from this range is associated with a higher failure rate and shorter implant survival. All included studies assessed the ConforMIS PSI, which applies the traditional mechanical alignment strategy. Indeed, two of these found that the proportion of outliers $> 3°$ deviation from the neutral axis in the coronal plane were lower in the PSI group than in the OTS implant group [16,19]. This is consistent with the findings of a case series by Levengood et al. [39] and Arnholdt et al. [40]. Whether the more precise alignment is actually a result of the patient-specific implants or rather the patient-specific instrumentation is questionable [41]. Furthermore, it is debatable to what extent patients benefit from the apparent better mechanical alignment of the implants, as recent studies have shown no detrimental influence of varus and valgus outliers $> 3°$ on implant survival after 10 and 20 years [42,43].

Indeed, the optimal realignment strategy is currently undergoing a paradigm shift away from a strict mechanical alignment and towards a more personalised alignment. Another PSI manufacturer Symbios (Yverdon-les-bains, Switzerland), which has not yet been included in comparative studies because of its quite recent entry on the market, applies a recently developed individualised alignment strategy. It is based on the restricted phenotype alignment, which allows a better reproduction of the patient-specific limb alignment in addition to the individual knee morphology [44]. Combining a patient-specific implant with a more individualised alignment strategy seems promising; however, long-term studies assessing the impact of this alignment on the clinical outcome are still lacking.

It is commonly accepted that the optimal rotational alignment of the implant components is crucial. Internal rotation of the tibial component has been shown to be associated with poorer clinical outcome and is considered a major cause of postoperative pain [45,46]. Schroeder et al. [23] simulated the compromise between adequate bone coverage and optimal rotation alignment that has to be made when using OTS tibial components, which is not the case with PSI due to their individualised design. Although intuitive, these results should be verified in comparative cohort studies on postoperative radiological exams.

The improved tibial bone coverage of the PSI was demonstrated in several studies included in the review as well as in case series [23,27,47]. It has been shown that the anteroposterior to mediolateral femoral condyle ratios are related to ethnicity and gender [48,49]. The use of PSI in patients who present less conventional anthropometric characteristics is expected to reduce femoral component overhang and undercoverage as well as the associated increased risks of postoperative pain and functional limitations [50,51]. The better bone coverage and potentially shorter surgery time with PSI could be seen as the reason for the lower blood loss and Hb drop [18,24]. Other beneficial effects of an optimal tibial fit are a decreased risk of subsidence and soft tissue impingement [52]. Furthermore, PSI allow a more precise rotational alignment of the femoral component in addition to recreating the individual trochlear groove matching the shape of the patella. This improves patellar tracking by maintaining its native alignment. Nevertheless, this aspect has not yet been assessed in comparative studies; thus, no conclusions can be drawn in this regard.

With rising healthcare costs worldwide and an increase in patients requiring TKA, there is concern that providing patients with PSI will result in higher costs compared to OTS implants. PSI indeed have higher upfront costs due to the required preoperative imaging and the customised manufacturing process [53]. However, Culler et al. [18] saw no difference in overall costs, and O'Conner et al. [21] even found significantly lower costs in the PSI group when looking at total postoperative costs up to one year after surgery. Possible reasons for the lower total costs seem to be the reduced length of hospital stay and fewer discharge to rehabilitation facilities compared to OTS implants [17,18]. However, this has to be taken with a grain of salt, as patients receiving PSI tend to be younger, healthier, and of a higher socioeconomic status.

The most relevant limitation of this systematic review is the heterogenic radiological endpoints and outcome assessment methods used in the included studies, which rendered a comparison difficult. In addition, the quality of these studies was rather low with an average MINORS of 17.7 (SD $\pm$ 2) and only few authors performing a sample size power calculation beforehand. Due to the higher upfront cost, it is suspected that many of these TKA with PSI were performed in private hospitals or at least on patients with additional insurance, which may lead to a selection bias. Moreover, the TKA were performed in Western countries, with a probably mostly Caucasian population, although it is suspected that PSI could be especially beneficial for patient with different anthropometric measurement (i.e., ethnic backgrounds). Lastly, since PSI were first introduced to the market about a decade ago and many single cohort studies show promising results, long-term comparative studies are still lacking. However, a paradigm shift in the field of knee arthroplasty towards a more personalised approach that combines enhanced surgical accuracy using patient-specific instrumentation, individualised alignment strategies, improved fit with customised implants and thus a better restoration the native knee joint seems ineluctable.

5. Conclusions

This study demonstrates inconclusive results and mostly non-significant differences in terms of clinical outcome between PSI and OTS implants. Although the use of PSI resulted in a better alignment as well as implant fit and positioning, these improved radiological findings remain of questionable clinical impact. The effective overall superiority of PSI has yet to be proven.

Author Contributions: Conceptualisation, B.L.S. and C.S.M.; methodology, B.L.S. and C.S.M.; data curation and synthesis, B.L.S. and C.S.M.; writing—original draft preparation, B.L.S. and C.S.M.; writing—review and editing, B.L.S., C.S.M. and M.T.H.; supervision, M.T.H.; All authors interpreted the data, critically reviewed the work, made important contributions to the manuscript with their suggestions for improvement, approved the published version, and agreed to be responsible for all aspects of the work. C.S.M. and B.L.S. have contributed equally to this work. All authors have read and agreed to the published version of the manuscript.

Funding: This research received no external funding.

Institutional Review Board Statement: Ethical review and approval were waived for this study, because, unlike primary research, no new personal, sensitive or confidential information were collected from participants. Only publicly available documents were used for the systematic reviewer.

Informed Consent Statement: Not applicable.

Data Availability Statement: Not applicable.

Conflicts of Interest: The authors declare no conflict of interest.

References

1. Lutzner, J.; Hubel, U.; Kirschner, S.; Gunther, K.P.; Krummenauer, F. Long-term results in total knee arthroplasty. A meta-analysis of revision rates and functional outcome. *Chirurg* **2011**, *82*, 618–624.
2. Callahan, C.M.; Drake, B.G.; A Heck, D.; Dittus, R.S. Patient outcomes following tricompartmental total knee replacement. A meta-analysis. *JAMA* **1994**, *271*, 1349–1357. [CrossRef]
3. Cross, M.; Smith, E.; Hoy, D.; Nolte, S.; Ackerman, I.; Fransen, M.; Bridgett, L.; Williams, S.; Guillemin, F.; Hill, C.L.; et al. The global burden of hip and knee osteoarthritis: Estimates from the Global Burden of Disease 2010 study. *Ann. Rheum. Dis.* **2014**, *73*, 1323–1330. [CrossRef] [PubMed]
4. Vos, T.; Flaxman, A.D.; Naghavi, M.; Lozano, R.; Michaud, C.; Ezzati, M.; Shibuya, K.; A Salomon, J.; Abdalla, S.; Aboyans, V.; et al. Years lived with disability (YLDs) for 1160 sequelae of 289 diseases and injuries 1990–2010: A systematic analysis for the Global Burden of Disease Study 2010. *Lancet* **2012**, *380*, 2163–2196. [CrossRef]
5. Hofmann, S.; Seitlinger, G.; Djahani, O.; Pietsch, M. The painful knee after TKA: A diagnostic algorithm for failure analysis. *Knee Surg. Sports Traumatol. Arthrosc.* **2011**, *19*, 1442–1452. [CrossRef]
6. Mandalia, V.; Eyres, K.; Schranz, P.; Toms, A.D. Evaluation of patients with a painful total knee replacement. *J. Bone Jt. Surg. Br. Vol.* **2008**, *90*, 265–271. [CrossRef]
7. Toms, A.D.; Mandalia, V.; Haigh, R.; Hopwood, B.; Toms, A.D.; Mandalia, V.; Haigh, R.; Hopwood, B. The management of patients with painful total knee replacement. *J. Bone Jt. Surg. Br. Vol.* **2009**, *91*, 143–150. [CrossRef]
8. Beswick, A.D.; Wylde, V.; Gooberman-Hill, R.; Blom, A.W.; Dieppe, P. What proportion of patients report long-term pain after total hip or knee replacement for osteoarthritis? A systematic review of prospective studies in unselected patients. *BMJ Open* **2012**, *2*, e000435. [CrossRef]
9. Baker, P.N.; van der Meulen, J.H.; Lewsey, J.; Gregg, P.J.; National Joint Registry for England and Wales. The role of pain and function in determining patient satisfaction after total knee replacement. Data from the National Joint Registry for England and Wales. *J. Bone Jt. Surg. Br.* **2007**, *89*, 893–900. [CrossRef]
10. Vince, K.G.; Abdeen, A.; Sugimori, T. The unstable total knee arthroplasty: Causes and cures. *J. Arthroplast.* **2006**, *21*, 44–49. [CrossRef]
11. Sharkey, P.F.; Hozack, W.J.; Rothman, R.H.; Shastri, S.; Jacoby, S.M. Why Are Total Knee Arthroplasties Failing Today? *Clin. Orthop. Relat. Res.* **2002**, *404*, 7–13. [CrossRef]
12. Sharkey, P.F.; Lichstein, P.M.; Shen, C.; Tokarski, A.T.; Parvizi, J. Why Are Total Knee Arthroplasties Failing Today—Has Anything Changed After 10 Years? *J. Arthroplast.* **2014**, *29*, 1774–1778. [CrossRef]
13. Budhiparama, N.C.; Lumban-Gaol, I.; Ifran, N.N.; De Groot, P.C.; Nelissen, R.G. Anthropometric Measurement of Caucasian and Asian Knees, Mismatch with Knee Systems? *Orthop. J. Sports Med.* **2020**, *8*, 8. [CrossRef]
14. Noble, P.C.; Scuderi, G.R.; Brekke, A.C.; Sikorskii, A.; Benjamin, J.B.; Lonner, J.H.; Chadha, P.; Daylamani, D.A.; Scott, N.W.; Bourne, R.B. Development of a New Knee Society Scoring System. *Clin. Orthop. Relat. Res.* **2012**, *470*, 20–32. [CrossRef]
15. Slim, K.; Nini, E.; Forestier, D.; Kwiatkowski, F.; Panis, Y.; Chipponi, J. Methodological Index for Non-Randomized Studies (MINORS): Development and Validation of a New Instrument. *ANZ J. Surg.* **2003**, *73*, 712–716. [CrossRef]
16. Arbab, D.; Reimann, P.; Brucker, M.; Bouillon, B.; Lüring, C. Alignment in total knee arthroplasty—A comparison of patient-specific implants with the conventional technique. *Knee* **2018**, *25*, 882–887. [CrossRef]
17. Buch, R.; Schroeder, L.; Buch, R.; Eberle, R. Does Implant Design Affect Hospital Metrics and Patient Outcomes? TKA Utilizing a "Fast-Track" Protocol. *Reconstr. Rev.* **2019**, *9*. [CrossRef]

18. Culler, S.D.; Martin, G.M.; Swearingen, A. Comparison of adverse events rates and hospital cost between customized individually made implants and standard off-the-shelf implants for total knee arthroplasty. *Arthroplast. Today* **2017**, *3*, 257–263. [CrossRef] [PubMed]
19. Ivie, C.B.; Probst, P.J.; Bal, A.K.; Stannard, J.T.; Crist, B.D.; Bal, B.S. Improved Radiographic Outcomes With Patient-Specific Total Knee Arthroplasty. *J. Arthroplast.* **2014**, *29*, 2100–2103. [CrossRef] [PubMed]
20. Meheux, C.J.; Park, K.J.; Clyburn, T.A. A Retrospective Study Comparing a Patient-specific Design Total Knee Arthroplasty With an Off-the-Shelf Design: Unexpected Catastrophic Failure Seen in the Early Patient-specific Design. *JAAOS Glob. Res. Rev.* **2019**, *3*, e19.00143. [CrossRef] [PubMed]
21. O'Connor, M.I.; Blau, B.E. The Economic Value of Customized versus Off-the-Shelf Knee Implants in Medicare Fee-for-Service Beneficiaries. *Am. Health Drug Benefits* **2019**, *12*, 66–73. [PubMed]
22. Reimann, P.; Brucker, M.; Arbab, D.; Lüring, C. Patient satisfaction—A comparison between patient-specific implants and conventional total knee arthroplasty. *J. Orthop.* **2019**, *16*, 273–277. [CrossRef] [PubMed]
23. Schroeder, L.; Martin, G. In Vivo Tibial Fit and Rotational Analysis of a Customized, Patient-Specific TKA versus Off-the-Shelf TKA. *J. Knee Surg.* **2018**, *32*, 499–505. [CrossRef] [PubMed]
24. Schwarzkopf, R.; Brodsky, M.; Garcia, G.A.; Gomoll, A.H. Surgical and Functional Outcomes in Patients Undergoing Total Knee Replacement With Patient-Specific Implants Compared With "Off-the-Shelf" Implants. *Orthop. J. Sports Med.* **2015**, *3*. [CrossRef]
25. Wheatley, B.; Nappo, K.; Fisch, J.; Rego, L.; Shay, M.; Cannova, C. Early outcomes of patient-specific posterior stabilized total knee arthroplasty implants. *J. Orthop.* **2019**, *16*, 14–18. [CrossRef]
26. White, P.B.; Ranawat, A.S. Patient-Specific Total Knees Demonstrate a Higher Manipulation Rate Compared to "Off-the-Shelf Implants". *J. Arthroplast.* **2016**, *31*, 107–111. [CrossRef]
27. Demange, M.K.; Von Keudell, A.; Probst, C.; Yoshioka, H.; Gomoll, A.H. Patient-specific implants for lateral unicompartmental knee arthroplasty. *Int. Orthop.* **2015**, *39*, 1519–1526. [CrossRef]
28. Mayer, C.; Bittersohl, B.; Haversath, M.; Franz, A.; Krauspe, R.; Jäger, M.; Zilkens, C. The learning curve of patient-specific unikondylar arthroplasty may be advantageous to off-the-shelf implants: A preliminary study. *J. Orthop.* **2020**, *22*, 256–260. [CrossRef]
29. Steinert, A.F.; Sefrin, L.; Jansen, B.; Schröder, L.; Holzapfel, B.M.; Arnholdt, J.; Rudert, M. Patient-specific cruciate-retaining total knee replacement with individualized implants and instruments (iTotal™ CR G2). *Oper. Orthop. Traumatol.* **2021**, *33*, 170–180. [CrossRef]
30. Neginhal, V.; Kurtz, W.; Schroeder, L. Patient Satisfaction, Functional Outcomes, and Survivorship in Patients with a Customized Posterior-Stabilized Total Knee Replacement. *JBJS Rev.* **2020**, *8*, e19.00104. [CrossRef] [PubMed]
31. Huber, B.; Tait, R.; Kurtz, W.; Burkhardt, J.; Swanson, T.; Clyburn, T. Outcomes after Customized Individually Made Total Knee Arthroplasty. In Proceedings of the ICJR Pan Pacific Congress 2016, Waikoloa, HI, USA, 10–13 August 2016.
32. Kaelin, R.; Vogel, N.; Arnold, M.P. Clinical and Patient-Reported Short-Term Results after Customized Individually Made Total Knee Arthroplasty. *Swiss Med. Wkly.* **2019**, *149*, 62s.
33. Zeller, I.M.; Sharma, A.; Kurtz, W.B.; Anderle, M.R.; Komistek, R.D. Customized versus Patient-Sized Cruciate-Retaining Total Knee Arthroplasty: An InVivo Kinematics Study Using Mobile Fluoroscopy. *J. Arthroplast.* **2017**, *32*, 1344–1350. [CrossRef] [PubMed]
34. Patil, S.; Bunn, A.; Bugbee, W.D.; Colwell, C.W.; D'Lima, D.D. Patient-specific implants with custom cutting blocks better approximate natural knee kinematics than standard TKA without custom cutting blocks. *Knee* **2015**, *22*, 624–629. [CrossRef]
35. Katthagen, B.-D.; Chatziandreou, I. Comparison of Hospital Metrics and Patient Reported Outcomes for Patients with Customized, Individually Made Vs. Conventional TKA. In Proceedings of the 2015 World Arthroplasty Congress (WAC), Paris, France, 16–18 April 2015.
36. Kay, A.B.; Kurtz, W.B.; Martin, G.M.; Huber, B.M.; Tait, R.J.; A Clyburn, T. Manipulation Rate Is Not Increased After Customized Total Knee Arthroplasty. *Reconstr. Rev.* **2018**, *8*, 8. [CrossRef]
37. Ritter, M.A.; Davis, K.E.; Meding, J.B.; Pierson, J.L.; Berend, M.E.; Malinzak, R.A. The Effect of Alignment and BMI on Failure of Total Knee Replacement. *J. Bone Jt. Surg. Am. Vol.* **2011**, *93*, 1588–1596. [CrossRef]
38. Fang, D.M.; Ritter, M.A.; Davis, K.E. Coronal Alignment in Total Knee Arthroplasty Just How Important is it? *J. Arthroplast.* **2009**, *24*, 39–43. [CrossRef] [PubMed]
39. Levengood, G.A.; Dupee, J. Accuracy of Coronal Plane Mechanical Alignment in a Customized, Individually Made Total Knee Replacement with Patient-Specific Instrumentation. *J. Knee Surg.* **2018**, *31*, 792–796. [CrossRef]
40. Arnholdt, J.; Kamawal, Y.; Holzapfel, B.M.; Ripp, A.; Rudert, M.; Steinert, A.F. Evaluation of implant fit and frontal plane alignment after bi-compartmental knee arthroplasty using patient-specific instruments and implants. *Arch. Med. Sci.* **2018**, *14*, 1424–1431. [CrossRef]
41. Thienpont, E.; Schwab, P.E.; Fennema, P. Efficacy of Patient-Specific Instruments in Total Knee Arthroplasty: A Systematic Review and Meta-Analysis. *J. Bone Jt. Surg. Am.* **2017**, *99*, 521–530. [CrossRef]
42. Abdel, M.P.; Ollivier, M.; Parratte, S.; Trousdale, R.T.; Berry, D.J.; Pagnano, M.W. Effect of Postoperative Mechanical Axis Alignment on Survival and Functional Outcomes of Modern Total Knee Arthroplasties with Cement A Concise Follow-up at 20 Years. *J. Bone Jt. Surg. Am Vol.* **2018**, *100*, 472–478. [CrossRef] [PubMed]

43. Howell, S.M.; Shelton, T.J.; Hull, M.L. Implant Survival and Function Ten Years After Kinematically Aligned Total Knee Arthroplasty. *J. Arthroplast.* **2018**, *33*, 3678–3684. [CrossRef] [PubMed]
44. Bonnin, M.P.; Beckers, L.; Leon, A.; Chauveau, J.; Muller, J.H.; Tibesku, C.O.; Ait-Si-Selmi, T. Custom total knee arthroplasty facilitates restoration of constitutional coronal alignment. *Knee Surg. Sports Traumatol. Arthrosc.* **2020**. Online ahead of print. [CrossRef]
45. Panni, A.S.; Ascione, F.; Rossini, M.; Braile, A.; Corona, K.; Vasso, M.; Hirschmann, M.T. Tibial internal rotation negatively affects clinical outcomes in total knee arthroplasty: A systematic review. *Knee Surg. Sports Traumatol. Arthrosc.* **2017**, *26*, 1636–1644. [CrossRef] [PubMed]
46. Nicoll, D.; Rowley, D.I. Internal rotational error of the tibial component is a major cause of pain after total knee replacement. *J. Bone Jt. Surg. Br. Vol.* **2010**, *92*, 1238–1244. [CrossRef]
47. Carpenter, D.P.; Holmberg, R.R.; Quartulli, M.J.; Barnes, C.L. Tibial Plateau Coverage in UKA: A Comparison of Patient Specific and Off-The-Shelf Implants. *J. Arthroplast.* **2014**, *29*, 1694–1698. [CrossRef]
48. Mahoney, O.M.; Kinsey, T. Overhang of the Femoral Component in Total Knee Arthroplasty: Risk Factors and Clinical Consequences. *J. Bone Jt. Surg. Am. Vol.* **2010**, *92*, 1115–1121. [CrossRef]
49. Kim, T.K.; Phillips, M.; Bhandari, M.; Watson, J.; Malhotra, R. What Differences in Morphologic Features of the Knee Exist Among Patients of Various Races? A Systematic Review. *Clin. Orthop. Relat. Res.* **2017**, *475*, 170–182. [CrossRef]
50. Yue, B.; Varadarajan, K.M.; Ai, S.; Tang, T.; Rubash, H.E.; Li, G. Differences of Knee Anthropometry Between Chinese and White Men and Women. *J. Arthroplast.* **2011**, *26*, 124–130. [CrossRef] [PubMed]
51. Meier, M.; Zingde, S.; Steinert, A.; Kurtz, W.; Koeck, F.; Beckmann, J. What Is the Possible Impact of High Variability of Distal Femoral Geometry on TKA? A CT Data Analysis of 24,042 Knees. *Clin. Orthop. Relat. Res.* **2019**, *477*, 561–570. [CrossRef] [PubMed]
52. Hofmann, A.A.; Bachus, K.N.; Wyatt, R.W. Effect of the tibial cut on subsidence following total knee arthroplasty. *Clin. Orthop. Relat. Res.* **1991**, *269*, 63–69. [CrossRef]
53. Namin, A.T.; Jalali, M.S.; Vahdat, V.; Bedair, H.S.; O'Connor, M.I.; Kamarthi, S.; Isaacs, J.A. Adoption of New Medical Technologies: The Case of Customized Individually Made Knee Implants. *Value Health* **2019**, *22*, 423–430. [CrossRef] [PubMed]

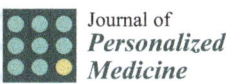

Article

Individual Revision Knee Arthroplasty Is a Safe Limb Salvage Procedure

Peter Savov *[ID], Lars-Rene Tuecking, Henning Windhagen and Max Ettinger

Department of Orthopedic Surgery, Hannover Medical School, Anna-von-Borries-Strasse 1–7, 30625 Hanover, Germany; lars-rene.tuecking@diakovere.de (L.-R.T.); henning.windhagen@diakovere.de (H.W.); max.ettinger@diakovere.de (M.E.)
* Correspondence: peter@savov-medizin.de

Abstract: Introduction: Revision total knee arthroplasty after multiple pre-surgeries is challenging. Due to severe bone defects, standard implants for metaphyseal and diaphyseal anchoring may no longer be suitable. The primary aim of this case series is to evaluate the early complication rate for individual knee implants with custom-made cones and stems after two-stage revision with severe bone defects. Methods: Ten patients who were treated with custom-made 3D-printed knee revision implants were included. Inclusion criteria were a two-stage revision due to late-onset or chronic periprosthetic joint infection as well as aseptic loosening. All severe bone defects were AORI type III. All procedure-related complications were evaluated. Postoperative range of motion after one year was measured. The time between the two surgeries was evaluated. Results: The mean follow-up was 21 months (range: 12–40). The mean time between the two-stage surgeries was 71.6 days. No fractures were observed intra- and postoperatively. Two patients were revised without changing metal components due to persistent hematoma (three weeks post-surgery) and persistent PJI (three months post-surgery). The mean passive postoperative range of motion was 92° (range: 80–110°). Conclusions: Individual custom-made implants for rTKA provide a safe procedure for patients with huge bone defects after several pre-surgeries. If standard knee systems with standard cones or sleeves are not suitable anymore, custom-made treatment offers the patient the last option for limb preservation. However, this is associated with increased costs.

Keywords: custom-made; rTKA; 3D-printed; individual; limb-salvage; cone

1. Introduction

Due to rising numbers of total knee arthroplasties (TKA) for the treatment of osteoarthritis (OA) of the knee joint, the numbers for revision total knee arthroplasty (rTKA) are analogously rising. In Germany, 14,462 revision surgeries were performed in 2019. At least one metal component was changed in 57.8% of the cases. This is an increase of 3% compared to 2018 [1]. A projection for the United States of America indicates an increase of 601% of rTKA between 2005 and 2030 [2]. In 31.2% of all revisions being performed in Germany in 2019, a condylar constrained knee (CCK) or rotating-hinge implant was needed to stabilize the knee. The correct diagnosis and the operative plan require a high amount of surgical experience. Likewise, the infrastructure is essential being able to address the reasons for the revision indication [3].

In the past, implant failure and polyethylene wear were the main reasons for rTKA. Currently, aseptic loosening, infections, and instability problems are the primary cause of revisions [1,4]. The primary aim of rTKA is restoring the natural joint line in the frontal and sagittal plane with sufficient anchoring. An elevation of the joint line of 4 mm already reduces significantly the maximal flexion [5–7]. Further, a loss of posterior condylar offset (PCO) is also associated with a reduction of the postoperative flexion of the knee joint [8,9].

Increasing numbers of rTKAs in younger patients due to the high amount of primary TKA in patients under the age of 65 leads to additional issues. In the case of aseptic

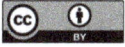

loosening, periprosthetic osteolysis (PROL) becomes a significant problem in the revision procedure. Increased accumulation of osteoclasts at the bone-implant interface, impaired osteoblast function, mechanical stresses, and increased production of synovial fluid lead to bone resorption and subsequent loosening of the implant. One of the main causes for PROL is the activity level of the patient [10].

In case of periprosthetic joint infection (PJI), one- or two-stage surgical revision with an exchange of the implant is needed. In addition to antibiotic therapy, a radical debridement of the situs is essential to ensure infection eradication. However, the preservation of good bone stock is the basis for a successful reimplantation of a new implant [11]. For fixation, two different zones should be used. The articular surface is in most cases insufficient for fixation. To provide good stability, the fixation is based on both the metaphysis and diaphysis. Cemented or cementless stems are used for the fixation in the diaphysis [11,12]. In recent years, sleeves and cones were established for augmentation of metaphysical defects and represent the new gold standard. With those modern techniques, AORI-type-IIb and III defects can be addressed very well [11,13]. In addition, metal augments and bone-impaction grafting are used to restore the native joint line [14].

However, standard instrumentation and implants have limitations when huge bone defects occur. Traditionally, megaprosthesis with a proximal tibial replacement, arthrodesis, or amputation were performed in those cases. With modern titanium alloy 3D printing technologies, CT-based individual implants could be used for major bony defects [15]. Both individual cones and stems can be manufactured. Those individual implants provide a homogeneously distributed bone stress [16]. The CT scan can be performed preoperatively before a one-stage revision or in the interval of a two-stage revision procedure. Thus, megaprostheses with the loss of the tuberosity tibiae with a high early and long-term revision rate can be avoided for those previously difficult to treat cases. For those megaprostheses, a complication rate of 52% is reported after a midterm follow-up [17].

Due to the lack of evidence, a case series was performed to analyze the complication rate for individual knee implants with custom-made cones and stems after two-stage revision with severe bone defects after aseptic loosening and PJI in a single center. The primary hypothesis is that the treatment with individual custom-made knee implants is a safe procedure and provides low complication rates.

2. Methods
2.1. Patients

Ten patients who were treated with individual custom-made 3D-printed knee revision implants were included. The basis of the knee system was the Link® Endo-Modell rotating-hinge system (RTH) and Megasystem-C distal femoral replacement (DFR) (Waldemar Link GmbH & Co. KG, Hamburg, Germany). All patients were treated between March 2019 and May 2020. The minimum follow-up was 12 months. The mean patient age at the time of surgery was 68.4 years (range 59–79). Inclusion criteria were a two-stage revision due to late-onset or chronic PJI as well as severe bone defect after aseptic loosening. All bone defects were AORI type III and could not be treated with a standard cone or stem (Figure 1A). All patients were treated with an antibiotic static cement spacer in the two-stage revision interval. No aspirations were routinely performed before the second-stage revision. There were no exclusion criteria. All surgeries were performed by a single senior surgeon. Approval for this retrospective case series was given by the institution's review board (8439_BO_K_2019). Informed consent was obtained from all subjects involved in the study.

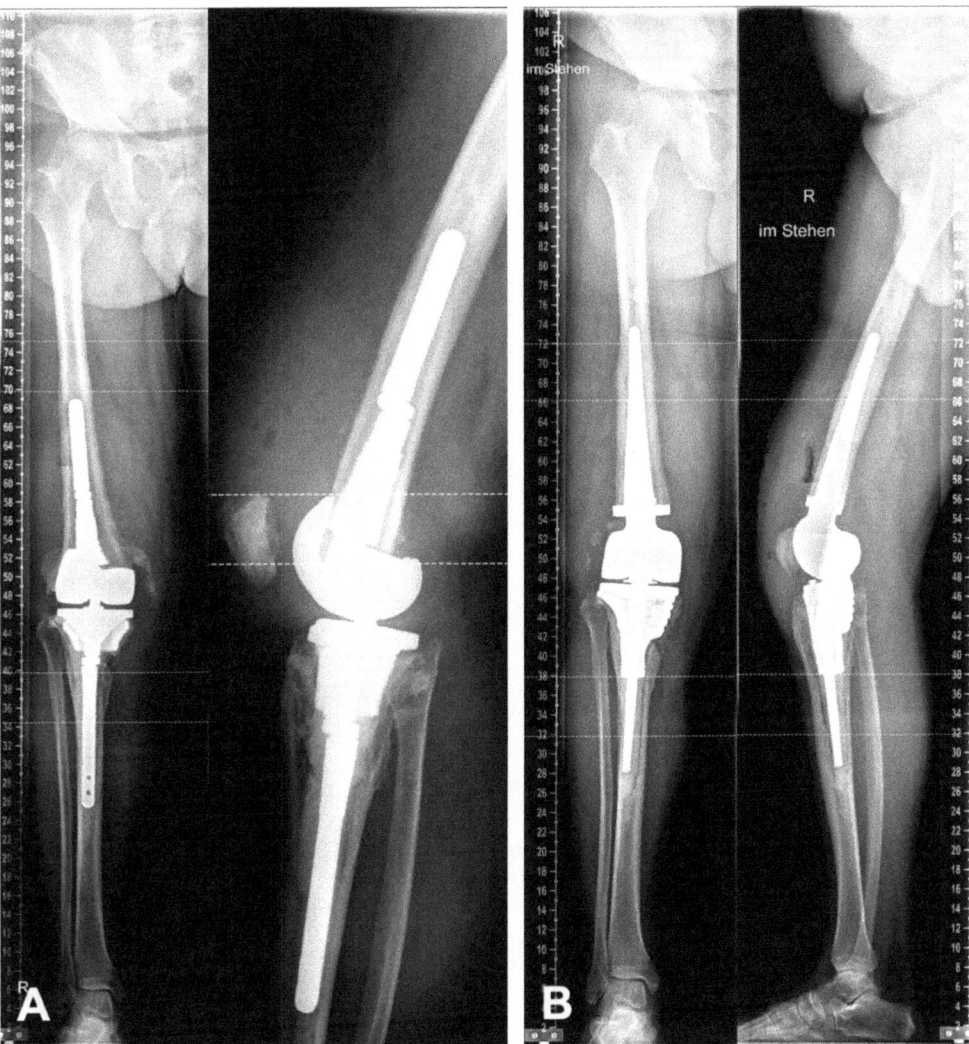

Figure 1. (**A**) Preoperative X-rays before explantation of the septic prosthesis. (**B**) Postoperative X-rays after reimplantation. The joint line and limb alignment are fully reconstructed. (R = right).

2.2. Parameters

The indications and characteristics of each implant are displayed in Table 1. The previous surgeries of the patients and all implant costs are displayed in Table 2. The time between the two surgeries was evaluated. All patients received pre- and postoperative standard long leg and true lateral radiographs. The hip–knee–ankle angle (HKA) was analyzed pre- and postoperatively. All procedure-related complications were evaluated including early revision due to seroma, hematoma, or wound healing disorder, intra- and postoperative fractures, early-onset (<4 weeks), and late-onset (>4 weeks) infections. Postoperative range of motion after one year was measured. The pre- and postoperative VAS scale was raised.

Table 1. Age, BMI, and the days of the interval between the two-stage procedures were listed as well as the number of pre-surgeries and pre-implants of each patient. Pre-surgeries comprise all procedures in the past including changes of metal components or soft tissue revisions. Pre-implants comprise all protheses including primary and revision TKA in the patient's past. (ID: patient number, PJI: periprosthetic joint infection, AL: aseptic loosening).

ID	Age	BMI	Interval (Days)	Pre-Surgeries	Pre-Implants	Indication
1	69	25.7	67	3	2	PJI
2	61	26.5	78	7	3	PJI
3	70	26.8	73	7	4	AL
4	62	34.1	110	5	3	PJI
5	60	28.7	50	4	4	AL
6	79	21.6	57	5	3	AL
7	77	35.2	83	3	2	PJI
8	59	34.1	70	8	3	PJI
9	72	40.4	44	7	4	PJI
10	75	29.0	84	3	2	AL
Mean	68.4	30.2	71.6	5.2	3	

Table 2. The knee system, the amount and type of the specific individual implants, and the total costs are listed. (ID: patient number, DFR: distal femoral replacement, RTH: rotating hinge prosthesis, Ind: individual, Std: standard).

	Knee System		Femur Implants		Tibia Implants		Total Costs €
ID	Femur	Tibia	Ind. Cone	Ind. Stem	Ind. Cone	Std. Cone	
1	DFR	RTH	No	Yes	No	Yes	12.039,45
2	DFR	RTH	Yes	No	Yes	No	13.166,58
3	DFR	RTH	No	Yes	Yes	No	16.476,88
4	RTH	RTH	No	Yes	Yes	No	9.969,62
5	RTH	RTH	No	No	Yes	No	5.131,78
6	DFR	RTH	No	No	Yes	No	8.772,03
7	RTH	RTH	Yes	No	Yes	No	11.842,35
8	DFR	RTH	No	Yes	Yes	No	19.900,82
9	RTH	RTH	No	No	Yes	No	4.321,53
10	RTH	RTH	No	No	Yes	No	5.778,14
Mean							10.739,92

2.3. Manufacturing

The planning and manufacturing of each implant is based on a CT scan. Close cooperation with the respective engineer of the manufacturer is necessary. Nonmetallic static spacers are recommended for use to increase the quality of the scan with fewer image artifacts. One-stage revisions are possible as well. In those cases, a metal artifact reduction sequence (MARS) should be used.

For severe metaphyseal tibial and femoral defects, hybrid cones are individually manufactured from titanium alloy (TiAl6V4). For the 3D printing process, the electronic beam melting (EBM) or selective laser melting (SLM) technique are used. This is followed by a hot isostatic pressing (HIP) to close unwanted cavities. To achieve improved osteointegration, the cone is coated with calcium phosphate. The surface is highly porous with a structural depth of 2 mm and a pore size of 610–820 µm.

To provide additional stability, individual stems for the femur or tibia with an oval shape can be used. Thus, an almost form-fit anchoring is possible over the entire length of the stem with an additional degree of rotational stability. These stems are usually provided with a taper that allows coupling with a component of a standard implant. An individual printed or standard collar with calcium phosphate coating can be used for the femur implant. Each custom-made stem is made by a CNC machine and comes with an individual rasp. Both cemented and cementless fixation is possible. Further, the implants can be coated with silver by the manufacturer.

2.4. Planning and Surgical Technique

After segmentation, the first step of planning is the analysis of the bone defect (Figure 2). If the defect of the distal femur is too devastating, resection of the distal femur may be necessary. In such a scenario, the use of a conical oval stem is advisable (Figure 3). If the tibial tuberosity is still intact, proximal tibial replacement may not be required. With the help of a tibial cone, a standard tibial implant can be used. The cone provides a bearing surface to reconstruct the joint line (Figure 4). If iatrogenic fractures occurred during the first operation, this should be taken into account when planning the stem length. Features such as notches for cerclages or additional attachment options for the extensor mechanism are possible after consultation with the engineers (Figures 5 and 6D).

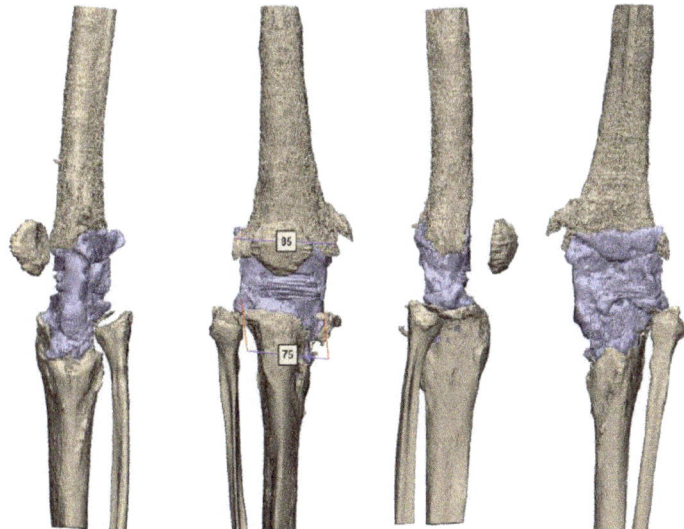

Figure 2. CT scan after the explantation of the septic prosthesis with a huge bone defect on the metaphysis of the tibia and femur. The tuberositas tibiae is still intact. However, the medial tibia plateau is loss. AO fixature bars are used for the rigid spacer. The mediolateral size for the femur is 85 mm and for the tibia 75 mm.

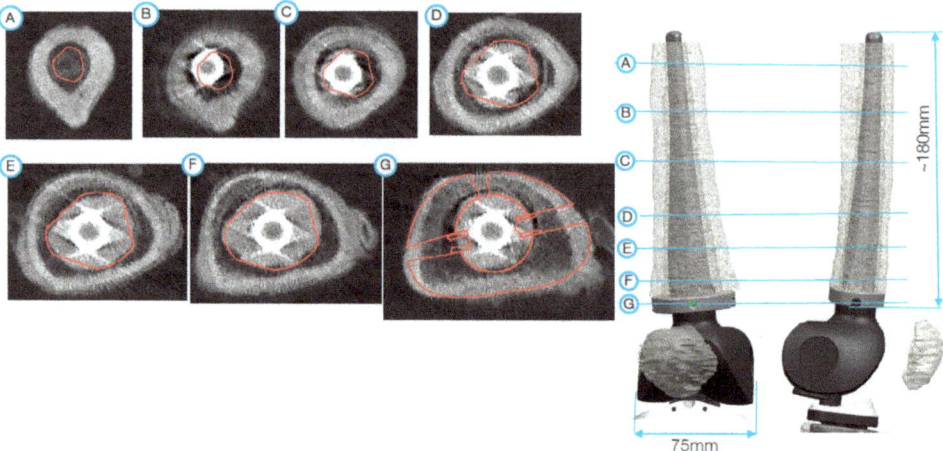

Figure 3. Planning of the femur component. For the diaphysis, an individual stem was planned. This is oval and takes up the natural curvature of the femur. Because of the defect of the metaphysis, a distal femoral replacement is used. The subfigures on the left side (A, B, C, ... , G) demonstrate the axial view of the femur from the corresponding markings on the right side.

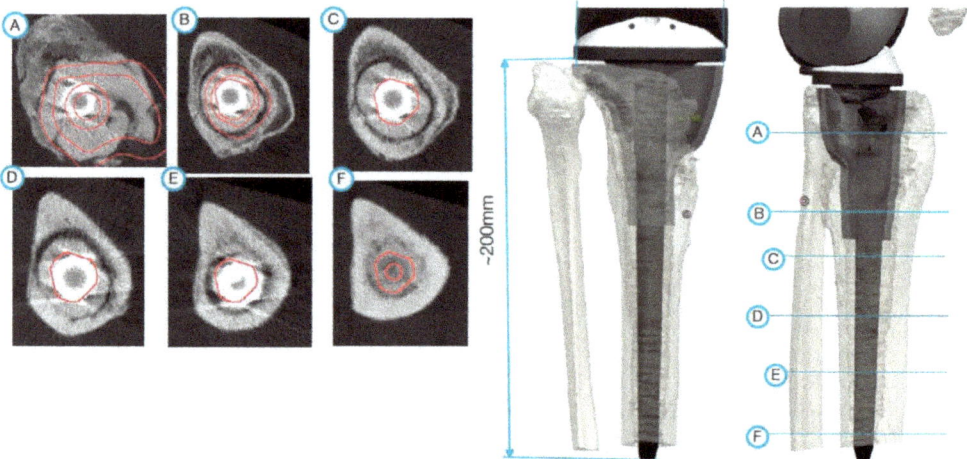

Figure 4. During planning, special consideration had to be given to the large defect of the medial tibial plateaus. The subfigures on the left side (A, B, C, ... , F) demonstrate the axial view of the tibia from the corresponding markings on the right side.

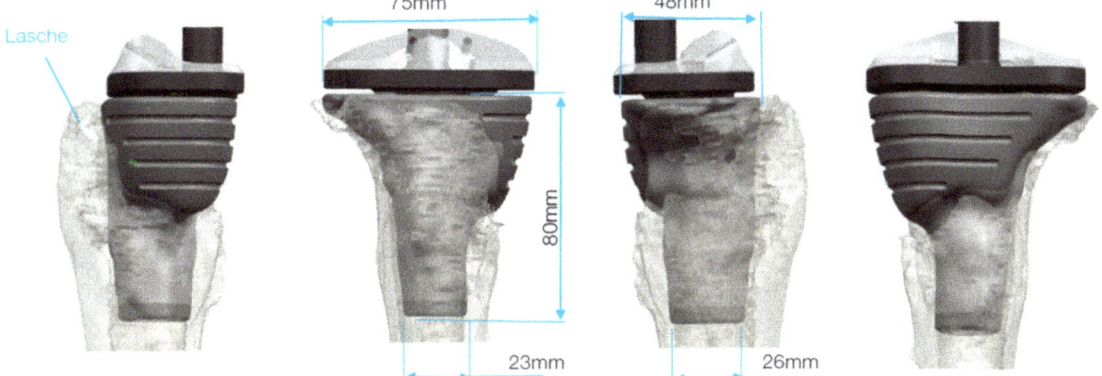

Figure 5. The customized cone has a porous structure in the area of bone contact and prefabricated grooves for possible osteosynthesis using cerclages.

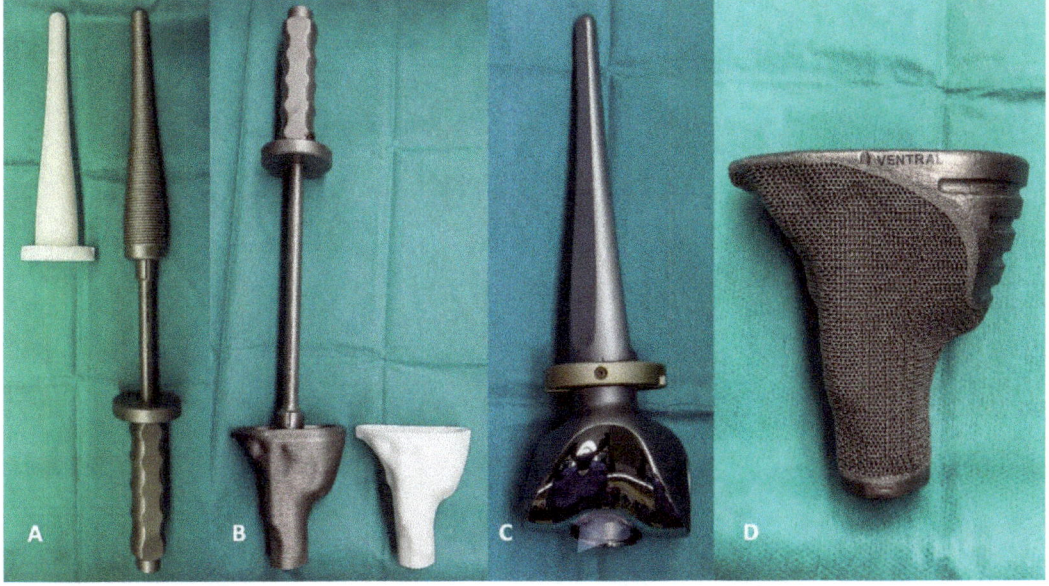

Figure 6. (**A,B**) A special rasp or impactor is supplied with each implant. The fit of the implant can be tested with a 3D dummy. (**C**) In planning, attention should be paid to the method of fixing the shafts. In this case, a cemented version was chosen. (**D**) Individual cones show improved biomechanics, as the force application into the bone is much more homogeneous. Each implant can be equipped with special features, such as fixation guides for osteosyntheses.

During the surgery, the bone bed is prepared with custom-made rasps, respectively, and impactors (Figure 6A,B). Trial implants can be used to check the position and progress of the preparation. The bone surface must be cleaned of any soft tissue such as pseudomembranes or cement residues to enable the best possible osteointegration to the cone surface. Bone-impaction grafting can be used to fill the remaining defects (Figure 7). The stems are usually cemented (Figure 1B).

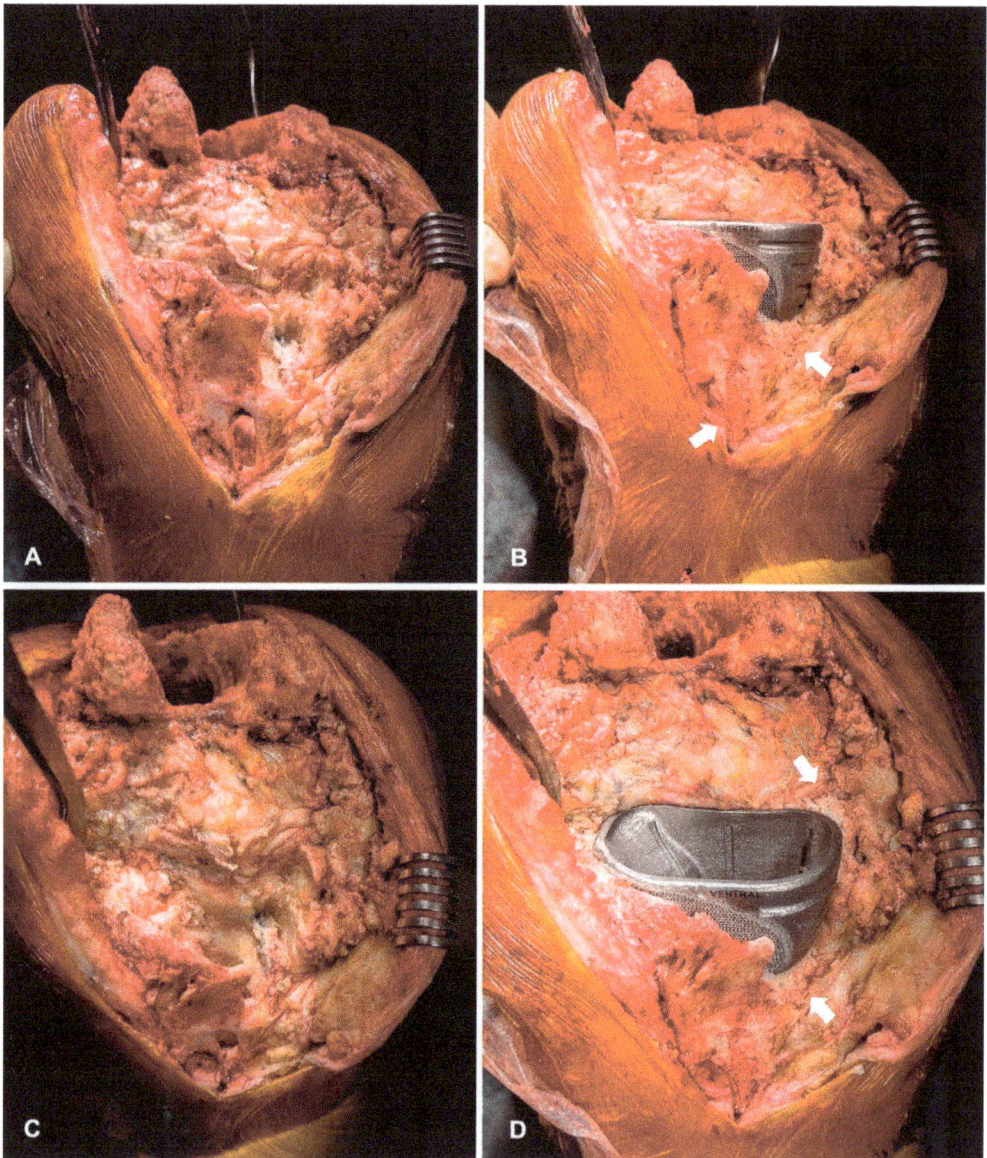

Figure 7. (**A,C**) Intraoperative findings of severe defect of the tibial metaphysis. The complete medial plateau is loss. (**B,D**) After cementless implantation of the cone, defects are filled with bone-impaction grafting (arrows). This leads to secondary osteointegration and partial reconstruction of the bone defect.

3. Results

All demographics and indications are shown in Table 1. Six patients had a PJI and four an aseptic loosening (AL). The mean follow-up was 21 months (range: 12–40). The mean time between the two-stage surgeries was 71.6 days. No fractures were observed intra- and postoperatively. One patient was revised due to persistent hematoma (three weeks post-surgery) and one patient due to persistent PJI. This patient was treated with a change of polyethylene (three months post-surgery) and permanent antibiotic suppression therapy (cotrimoxazole). The type of implants, the postoperative range of motion, and the individual costs are listed in Table 2. Five patients received a distal femoral replacement (DFR) and no one needed a proximal tibial replacement. The mean preoperative VAS scale was 8.1 points (range: 7–9) and the mean postoperative VAS scale was 2 points (range: 0–5). The mean preoperative HKA was 177.2° varus (range: 176–181°) and the mean postoperative HKA was 179.2° varus (range: 178–180°). The mean passive postoperative range of motion was 92° (range: 80–110°). No extension deficit or extensor lag was observed.

4. Discussion

The most important finding of this study is that individual custom-made implants in rTKA are a safe procedure for limb salvage when standard implants are not suitable anymore. With the help of the individual tibial cones, the tuberosity tibiae with the extensor mechanism can be preserved. This leads to a good functional outcome and range of motion.

Megaprostheses have a high risk for early mechanical complications and infections followed by amputations [18]. We present an early revision rate of 20%. One patient was revised due to a persistent hematoma after three weeks and one due to a persistent PJI with the need for an exchange of the polyethylene and a permanent antibiotic suppression therapy. During the revision of this patient the same pathogen as in the previous surgeries was detected (multi-resistant *Staphylococcus capitis* and *Proteus mirabilis*). This is comparable to the current literature of outcome after implanting megaprostheses. Fraser et al. reported a revision-free survival of 58% after eight years in 247 cases with a rotating-hinge megaprosthesis [19]. Höll et al. reported a mid-term revision rate of 55% after a mean follow-up of 34 months (range: 10–84 months) [17]. Vertesich et al. reported a revision-free survival of distal femoral replacement of 74.8% at one year, 62.5% at three years, and 40.9% at ten years postoperatively [20]. Smith et al. demonstrated a complication rate at two years follow-up of 34% in a septic and aseptic mixed cohort [21]. Von Hintze et al. reported that PJI was the most common cause for revision after implanting rotating-hinge prostheses at a mid-term follow-up [22]. It is known that silver coating can reduce the revision rate after implanting megaprostheses in the case of PJI [23]. However, no anti-septic coatings were used in this study. The long-term results of our cohort concerning loosening rate remain to be seen. Evidence for superiority in terms of stability or survival of oval cemented stems over standard stems is not currently available. However, an advantage over standard implants is certainly possible.

The rate of intraoperative fractures regarding cone preparation and insertion for standard implants is very low. In a systematic review from 2018, Divano et al. observed an intraoperative fracture cones-related rate of 0.89% [13]. A recent systematic review from 2020 evaluated 927 cones and reported an intraoperative fracture rate of 1.2 ± 4.8% [24]. This suggests that those types of implants are safe to use in principle. Burastero et al. evaluated eleven patients with 16 custom-made cones regarding the clinical and biomechanical outcome. They reported no intraoperative fractures and no component migration after a mean follow-up of 26 months. Further, the authors demonstrated that custom-made cones induce a more homogeneously distributed bone stress compared to standard cemented or cementless stems in a finite element analysis [16]. We observed comparable results and had no fractures in this case series.

In severe metaphyseal tibial bone defects, proximal tibial replacement (PTR) has to be taken into account. One of the major issues of this treatment method is the comparatively poor function, especially a possible extensor lag. Fram et al. reported in a small case series an extensor lag in almost all patients [25]. Biau et al. reported a failure of the extensor mechanism in 26% of all patients with PTR after bone tumor resection [26]. However, the comparability between tumor resection and condition after failed knee replacement is not given. We could demonstrate a good postoperative function with a mean passive flexion of 92° and no extension deficit or extensor lag due to the preservation of the tuberosity tibiae and the natural extensor mechanism. There is good evidence for reducing the infection rate with the help of medial gastrocnemius muscle flap after PTR [27–29]. This primarily refers to PTR after malignant bone tumors, however, these results can be drawn with severe defects especially in the medial proximal tibia area after revision arthroplasty. In the present study, flap coverage was not necessary, but this should always be considered and evaluated individually.

A major point of criticism of custom-made implants is the prolonged time between the two procedures to plan and manufacture the implant. The mean interval between the removal and replacement was 71.6 days (range: 44–110 days). From our point of view, this correlates with the extent of bone loss, the number of implants to be fabricated, and the complexity of the case. In a case as described in 2.4. (Figures 1 and 2), an intensive dialogue with the corresponding engineer is necessary. If only a tibial conus is needed, a six-week interval is possible (Table 2). Thus, the recommended six- to eight-week interval cannot always been adhered to [30]. However, due to the primary goal of joint preservation, this is accepted from the authors' point of view. Nevertheless, the period from the removal procedure to the CT scan and production of the implant has the greatest potential for improvement in the future. Despite the extended interval, the results of this study are comparable to those in the literature. Winkler et al. reported a mean interval from explantation to implantation in a long-interval group of 63 days (range: 28–204 days) [31].

Another crucial point are the high implant costs. The mean implant cost in this study was EUR 10.739,92 per patient. However, the range is wide (EUR 4.321,53 to 19.900,82) and depends on the individual bone defect with the need for different implants such as cones or stems. However, these costs also include custom-made instruments such as raps or impactors (Figure 6A,B) that can only be used for the specific case.

There are several limitations to this study. This is a case series with a low volume of patients. Due to the very modern and young procedure of 3D printing with high costs, the extent of usage is limited. However, the caseload has been increasing in the past few years. Another reason for the low number of patients is the cost factor of implants. These are not fully reflected by the DRG of the national health insurance, which makes the use of such implants the last resort. Another point of criticism is the lack of a control group. However, due to the strict inclusion criteria with major bone defects, standard megaprostheses with a proximal tibial replacement have a severe functional disadvantage and randomization cannot be performed based on the ethical standards. Due to low volume of patients, we did not compare different types of implant coating. Especially in case of PJI, an antiseptic coating like silver could reduce the revision rate. Furthermore, we presented an early follow-up with no clinical data and no patient reported outcome parameters. However, the primary aim of this study was to investigate the early revision rate of these limb-salvage procedures. Further prospective studies are required to analyze the clinical outcomes and mid- and long term follow-up.

5. Conclusions

Individual custom-made implants for rTKA provide a safe procedure for patients with huge bone defects after several pre-surgeries. If standard knee systems with standard cones or sleeves are not suitable anymore, custom-made treatment offers the patient the last option for limb preservation. However, this is associated with increased costs.

Author Contributions: Conceptualization and methodology, P.S., L.-R.T., H.W. and M.E.; validation, P.S., H.W. and M.E.; data curation, L.-R.T.; writing—original draft preparation, P.S.; writing—review and editing, M.E., L.-R.T. and H.W.; visualization, P.S. and L.-R.T.; supervision, H.W.; project administration, M.E.; All authors have read and agreed to the published version of the manuscript.

Funding: This research received no external funding.

Institutional Review Board Statement: The study was conducted according to the guidelines of the Declaration of Helsinki, and approved by the Institutional Review Board (8439_BO_K_2019, date of approval: 26.04.2019).

Informed Consent Statement: Informed consent was obtained from all subjects involved in the study.

Data Availability Statement: The data presented in this study are available in this article. Further datasets of this study are available from the corresponding author on reasonable request.

Conflicts of Interest: M.E. is an educational consultant for Stryker, and Smith and Nephew. H.W. is an educational consultant for Stryker, Medacta, Aesculap, and Smith and Nephew.

References

1. Grimberg, A.; Jansson, V.; Lützner, J.; Melsheimer, O.; Morlock, M.; Steinbrück, A. *German Arthroplasty Registry (Endoprothesenregister Deutschland—EPRD)—Annual Report 2020*; German Arthroplasty Registry EPRD: Berlin, Germany, 2020. [CrossRef]
2. Patel, A.; Pavlou, G.; Mujica-Mota, R.E.; Toms, A.D. The epidemiology of revision total knee and hip arthroplasty in England and Wales: A comparative analysis with projections for the United States. A study using the National Joint Registry dataset. *Bone Jt. J.* **2015**, *97-B*, 1076–1081. [CrossRef]
3. Halder, A.M.; Gehrke, T.; Gunster, C.; Heller, K.D.; Leicht, H.; Malzahn, J.; Niethard, F.U.; Schrader, P.; Zacher, J.; Jeschke, E. Low Hospital Volume Increases Re-Revision Rate Following Aseptic Revision Total Knee Arthroplasty: An Analysis of 23,644 Cases. *J. Arthroplast.* **2020**, *35*, 1054–1059. [CrossRef] [PubMed]
4. Delanois, R.E.; Mistry, J.B.; Gwam, C.U.; Mohamed, N.S.; Choksi, U.S.; Mont, M.A. Current Epidemiology of Revision Total Knee Arthroplasty in the United States. *J. Arthroplast.* **2017**, *32*, 2663–2668. [CrossRef]
5. Han, H.S.; Yu, C.H.; Shin, N.; Won, S.; Lee, M.C. Femoral joint line restoration is a major determinant of postoperative range of motion in revision total knee arthroplasty. *Knee Surg. Sports Traumatol. Arthrosc.* **2019**, *27*, 2090–2095. [CrossRef] [PubMed]
6. Clave, A.; Le Henaff, G.; Roger, T.; Maisongrosse, P.; Mabit, C.; Dubrana, F. Joint line level in revision total knee replacement: Assessment and functional results with an average of seven years follow-up. *Int. Orthop.* **2016**, *40*, 1655–1662. [CrossRef] [PubMed]
7. van Lieshout, W.A.M.; Valkering, K.P.; Koenraadt, K.L.M.; van Etten-Jamaludin, F.S.; Kerkhoffs, G.; van Geenen, R.C.I. The negative effect of joint line elevation after total knee arthroplasty on outcome. *Knee Surg. Sports Traumatol. Arthrosc.* **2019**, *27*, 1477–1486. [CrossRef]
8. Ettinger, M.; Savov, P.; Balubaid, O.; Windhagen, H.; Calliess, T. Influence of stem length on component flexion and posterior condylar offset in revision total knee arthroplasty. *Knee* **2018**, *25*, 480–484. [CrossRef]
9. Clement, N.D.; MacDonald, D.J.; Hamilton, D.F.; Burnett, R. Posterior condylar offset is an independent predictor of functional outcome after revision total knee arthroplasty. *Bone Jt. Res.* **2017**, *6*, 172–178. [CrossRef]
10. Gallo, J.; Goodman, S.B.; Konttinen, Y.T.; Wimmer, M.A.; Holinka, M. Osteolysis around total knee arthroplasty: A review of pathogenetic mechanisms. *Acta Biomater.* **2013**, *9*, 8046–8058. [CrossRef]
11. Kim, H.J.; Lee, O.S.; Lee, S.H.; Lee, Y.S. Comparative Analysis between Cone and Sleeve in Managing Severe Bone Defect during Revision Total Knee Arthroplasty: A Systematic Review and Meta-Analysis. *J. Knee Surg.* **2018**, *31*, 677–685. [CrossRef]
12. Wang, C.; Pfitzner, T.; von Roth, P.; Mayr, H.O.; Sostheim, M.; Hube, R. Fixation of stem in revision of total knee arthroplasty: Cemented versus cementless—A meta-analysis. *Knee Surg. Sports Traumatol. Arthrosc.* **2016**, *24*, 3200–3211. [CrossRef] [PubMed]
13. Divano, S.; Cavagnaro, L.; Zanirato, A.; Basso, M.; Felli, L.; Formica, M. Porous metal cones: Gold standard for massive bone loss in complex revision knee arthroplasty? A systematic review of current literature. *Arch. Orthop. Trauma Surg.* **2018**, *138*, 851–863. [CrossRef] [PubMed]
14. Lei, P.F.; Hu, R.Y.; Hu, Y.H. Bone Defects in Revision Total Knee Arthroplasty and Management. *Orthop. Surg.* **2019**, *11*, 15–24. [CrossRef] [PubMed]
15. McNamara, C.A.; Gosthe, R.G.; Patel, P.D.; Sanders, K.C.; Huaman, G.; Suarez, J.C. Revision total knee arthroplasty using a custom tantalum implant in a patient following multiple failed revisions. *Arthroplast. Today* **2017**, *3*, 13–17. [CrossRef]
16. Burastero, G.; Pianigiani, S.; Zanvettor, C.; Cavagnaro, L.; Chiarlone, F.; Innocenti, B. Use of porous custom-made cones for meta-diaphyseal bone defects reconstruction in knee revision surgery: A clinical and biomechanical analysis. *Arch. Orthop. Trauma Surg.* **2020**, *140*, 2041–2055. [CrossRef]
17. Höll, S.; Schlomberg, A.; Gosheger, G.; Dieckmann, R.; Streitbuerger, A.; Schulz, D.; Hardes, J. Distal femur and proximal tibia replacement with megaprosthesis in revision knee arthroplasty: A limb-saving procedure. *Knee Surg. Sports Traumatol. Arthrosc.* **2012**, *20*, 2513–2518. [CrossRef] [PubMed]
18. Huten, D. Femorotibial bone loss during revision total knee arthroplasty. *Orthop. Traumatol. Surg. Res.* **2013**, *99*, S22–S33. [CrossRef]
19. Fraser, J.F.; Werner, S.; Jacofsky, D.J. Wear and loosening in total knee arthroplasty: A quick review. *J. Knee Surg.* **2015**, *28*, 139–144. [CrossRef]
20. Vertesich, K.; Puchner, S.E.; Staats, K.; Schreiner, M.; Hipfl, C.; Kubista, B.; Holinka, J.; Windhager, R. Distal femoral reconstruction following failed total knee arthroplasty is accompanied with risk for complication and reduced joint function. *BMC Musculoskelet. Disord.* **2019**, *20*, 47. [CrossRef]
21. Smith, E.L.; Shah, A.; Son, S.J.; Niu, R.; Talmo, C.T.; Abdeen, A.; Ali, M.; Pinski, J.; Gordon, M.; Lozano-Calderon, S.; et al. Survivorship of Megaprostheses in Revision Hip and Knee Arthroplasty for Septic and Aseptic Indications: A Retrospective, Multicenter Study with Minimum 2-Year Follow-Up. *Arthroplast. Today* **2020**, *6*, 475–479. [CrossRef]
22. von Hintze, J.; Niemeläinen, M.; Sintonen, H.; Nieminen, J.; Eskelinen, A. Outcomes of the rotating hinge knee in revision total knee arthroplasty with a median follow-up of 6.2 years. *BMC Musculoskelet. Disord.* **2021**, *22*, 336. [CrossRef] [PubMed]

23. Zajonz, D.; Birke, U.; Ghanem, M.; Prietzel, T.; Josten, C.; Roth, A.; Fakler, J.K.M. Silver-coated modular Megaendoprostheses in salvage revision arthroplasty after periimplant infection with extensive bone loss—A pilot study of 34 patients. *BMC Musculoskelet. Disord.* **2017**, *18*, 383. [CrossRef] [PubMed]
24. Zanirato, A.; Formica, M.; Cavagnaro, L.; Divano, S.; Burastero, G.; Felli, L. Metaphyseal cones and sleeves in revision total knee arthroplasty: Two sides of the same coin? Complications, clinical and radiological results—A systematic review of the literature. *Musculoskelet. Surg.* **2020**, *104*, 25–35. [CrossRef]
25. Fram, B.; Smith, E.B.; Deirmengian, G.K.; Abraham, J.A.; Strony, J.; Cross, M.B.; Ponzio, D.Y. Proximal tibial replacement in revision knee arthroplasty for non-oncologic indications. *Arthroplast. Today* **2020**, *6*, 23–35. [CrossRef]
26. Biau, D.; Faure, F.; Katsahian, S.; Jeanrot, C.; Tomeno, B.; Anract, P. Survival of total knee replacement with a megaprosthesis after bone tumor resection. *J. Bone Jt. Surg. Am.* **2006**, *88*, 1285–1293. [CrossRef]
27. Myers, G.J.; Abudu, A.T.; Carter, S.R.; Tillman, R.M.; Grimer, R.J. The long-term results of endoprosthetic replacement of the proximal tibia for bone tumours. *J. Bone Jt. Surg. Br.* **2007**, *89*, 1632–1637. [CrossRef]
28. Buchner, M.; Zeifang, F.; Bernd, L. Medial gastrocnemius muscle flap in limb-sparing surgery of malignant bone tumors of the proximal tibia: Mid-term results in 25 patients. *Ann. Plast. Surg.* **2003**, *51*, 266–272. [CrossRef] [PubMed]
29. Guo, W.; Ji, T.; Yang, R.; Tang, X.; Yang, Y. Endoprosthetic replacement for primary tumours around the knee: Experience from Peking University. *J. Bone Jt. Surg. Br.* **2008**, *90*, 1084–1089. [CrossRef]
30. Burnett, R.S.; Kelly, M.A.; Hanssen, A.D.; Barrack, R.L. Technique and timing of two-stage exchange for infection in TKA. *Clin. Orthop. Relat. Res.* **2007**, *464*, 164–178. [CrossRef]
31. Winkler, T.; Stuhlert, M.G.W.; Lieb, E.; Müller, M.; von Roth, P.; Preininger, B.; Trampuz, A.; Perka, C.F. Outcome of short versus long interval in two-stage exchange for periprosthetic joint infection: A prospective cohort study. *Arch. Orthop. Trauma Surg.* **2019**, *139*, 295–303. [CrossRef]

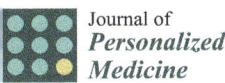 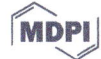

Article

Comparison of Postoperative Coronal Leg Alignment in Customized Individually Made and Conventional Total Knee Arthroplasty

Felix Wunderlich [1,*], Maheen Azad [2], Ruben Westphal [3], Thomas Klonschinski [1], Patrick Belikan [1], Philipp Drees [1] and Lukas Eckhard [1]

[1] Department of Orthopedics and Traumatology, University Medical Center of the Johannes Gutenberg University Mainz, 55131 Mainz, Germany; thomas.klonschinski@unimedizin-mainz.de (T.K.); patrick.belikan@unimedizin-mainz.de (P.B.); philipp.drees@unimedizin-mainz.de (P.D.); lukas.eckhard@unimedizin-mainz.de (L.E.)

[2] Clinic for Traumatology and Orthopedics, Heilig-Geist-Hospital Bingen, 55411 Bingen, Germany; maheen.azad@marienhaus.de

[3] Institute of Medical Biostatistics, Epidemiology and Informatics, University Medical Center of the Johannes Gutenberg University Mainz, 55131 Mainz, Germany; ruben.westphal@unimedizin-mainz.de

* Correspondence: felix.wunderlich@unimedizin-mainz.de; Tel.: +49-6131-177302

Abstract: Neutral coronal leg alignment is known to be important for postoperative outcome in total knee arthroplasty (TKA). Customized individually made implants (CIM) instrumented with patient-specific cutting guides are an innovation aiming to increase the precision and reliability of implant positioning and reconstruction of leg alignment. We aimed to compare reconstruction of the hip–knee–ankle angle (HKA) of the novel CIM system iTotal™ CR G2 (ConforMIS Inc.) to a matched cohort of the off-the-shelf (OTS) knee replacement system Vanguard™ CR (Zimmer Biomet). Retrospective analysis of postoperative coronal full-leg weight-bearing radiographs of 562 TKA (283 CIM TKA, 279 OTS TKA) was conducted. Via a medical planning software, HKA and rotation of the leg were measured in postoperative radiographs. HKA was then adjusted for rotational error, and 180° ± 3° varus/valgus was defined as the target zone HKA. Corrected postoperative HKA in the CIM group was 179.0° ± 2.8° and 179.2° ± 3.1° in the OTS group ($p = 0.34$). The rate of outliers, outside of the ±3° target zone, was equal in both groups (32.9%). Our analysis showed that TKA using patient-specific cutting guides and implants and OTS TKA implanted with conventional instrumentation resulted in equally satisfying restoration of the coronal leg alignment with less scattering in the CIM group.

Keywords: total knee arthroplasty; leg alignment; patient-specific instruments; custom-made implant; rotational correction

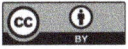

1. Introduction

Total knee arthroplasty is a common and reliable procedure for successfully treating end-stage osteoarthritis (OA) of the knee. Although continued development of implant design, surgical technique, and postoperative follow-up treatment has improved the overall outcome of the procedure, there is still a noticeable number of patients who remain partially unsatisfied after TKA [1]. Amongst other factors, correct fitting and position of the TKA components with consecutive restoration of the axial alignment and mechanical axis of the limb lead to a good postoperative outcome and longer implant survival [2–5]. To maximize the capabilities of TKA regarding these factors, patient-specific customized implants have been developed in the recent past [6,7]. One of these implants is the patient-specific cruciate retaining knee replacement system iTotal™ CR G2 with custom-made implants and instruments, using computer-aided design and manufacturing (CAD/CAM) based on computed tomography (CT) scans of the patients' leg. The goal of this implant is to restore a neutral postoperative mechanical axis, reduce bone resection, and optimize component fit. Previously published results are promising [8,9], although studies comparing CIM TKA to off-the-shelf implants implanted using conventional instrumentation are scarce, while most existing studies focus on patient-specific instrumentation rather than patient-specific implants. We therefore aimed to compare restoration of the hip–knee–ankle angle of the novel patient-specific knee replacement system iTotal CR G2 (ConforMIS Inc.; Burlington, MA, USA) to a matched cohort of the traditional knee replacement system Vanguard™ CR (Zimmer Biomet; Warsaw, IN, USA).

2. Materials and Methods

In total, 562 patients undergoing TKA (right: 235; left: 205; bilateral: 122) were included in the retrospective analysis with a distribution of 283 patient-specific knee replacement systems, iTotal™ CR G2, and a matched cohort of 279 traditional knee replacement systems, Vanguard™ CR. Both products match the country product clearances for Germany and are approved by the United States Food and Drug Administration (FDA).

All surgeries were conducted from 2015 to 2020 by the endoprosthetics team of the Department of Orthopedics and Traumatology of the University Medical Center of the Johannes Gutenberg University, containing four primary surgeons. Indication for TKA was end-stage primary or posttraumatic OA of the knee with no signs of ligamentous instability. Patients with varus or valgus deformity >15° were excluded due to eligibility criteria of the implants. For preoperative planning, all patients received coronal full-leg weight-bearing radiographs as well as antero-posterior lateral, and patella tangential conventional radiographs of the affected knee. Planning of the OTS Vanguard™ CR system was conducted via the mediCAD 2D Knee planning software (mediCAD Hectec GmbH, Altdorf, BY, Germany). In the case of a planned implantation of the iTotal™ CR G2 system, a CT-scan of the affected leg was conducted with a standard protocol and the CIM was designed and manufactured using the iFit software algorithm and 3D CAD/CAM technology as previously described by Arnholdt et al. [8]. We used a standard midline incision and medial parapatellar capsulotomy in all patients, adding local infiltration analgesia containing ropivacaine and adrenalin as well as i.v. and intraarticular tranexamic acid at the end of each surgery. No tourniquet or drainage was used. Postoperative radiological control of implant fit and leg axis was conducted via ap and lateral knee radiographs and coronal full-leg weight-bearing radiographs as soon as the patient was able to walk stairs and a full extension of the operated knee was possible.

Radiographic analysis of the postoperative coronal leg alignment was executed using the mediCAD 2D planning software on postoperative coronal full-leg weight-bearing radiographs. The radiographs were first checked for eligibility according to the following quality criteria: missing postoperative pictures, minor quality with incomplete imaging of the operated leg or poor image quality, and excessive rotational error. For determination of the leg axis, the HKA was measured using the angle between the mechanical axis of the femur (FMA) and tibia (TMA) (Figure 1). The operation aimed to restore a neutral mechanical alignment (180° ± 3° varus/valgus). For further improvement of the measurement accuracy, we calculated rotational correction for the measured HKA using the formula published by Maderbacher et al. in 2014 and 2021 [10,11], which is based on the proximal tibio-fibular overlap in long leg radiographs measured via the mediCAD 2D planning software (Figure 2).

Microsoft Excel 2007 (Microsoft Corporation, Redmond, USA) was used for descriptive analysis (mean ± standard deviation). R version 4.0.2 with ggplot2 version 3.3.3 was used to create histograms and for all hypothesis tests. Group mean angles were compared with two-sided Welch two-sample t-tests for equality of means, and group proportions were compared using chi-squared tests for equal proportions. For all statistical analyses, single knees were treated as independent observations.

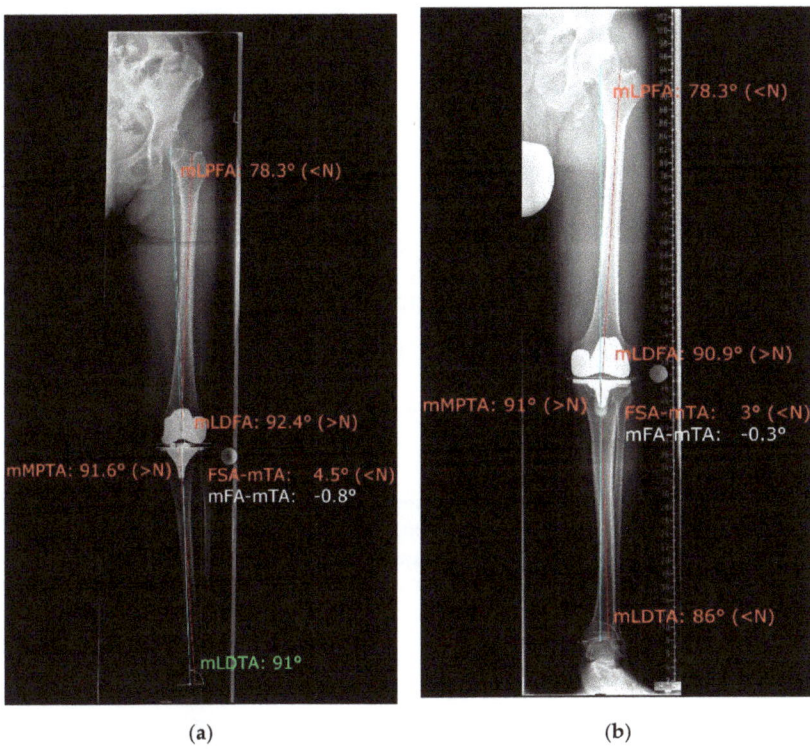

Figure 1. Measuring the HKA angle in mediCAD 2D planning software (**a**) iTotal CR G2 patient specific implant; (**b**) Vanguard CR conventional implant.

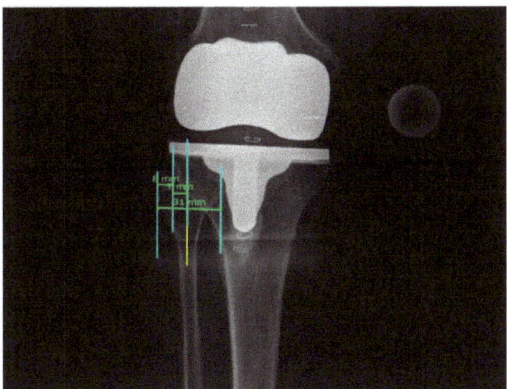

Figure 2. Detail of rotational analysis of a full-leg weight-bearing radiograph using the proximal tibio-fibular overlap.

3. Results

All 562 postoperative full-leg weight-bearing radiographs could be included in the analysis according to the above-mentioned quality criteria. Mean age at time of surgery in the CIM group was 69.4 ± 10.31 years (range 24–89 years) with a gender distribution of 149 male and 134 female patients. Mean age at time of surgery in the OTS group was 71.7 ± 10.43 years (range 35–92 years) with a gender distribution of 105 male and 174 female patients. In all, 8.5% (24/283) and 5.3% (15/279) of patients had prior surgery on the affected knee in the CIM and OTS group, respectively. Baseline characteristics are shown in Table 1.

Table 1. Baseline characteristics.

Variable	CIM (iTotal CR G2)	OTS (Vanguard CR)
Age (years) (mean (SD))	69.5 (10.3)	71.7 (10.4)
Gender		
male	149	105
female	134	174
Side of Surgery		
left	90	115
right	108	127
both	85	37
Previous operation on affected leg (%)	24 (8.5%)	15 (5.3%)

3.1. Rotational Correction

Calculated rotation in coronal full-leg weight-bearing radiographs in the CIM group ranged from $-32.05°$ internal to $22.57°$ external rotation of the leg (mean $-3.56°$, SD $9.65°$). Rotation in the OTS group ranged from $-1.51°$ to $23.49°$ (mean $-5.29°$, SD $9.10°$). Derived correctional factors for HKA ranged from $-2.23°$ varus to $1.57°$ valgus correction (mean $-0.25°$, SD $0.67°$) in the CIM, and $-2.20°$ to $1.64°$ correction (mean $-0.37°$, SD $0.63°$) in the OTS group, respectively.

3.2. Coronal Alignment

The postoperative radiologically measured corrected and uncorrected HKAs with SD in all 562 patients who underwent TKA are displayed in Table 2.

Table 2. Postoperative uncorrected and corrected mean HKA ± SD after iTotal™ CR G2 and Vanguard™ CR implantation.

	iTotal™ CR G2 (n = 283)	Vanguard™ CR (n = 279)
HKA uncorrected	179.2° ± 2.9°	179.6° ± 3.1°
HKA corrected	179.0° ± 2.8°	179.2° ± 3.1°

Maximum varus and valgus HKAs were 171.2° (171.2° corrected) and 190.1° (189.2° corrected) in the OTS group and 168.6° (169.3° corrected) and 187.7° (188.21° corrected) in the CIM group, respectively. The distribution of corrected HKAs in both groups is shown in Figure 3. Outliers, outside the $180° \pm 3°$ target zone, were 32.9% in both implant groups (93/283 CIM group; 92/279 OTS group) with a trend toward varus alignment in both groups (CIM group: 71/283 varus; OTS group: 62/279 varus).

The Welch two-sample test for mean corrected HKA between both groups showed no significance, with $p = 0.34$. Further analysis for corrected HKA range $+/-1°$ and $+/-3°$ degrees showed no significant differences between the OTS and CIM group, with p-values $p = 0.56$ and $p = 1.00$, respectively.

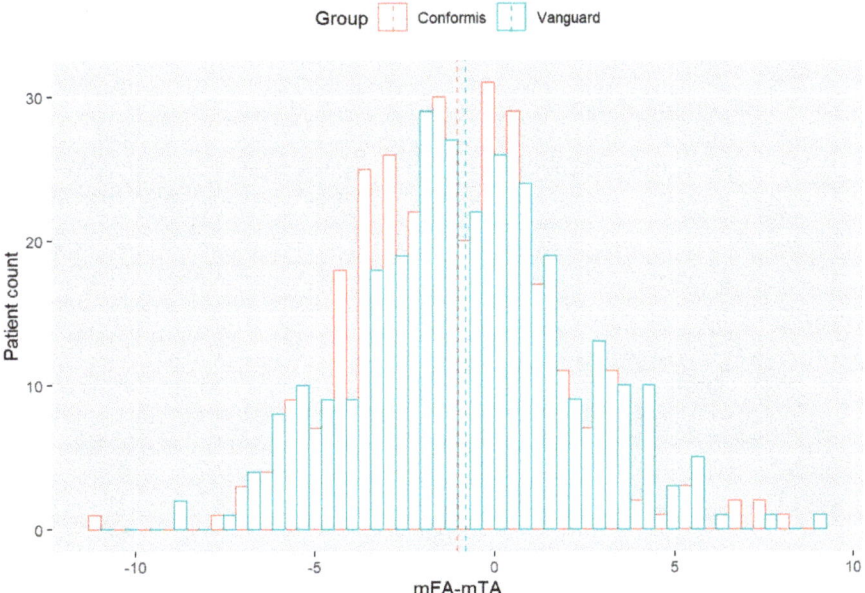

Figure 3. Distribution of corrected postoperative HKA angle in CIM (ConforMIS) and OTS (Vanguard) groups (0 on x-axis corresponds to 180°, dotted lines indicate group mean).

4. Discussion

In this study, analysis of the up-to-now largest cohort of postoperative coronal leg alignment after implantation of CIM TKA using patient-specific cutting guides and OTS TKA implanted with conventional instrumentation showed equally satisfying results in restoring the HKA angle toward neutral alignment.

To improve surgical technique toward better postoperative leg alignment, computer-aided surgery as well as patient-specific instruments and implants have been developed, especially while conventional techniques using intramedullary guides show high liability to failure due to anatomic variability or surgical error [12]. Although there were no significant differences between leg alignments in both of our groups, we noticed a lower scattering range of leg axis in the CIM group. The rate of outliers in both groups (32.9% with more than ± 3° deviation) was in line with the rates described in other studies [13–16]. As postoperative leg malalignment and malpositioning of the implant are known to have a high impact on overall outcome and survivorship of TKA [3,13], it is of paramount interest to restore these entities precisely. Whilst computer-aided surgery proved to be superior in restoring leg axis than conventional techniques [17], patient-specific instruments such as cutting guides showed no improvement [18]. Even though patient-specific surgery in TKA is relatively well studied, comparison of CIM and OTS implants and their restoration of leg axis is scarce. Arbab et al. [9] showed no significant difference in pre- and postoperative leg axis change between conventional and patient-specific implants but noticed a trend toward fewer outliers in their CIM group. Steinert et al. [8] detected proper fitting and positioning of the patient-specific implant and a good restoration of leg axis toward neutral alignment. In both studies, coronal full-leg weight-bearing radiographs were used to determine the postoperative leg axis. Because of its complex provision and high liability to failure especially in malrotation [19,20], this radiograph shows a high variability in its reproducibility and therefore in determination of the leg axis. Further, weight-bearing full-leg radiographs are costly and expose the patient's pelvis to ionizing radiation, which makes correct analysis of the radiographs even more important to reduce recurrent imaging.

Various studies have shown alternatives for measuring the long leg axis, but long limb radiographs remain the gold standard [9,20,21]. To further exceed the analyzability of these radiographs, Maderbacher et al. [10,11] published a formula to predict knee rotation via tibio-fibular overlap and to calculate the influence of rotation on the measured alignment parameters. However, this method is limited by the uncertainty of knee flexion during the radiograph, which is common in the early postoperative long-leg radiograph due to painful or mechanical extension deficits. Nevertheless, surgeons should be aware of this method when regularly assessing postoperative long leg radiographs after TKA to prevent incorrect measurement.

The strengths of this study are that it is the largest analysis of custom TKA implants on leg axis and that it considers the rotation in all radiographs as well as its influence on coronal leg alignment. However, we did not take a possible extension deficit after surgery into account. Although full extension of the operated knee was a benchmark for postoperative long leg radiograph in our setting, a bias due to flexion of the knee during X-ray cannot be excluded. Furthermore, due to the retrospective nature of this comparative analysis, a bias for implant selection cannot be excluded. Lastly, we only assessed the ConforMIS iTotal™ CR G2 CIM, and our findings might not be transferable to other patient-specific customized implants.

5. Conclusions

TKA using patient-specific cutting guides and implants and OTS TKA implanted with conventional instrumentation resulted in equally satisfying restoration of the coronal leg alignment. When using coronal full-leg weight-bearing radiographs to assess the postoperative leg axis, the modifiers through rotational correction should be taken into account.

Author Contributions: All authors contributed to the study conception and design. F.W., M.A., R.W., P.B. and L.E. performed data collection, radiographic analysis, graphics production, and statistical analysis. The first draft of the manuscript was written by F.W., and all authors commented on previous versions of the manuscript. All authors have read and agreed to the published version of the manuscript.

Funding: This publication was supported by the Open Access Publication Fund of the University Medical Center of the Johannes Gutenberg University Mainz.

Institutional Review Board Statement: Not applicable.

Informed Consent Statement: Not applicable.

Data Availability Statement: The datasets used and/or analyzed during the current study are available from the corresponding author on reasonable request.

Acknowledgments: Data used in this study were derived from the doctoral thesis of M.A.

Conflicts of Interest: The authors declare no conflict of interest.

References

1. Bourne, R.B.; Chesworth, B.M.; Davis, A.M.; Mahomed, N.N.; Charron, K.D.J. Patient Satisfaction after Total Knee Arthroplasty: Who is Satisfied and Who is Not? *Clin. Orthop. Relat. Res.* **2010**, *468*, 57–63. [CrossRef] [PubMed]
2. Jeffery, R.S.; Morris, R.W.; A Denham, R. Coronal alignment after total knee replacement. *J. Bone Jt. Surg. Ser. B* **1991**, *73*, 709–714. [CrossRef] [PubMed]
3. Sikorski, J.M. Alignment in total knee replacement. *J. Bone Jt. Surgery. Br. Vol.* **2008**, *90*, 1121–1127. [CrossRef]
4. Sharkey, P.F.; Lichstein, P.M.; Shen, C.; Tokarski, A.T.; Parvizi, J. Why Are Total Knee Arthroplasties Failing Today—Has Anything Changed After 10 Years? *J. Arthroplast.* **2014**, *29*, 1774–1778. [CrossRef]
5. Collier, M.B.; Engh, C.A.; McAuley, J.P.; Engh, G.A. Factors associated with the loss of thickness of polyethylene tibial bearings after knee arthroplasty. *J. Bone Jt. Surg.Ser. A* **2007**, *89*, 1306–1314. [CrossRef]
6. Steinert, A.F.; Sefrin, L.; Jansen, B.; Schroder, L.; Horzapfel, B.M.; Arnholdt, J.; Rudert, M. Patient-specific cruciate-retaining total knee replacement with individualized implants and instruments (iTotalTM CR G2). *Oper. Orthop. Traumatol.* **2021**, *33*, 170–180. [CrossRef]

7. Schwechter, E.M.; Fitz, W. Design rationale for customized TKA: A new idea or revisiting the past? *Curr. Rev. Musculoskelet. Med.* **2012**, *5*, 303–308. [CrossRef]
8. Arnholdt, J.; Kamawal, Y.; Horas, K.; Holzapfel, B.M.; Gilbert, F.; Ripp, A.; Rudert, M.; Steinert, A.F. Accurate implant fit and leg alignment after cruciate-retaining patient-specific total knee arthroplasty. *BMC Musculoskelet. Disord.* **2020**, *21*, 1–8. [CrossRef]
9. Arbab, D.; Reimann, P.; Brucker, M.; Bouillon, B.; Lüring, C. Alignment in total knee arthroplasty—A comparison of patient-specific implants with the conventional technique. *Knee* **2018**, *25*, 882–887. [CrossRef]
10. Maderbacher, G.; Schaumburger, J.; Baier, C.; Zeman, F.; Springorum, H.-R.; Dornia, C.; Grifka, J.; Keshmiri, A. Predicting knee rotation by the projection overlap of the proximal fibula and tibia in long-leg radiographs. *Knee Surgery, Sports Traumatol. Arthrosc.* **2014**, *22*, 2982–2988. [CrossRef] [PubMed]
11. Maderbacher, G.; Matussek, J.; Greimel, F.; Grifka, J.; Schaumburger, J.; Baier, C.; Keshmiri, A. Lower Limb Malrotation Is Regularly Present in Long-Leg Radiographs Resulting in Significant Measurement Errors. *J. Knee Surg.* **2021**, *34*, 108–114. [CrossRef] [PubMed]
12. Reed, S.C.; Gollish, J. The accuracy of femoral intramedullary guides in total knee arthroplasty. *J. Arthroplast.* **1997**, *12*, 677–682. [CrossRef]
13. Chauhan, S.K.; Scott, R.G.; Breidahl, W. Computer-assisted knee arthroplasty versus a conventional jig-based technique. A randomised, prospective trial. *J. Bone Jt. Surg. Ser. B* **2004**, *86*, 372–377. [CrossRef] [PubMed]
14. Hart, R.; Janecek, M.; Chaker, A. Total knee arthroplasty implanted with and without kinematic navigation. *Int. Orthop.* **2003**, *27*, 366–369. [CrossRef]
15. Matsumoto, T.; Tsumura, N.; Kurosaka, M.; Muratsu, H.; Kuroda, R.; Ishimoto, K.; Tsujimoto, K.; Shiba, R. Prosthetic alignment and sizing in computer-assisted total knee arthroplasty. *Int. Orthop.* **2004**, *28*, 282–285. [CrossRef]
16. Noriega-Fernandez, A.; Hernández-Vaquero, D.; Suarez-Vazquez, A.; Sandoval-Garcia, M.A. Computer Assistance Increases Precision of Component Placement in Total Knee Arthroplasty with Articular Deformity. *Clin. Orthop. Relat. Res.* **2010**, *468*, 1237–1241.
17. Bäthis, H.; Perlick, L.; Tingart, M.; Lüring, C.; Zurakowski, D.; Grifka, J. Alignment in total knee arthroplasty. A comparison of computer-assisted surgery with the conventional technique. *J. Bone Jt. Surg. Ser. B* **2004**, *86*, 682–687. [CrossRef]
18. Nam, D.; Park, A.; Stambough, J.B.; Johnson, S.R.; Nunley, R.M.; Barrack, R.L. The Mark Coventry Award: Custom Cutting Guides Do Not Improve Total Knee Arthroplasty Clinical Outcomes at 2 Years Followup. *Clin. Orthop. Relat. Res.* **2016**, *474*, 40–46. [CrossRef]
19. Lonner, J.H.; Laird, M.T.; Stuchin, S.A. Effect of Rotation and Knee Flexion on Radiographic Alignment in Total Knee Arthroplasties. *Clin. Orthop. Relat. Res.* **1996**, *331*, 102–106. [CrossRef]
20. Maderbacher, G.; Baier, C.; Benditz, A.; Wagner, F.; Greimel, F.; Grifka, J.; Keshmiri, A. Presence of rotational errors in long leg radiographs after total knee arthroplasty and impact on measured lower limb and component alignment. *Int. Orthop.* **2017**, *41*, 1553–1560. [CrossRef]
21. Hinman, R.S.; May, R.L.; Crossley, K.M. Is There an Alternative to the Full-Leg Radiograph for Determining Knee Joint Alignment in Osteoarthritis? *Arthritis Care Res.* **2006**, *55*, 306–313. [CrossRef] [PubMed]

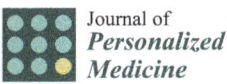

Article

Automatic Hip Detection in Anteroposterior Pelvic Radiographs—A Labelless Practical Framework

Feng-Yu Liu [1,†], Chih-Chi Chen [2,†], Chi-Tung Cheng [3,4], Cheng-Ta Wu [5], Chih-Po Hsu [3], Chih-Yuan Fu [3], Shann-Ching Chen [1,*], Chien-Hung Liao [3,4,*] and Mel S. Lee [5]

1. Compal Electronics, Smart Device Business Group, Taipei 114, Taiwan; ryk_liu@compal.com
2. Department of Physical Medicine and Rehabilitation, Chang Gung Memorial Hospital, Chang Gung University, Linkou, Taoyuan 333, Taiwan; claudia5477@gmail.com
3. Department of Trauma and Emergency Surgery, Chang Gung Memorial Hospital, Chang Gung University, Linkou, Taoyuan 333, Taiwan; atong89130@gmail.com (C.-T.C.); m7831@cgmh.org.tw (C.-P.H.); drfu5564@yahoo.com.tw (C.-Y.F.)
4. Center for Artificial Intelligence in Medicine, Chang Gung Memorial Hospital, Linkou, Taoyuan 333, Taiwan
5. Department of Orthopedic Surgery, Kaohsiung Chang Gung Memorial Hospital, Kaohsiung 833, Taiwan; oliverwu429@cgmh.org.tw (C.-T.W.); mellee@cgmh.org.tw (M.S.L.)
* Correspondence: ShannC_Chen@compal.com (S.-C.C.); surgymet@gmail.com (C.-H.L.)
† Feng-Yu Liu and Chih-Chi Chen contributed equally to this manuscript.

Abstract: Automated detection of the region of interest (ROI) is a critical step in the two-step classification system in several medical image applications. However, key information such as model parameter selection, image annotation rules, and ROI confidence score are essential but usually not reported. In this study, we proposed a practical framework of ROI detection by analyzing hip joints seen on 7399 anteroposterior pelvic radiographs (PXR) from three diverse sources. We presented a deep learning-based ROI detection framework utilizing a single-shot multi-box detector with a customized head structure based on the characteristics of the obtained datasets. Our method achieved average intersection over union (IoU) = 0.8115, average confidence = 0.9812, and average precision with threshold IoU = 0.5 (AP50) = 0.9901 in the independent testing set, suggesting that the detected hip regions appropriately covered the main features of the hip joints. The proposed approach featured flexible loose-fitting labeling, customized model design, and heterogeneous data testing. We demonstrated the feasibility of training a robust hip region detector for PXRs. This practical framework has a promising potential for a wide range of medical image applications.

Keywords: deep learning; hip detection; deep convolutional neural network; radiography

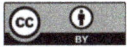

1. Introduction

The deep convolutional neural network (DCNN) has shown a significant breakthrough in many aspects of commercial image differentiation and identification. In recent years, DCNNs have also played important roles in medical image analysis [1,2]. For example, the ChestX-ray8 [3] and MURA [4] are two representative studies utilizing the state-of-the-art DCNN classification and visualization models to detect and locate disease patterns in the chest and musculoskeletal radiographs.

Some studies employ a more delicate "two-step" classification strategy, which first detects specific ROIs [5–9], followed by conventional classification methods [10–12]. A seminal work is the automatic knee osteoarthritis diagnosis in lateral knee radiographs, where knee regions are first identified [13], followed by classification and heatmap visualization [14]. The advantage of this "two-step" approach is the capability to identify subtle localized abnormalities and has gradually become the mainstream technology, especially for the analysis of PXRs, including fracture subclass identification [15], hip osteoarthritis grading [16], and avascular necrosis detection [17]. Nonetheless, the above studies barely mentioned the model parameter settings and selection criteria, and none of them reported the confidence score for the detected ROIs, which the confidence score is a crucial metric indicating the likelihood that the predicated ROI contains the correct object.

A critical component for a successful "two-step" classification system is accurate ROI detection, which falls into computer vision object detection tasks [18], usually tackled by different strategies [19]. Among these methods, the bounding-box-based methodology is advantageous for its lower annotation workload and simple implementation, which is proven to be effective in popular computer vision applications in other sectors. In order to identify multiple objects across different scales in one image, one must generate anchor boxes of varied sizes and aspect ratios for hyper-parameter optimization. However, there is usually a small number of non-overlapping objects in medical images. It is not optimal to apply the same object detection parameters on different underlying applications.

In this work, we propose a labor-less practical framework of ROI detection and parameter selection in medical images. To the best of our knowledge, this is the first work that provides a systematic guideline for parameter selection based on the obtained datasets and has a promising potential for a wide range of medical image applications for further personalized medicine.

2. Materials and Methods

2.1. Dataset Acquisition

This retrospective study analyzed hip joints seen on 7399 PXRs from three diverse sources, including the Chang Gung Memorial Hospital Osteoarthritis (CGOA) dataset containing 4290 high-resolution radiographs, the second Osteoarthritis Initiative Hip (OAIH, pelvic radiograph dataset extracted from a subset of data from the OAI [20]) dataset containing 3008 radiographs with relatively lower resolutions, and the third Google Image Search (GIS) dataset containing 101 heterogeneous radiographs. Table 1 lists the summary statistics of these datasets. This experimental design, which utilizes radiographs generated from diverse sources of different imaging protocols, resolutions, and ethnicities, ensures that model generalization can be achieved. Details of these three datasets can be found in Table 1.

Table 1. Summary statistics of the three datasets used in this study.

Datasets	Number of Images	Max (Pixels)	Min (Pixels)	Median (Pixels)	Mean (Pixels)	Standard Deviation	Recruit Year
CGOA	4290	4280	1616	2688	2635.8	201.1	2008–2017
OAIH	3008	1080	466	535	571.3	97.0	2004–2014
GIS	101	4256	225	258	515.3	626.6	N/A

2.2. Data Annotation

Figure 1 shows the overview of the proposed framework.

Clinical readings on etiology and grading of all CGOA images were performed by one physician with 15 years of clinical experience. To annotate hip regions of interest, we employed three annotators trained to place square bounding boxes approximately centered at the femoral head or the artificial hip joint with customized GUI software. It is noted that identifying a complete round femoral head in healthy hips is relatively straightforward; however, for cases with disrupted hip conditions with collapsed femoral heads, we employed a loose-fitting manner to make sure every hip joint lay appropriately in the bounding box. All the labeled ROIs in the CGOA dataset were visually reviewed by physicians, and the ROI annotators used the same rules to annotate the remaining OAIH and GIS datasets.

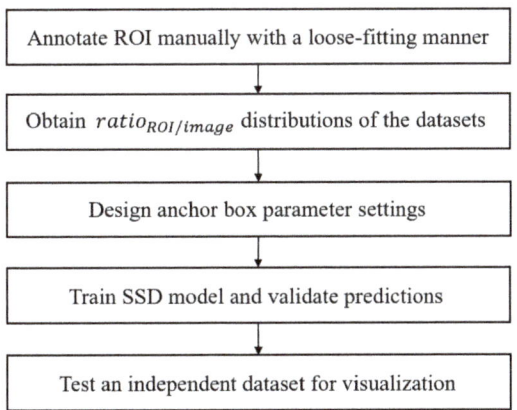

Figure 1. Overview of the proposed framework for hip ROI detection.

2.3. Proposed SSD Model Architecture for ROI Detection in Hip Radiographs

The proposed hip region detection architecture simplifies existing SSD model architecture (as Figure 2) [9], which was originally developed for detecting multiple objects with different sizes and aspect ratios in applications.

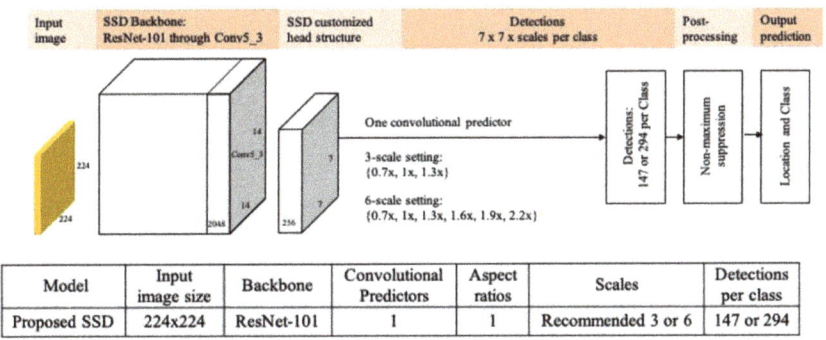

Model	Input image size	Backbone	Convolutional Predictors	Aspect ratios	Scales	Detections per class
Proposed SSD	224x224	ResNet-101	1	1	Recommended 3 or 6	147 or 294

Figure 2. Comparison of SSD model architectures. Proposed architecture with ResNet-101 backbone and other customized settings.

For ROI detection in medical images, we replaced the SSD VGG-16 backbone by ResNet-101 [11] backbone, which was pre-trained on ImageNet [21]. All these modifications could reduce ROI detections from several thousands to a few hundreds, decreasing training time and complexity as well as increasing detection accuracy and confidence.

To best determine the anchor box parameter settings, we first defined the size of the square ROI divided by the length of the long side of the input image (zero padding to a square if needed). This ratio is designed as a normalizer, making the anchor boxes and ROI instances compatible across different datasets. Next, we analyzed image size distributions (Figure 3A) and distributions (Figure 3B) of the three available heterogeneous datasets, where the ratios lie mostly between 10% to 30%.

We specified the input image size of 224×224 pixels split by 7×7 grid cells, where each grid cell is of size 32×32 pixels. We set 6 equally spaced scales parameters {0.7, 1.0, 1.3, 1.6, 1.9, 2.2} (Figure 3C) so that the smallest and largest anchor boxes could cover 10% and 31.4% of the images, respectively. This design ensures that the designed anchor boxes can identify appropriate hip ROIs in the datasets.

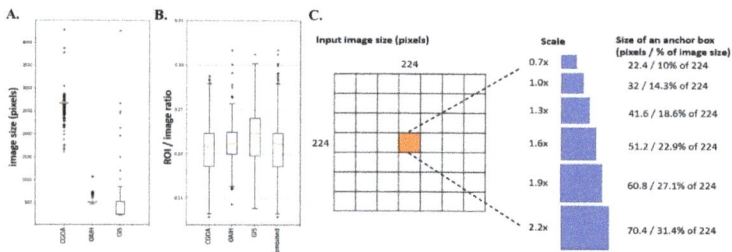

Figure 3. Comparison of three radiographic dataset distributions and generation of anchor boxes. (**A**) The image size distributions of the three datasets. (**B**) The distributions of three datasets. (**C**) Generation of anchor boxes for the one feature layer of the customized SSD head structure. With an input square image with 224 × 224 pixels, there are 7 × 7 grid cells with 32 × 32 pixels with scale = 1, and each grid cell can use different scale parameters to generate various sizes of anchor boxes covering 10% to 31.4% of the input image size, depending on the training image size distributions.

2.4. Data Preprocessing, Training, and Evaluation

For data preprocessing, each radiograph was zero padding to a square image and resized to 224 × 224 pixels with 8-bit grayscale before feeding into the model. The model was implemented by fastai v0.7 library [22] with Python 3.6.4, and we randomly split the combined CGOA and OAIH dataset into 90% for training and 10% for validation once, and used all 101 GIS radiographs as the independent test dataset. We fixed the same training and validation images in either the combined dataset or each individual dataset in all experiments for fair comparison. For evaluation, we used the standard IoU metric for comparing the predicted bounding box B_{pred} and ground truth bounding box B_{gt}:

$$IoU = \frac{B_{pred} \cap B_{gt}}{B_{pred} \cup B_{gt}}$$

where ∩ and ∪ denote intersection and union, respectively. We reported the associated confidence, which denotes the likelihood that the anchor box contains an object, for each predicted bounding box, average IoU, average confidence, minimal confidence, and AP50, as the 0.5 cutoff indicates poor ROI detection, which may cause issues for downstream analysis.

3. Results

3.1. Demographics of the Study Population

The original CGOA cohort contained 4643 high resolution radiographs, including 3013 patients who underwent hip surgery with an average age of 63.06 ± 15.72 years and 40.8% being male, and 1630 control cases from emergency room without undergoing hip surgery with an average age of 44.88 ± 20.46 years and 68.2% being male. Among the 3013 surgical patients, 353 cases with severe fractures were excluded due to completely different morphology and treatment options. The remaining 2660 trauma patients including hundreds of occult fracture cases and 1630 control cases constructed the COGA dataset. The second OAIH dataset was a consolidated pelvic radiograph dataset extracted from subset of data from the OAI project, which recruited 4796 participants from February 2004 to May 2006 to form a baseline cohort (58% female and ranged in age from 45 to 79 years at time of recruitment). The third GIS dataset was acquired through Google image search engine, and the demographics are not available.

3.2. Model Performance and Visualization

In Table 2, we take a closer look at the best performance results and carefully examine those cases where hip ROIs had IoU < 0.5. As AP50 metrics were 1 in both training and validation set and 0.9901 in the independent GIS test set, we only identified two cases below IoU 0.5 cutoff, which may indicate poor ROI detection and cause issues for downstream analysis.

Table 2. Detailed performance metrics with the optimal parameters using the proposed hip region detection architecture.

Datasets	Number of Images	Number of Hip ROIs	Avg IoU	Avg Confidence	Minimal IoU	Number of Hip ROIs with IoU < 0.5	AP50
All: CGOA & OAIH & GIS	7399	14,798	0.9176	0.9688	0.3861	2	0.9999
Train: 90% CGOA & OAIH	6568	13,136	0.9260	0.9698	0.5955	0	1
Valid: 10% CGOA & OAIH	730	1460	0.8571	0.9582	0.5907	0	1
Test: GIS	101	202	0.8115	0.9812	0.3861	2	0.9901

We further examined other radiographs in the heterogeneous test set, and the hip ROI detection showed several representative results, as Figure 4 presents. Figure 4A shows a radiograph with some text outside the key hip area. Figure 4B shows the dislocation on the left hip, but the detected hip ROI covers most key features of the left hip. Figure 4C shows a radiograph with plates on the left pubic ramus and acetabulum, and ROI can detect the hips correctly. Figure 4D shows a radiograph with pediatric patients. Figure 4E shows left hip artificial can be detected correctly. Figure 4F hip ROI indicated right proximal femoral fracture. Figure 4G shows right temporal cemented prosthesis fracture and left total hip replacement, and the hip ROI can be detected. Finally, as shown in Figure 4H, the hip ROI was able to detect right acetabular fracture with plate fixation and destructed femoral head. These results suggest that our model with specially designed anchors and trained by diverse datasets is a general and robust hip region detector that can be applicable for a wide range of heterogeneous datasets with different qualities and resolutions and can be potentially useful for automated assessment of many hip bone conditions.

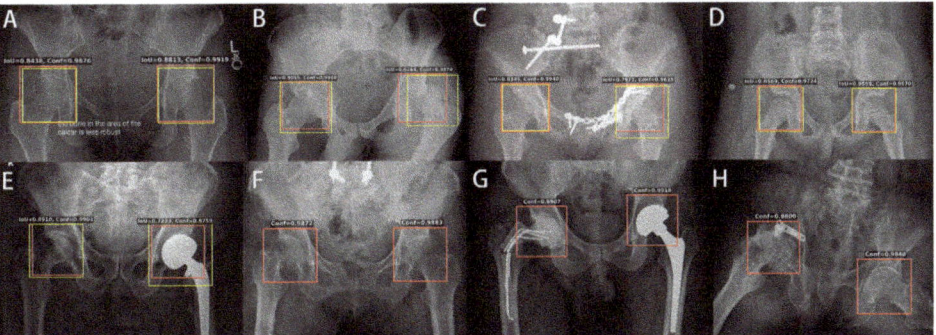

Figure 4. Visualization of hip ROI detection results on the testing dataset. Yellow boxes indicate manual labels, and red boxes indicate detected hip ROIs. In all scenarios, the ROI could be detected well in both hips. (**A**) A radiograph with some text outside the key hip area. (**B**) A radiograph with left hip dislocation. (**C**) A radiograph with plates on the left pubic ramus and acetabulum. The hips were detected correctly. (**D**) A radiograph of pediatric patients. (**E**) A radiograph showing left hip replacement and deformity of the right hip. (**F**) Right proximal femoral fracture. (**G**) The right hip showing a fracture of a temporal cemented prosthesis and left total hip replacement. (**H**) Right acetabular fixation with plate with destructed femoral head.

4. Discussion

In this work, we have demonstrated a practical framework for detecting regions of interest in medical images. With the case study for hip detection in PXRs, we achieved average IoU over 80% and average confidence higher than 95%. These independent test set showed promising ROI detection results on GIS with heterogeneous resolutions and appearance. The proposed hip region detection architecture simplified existing SSD model architecture, which was originally developed for detecting multiple objects with different sizes and aspect ratios in applications. For ROI detection in medical images, there are usually one or two important organs in one radiograph. It is feasible to have a simplified SSD architecture with only one feature layer as the only convolutional predictor, with an appropriate receptive field size, one aspect ratio (1:1 in for hip ROI), and a small set of scales.

Compared to traditional object detection tasks, which need to recognize multiple objects with different sizes and aspect ratios in images and videos, the proposed SSD architecture has the advantages of simpler structure, higher IoU accuracy, and reliable confidence. The challenge of determining those empirical parameter settings now relies on the basic statistics on the available datasets to generate enough anchor boxes. Our results suggest that more anchors do not necessarily encourage higher IoU but may decrease the prediction performance. The proposed method provides a more effective approach for anchor design and parameter optimization.

Annotation by doctors is time-consuming and is usually the bottleneck for medical image analysis. The approximate identification of hip regions by automated and accurate ROI detection is critical for automated computer-assisted analysis for screening and diagnostics. The proposed framework provides a guideline for parameter settings in anchor-based object detection algorithms, and it is especially useful for applications such as joint identification in medical image problems. Several studies have reported good results [14–17]. However, heavy labeling workload and cost of physicians' label are another consideration that has limited this method from going global. Our study provided a method of manual annotation with approximation identification of hip regions that can be performed effectively and inexpensively.

Medical artificial intelligence is progressive in order to change the healthcare system, and various DCNNs have showed that it is feasible to detect lesions from pathologic images [23] and radiography [24]. These algorithms presented outstanding achievement in disease detection or prediction of whose performance is not inferior to that of the physicians [23–25]. These results inspire us in that DCNN might help individuals in the healthcare sector in different ways. However, the development of medical AI is not accessible due to some limitations. The data clearance and accurate label were considered fundamental for deep learning because of the limited size and data quality of medical images [19] and the high cost of a medical expert to perform labeling [26]. Moreover, the hip ROI detection system can help the physician to label the lesion in a weak supervision way, wherein we can pick out the hip regions and save time for the physician to crop and copy the images. The reduction of the barrier between an outliner and the way in which to attract more physicians and scientists to join a new rising technologic field are other issues to be considered in the real world. In this study, we developed the diagnostic assistance system and created a useful tool for reducing the workload during data collection and tuning. With our tool, we can simply label workload, minimize the calculation requirement, and eventually make the physician use it in the way they need. There are numerous existing programs [27,28] that can help orthopedics to plan the surgical strategy. Our algorithm might accelerate the speed of these programs by reducing calculation requirements in the future. The utility of such ROI detection approaches highly depends on the downstream applications. With input of clinical physicians' expertise, this automated hip ROI detection enables applications such as fracture identification, osteoarthritis assessment, osteoporosis, and even surgical prediction in the future. The evaluations of such applications and integrated systems remain to be investigated in future works and remain to be open research topics.

5. Limitation

Our study provided a feasible framework of automated ROI labeling. However, there are still some limitations in the existing method. First, the manual hip annotation with loose-fitting criteria is not unique and can be varied from person to person, especially for those cases with destructed hips. In these situations, a closer visual examination is needed. Because of the data distribution, we excluded most images from patients with endomedullary prostheses to make the training data solid. Therefore, we did not have these kinds of images for further validation, which might impact the usability of this algorithm. Lastly, limited medical image data might influence the performance of this algorithm. Increasing data from other sources might increase the performance and prevent the possibility of overfitting.

6. Conclusions

In conclusion, with the proposed DCNN framework, we can identify the hip joint with high accuracy, reliability, and reproducibility. It has a clear approach for ROI detection in plain X-ray and has practical usefulness for future applications in medical imaging. Increasing data and destructed hip analysis might improve the performance of this algorithm. However, the downstream application of hip ROI detection is a further research direction, and with our tool, we can simply label workload and eventually adjust the algorithm to fulfil the physicians' need to achieve the aim of personalized healthcare.

Author Contributions: F.-Y.L., S.-C.C. and C.-H.L. designed the experiments; C.-C.C., C.-T.C. and C.-H.L. acquired radiographics for use in the study and provided strategic support; F.-Y.L. and S.-C.C. wrote code to achieve different tasks and carried out all experiments; F.-Y.L. implemented the annotation tools for data annotation; F.-Y.L., S.-C.C., C.-P.H. and C.-H.L. provided labels for use in measuring algorithm performance; F.-Y.L., C.-Y.F. and C.-C.C. drafted the manuscript; S.-C.C. helped extensively with writing the manuscript; S.-C.C., M.S.L. and C.-H.L. supervised the project; C.-T.W., C.-H.L. and M.S.L. revised this manuscript. All authors have read and agreed to the published version of the manuscript.

Funding: This research was funded by the Ministry of Science and Technology, Taiwan, MOST109-2622-B-182A-001 (NCRPG3J0012), and Chang Gung Memorial Hospital, grant numbers CMRPG3K0801, CMRPG3L0381 and CIRPG3H0021.

Institutional Review Board Statement: The study was conducted according to the guidelines of the Declaration of Helsinki and approved by the Institutional Review Board of Chang Gung Memorial hospital, no. 201801897B0.

Informed Consent Statement: Not applicable.

Data Availability Statement: The data are partially available under the request of the audience.

Acknowledgments: The authors thank CMRPG1K0091 and CIRPG3H0021 for supporting the study and operative system.

Conflicts of Interest: The authors declare no conflict of interest. The funders had no role in the design of the study; in the collection, analyses, or interpretation of data; in the writing of the manuscript; or in the decision to publish the results.

References

1. Cheng, C.-T.; Ho, T.-Y.; Lee, T.-Y.; Chang, C.-C.; Chou, C.-C.; Chen, C.-C.; Chung, I.-F.; Liao, C.-H. Application of a deep learning algorithm for detection and visualization of hip fractures on plain pelvic radiographs. *Eur. Radiol.* **2019**, *29*, 5469–5477. [CrossRef] [PubMed]
2. Xue, Y.; Zhang, R.; Deng, Y.; Chen, K.; Jiang, T. A preliminary examination of the diagnostic value of deep learning in hip osteoarthritis. *PLoS ONE* **2017**, *12*, e0178992. [CrossRef] [PubMed]

3. Wang, X.; Peng, Y.; Lu, L.; Lu, Z.; Bagheri, M.; Summers, R.M. Chest X-ray 8: Hospital-scale chest X-ray database and benchmarks on weakly-supervised classification and localization of common thorax diseases. In Proceedings of the IEEE Conference on Computer Vision and Pattern Recognition, Las Vegas, NV, USA, 27–30 June 2016; pp. 2097–2106.
4. Rajpurkar, P.; Irvin, J.; Bagul, A.; Ding, D.; Duan, T.; Mehta, H.; Yang, B.; Zhu, K.; Laird, D.; Ball, R.L.; et al. MURA: Large dataset for abnormality detection in musculoskeletal radiographs. *arXiv* **2017**, arXiv:1712.06957.
5. Redmon, J.; Farhadi, A. YOLOv3: An incremental improvement. *arXiv* **2018**, arXiv:1804.02767.
6. Redmon, J.; Divvala, S.; Girshick, R.; Farhadi, A. You only look once: Unified, real-time object detection. In Proceedings of the IEEE Conference on Computer Vision and Pattern Recognition, Las Vegas, NV, USA, 27–30 June 2016; pp. 779–788.
7. Redmon, J.; Farhadi, A. YOLO9000: Better, Faster, Stronger. *arXiv* **2016**, arXiv:1506.02640.
8. Bochkovskiy, A.; Wang, C.-Y.; Liao, H.-Y.M. YOLOv4: Optimal speed and accuracy of object detection. *arXiv* **2020**, arXiv:2004.10934.
9. Liu, W.; Anguelov, D.; Erhan, D.; Szegedy, C.; Reed, S.; Fu, C.-Y.; Berg, A.C. SSD: Single shot multibox detector. In *Proceedings of the Computer Vision—ECCV 2016*; Springer: Berlin/Heidelberg, Germany, 2016; pp. 21–37.
10. Simonyan, K.; Zisserman, A. Very deep convolutional networks for large-scale image recognition. *arXiv* **2014**, arXiv:1409.1556.
11. He, K.; Zhang, X.; Ren, S.; Sun, J. Deep residual learning for image recognition. In Proceedings of the IEEE Conference on Computer Vision and Pattern Recognition, Las Vegas, NV, USA, 27–30 June 2016; pp. 770–778.
12. Xie, S.; Girshick, R.; Dollár, P.; Tu, Z.; He, K. Aggregated residual transformations for deep neural networks. In Proceedings of the IEEE Conference on Computer Vision and Pattern Recognition, Honolulu, HI, USA, 21–26 July 2017; pp. 1492–1500.
13. Tiulpin, A.; Thevenot, J.; Rahtu, E.; Saarakkala, S. A novel method for automatic localization of joint area on knee plain radiographs. In *Proceedings of the Image Analysis*; Springer: Berlin/Heidelberg, Germany, 2017; pp. 290–301.
14. Tiulpin, A.; Thevenot, J.; Rahtu, E.; Lehenkari, P.; Saarakkala, S. Automatic knee osteoarthritis diagnosis from plain radiographs: A deep learning-based approach. *Sci. Rep.* **2018**, *8*, 1727. [CrossRef] [PubMed]
15. Krogue, J.D.; Cheng, K.V.; Hwang, K.M.; Toogood, P.; Meinberg, E.G.; Geiger, E.J.; Zaid, M.; McGill, K.C.; Patel, R.; Sohn, J.H.; et al. Automatic hip fracture identification and functional subclassification with deep learning. *Radiol. Artif. Intell.* **2020**, *2*, e190023. [CrossRef]
16. von Schacky, C.E.; Sohn, J.H.; Liu, F.; Ozhinsky, E.; Jungmann, P.M.; Nardo, L.; Posadzy, M.; Foreman, S.C.; Nevitt, M.C.; Link, T.M.; et al. Development and validation of a multitask deep learning model for severity grading of hip osteoarthritis features on radiographs. *Radiology* **2020**, *295*, 136–145. [CrossRef]
17. Li, Y.; Li, Y.; Tian, H. Deep learning-based end-to-end diagnosis system for avascular necrosis of femoral head. *IEEE J. Biomed. Health Inform.* **2020**. [CrossRef] [PubMed]
18. Zhao, Z.-Q.; Zheng, P.; Xu, S.-T.; Wu, X. Object detection with deep learning: A review. *IEEE Trans. Neural Netw. Learn. Syst.* **2019**, *30*, 3212–3232. [CrossRef]
19. Esteva, A.; Chou, K.; Yeung, S.; Naik, N.; Madani, A.; Mottaghi, A.; Liu, Y.; Topol, E.; Dean, J.; Socher, R. Deep learning-enabled medical computer vision. *NPJ Digit. Med.* **2021**, *4*, 5. [CrossRef] [PubMed]
20. Joseph, G.B.; Hilton, J.F.; Jungmann, P.M.; Lynch, J.A.; Lane, N.E.; Liu, F.; McCulloch, C.E.; Tolstykh, I.; Link, T.M.; Nevitt, M.C. Do persons with asymmetric hip pain or radiographic hip OA have worse pain and structure outcomes in the knee opposite the more affected hip? Data from the Osteoarthritis Initiative. *Osteoarthr. Cartil.* **2016**, *24*, 427–435. [CrossRef] [PubMed]
21. Russakovsky, O.; Deng, J.; Su, H.; Krause, J.; Satheesh, S.; Ma, S.; Huang, Z.; Karpathy, A.; Khosla, A.; Bernstein, M.; et al. ImageNet large scale visual recognition challenge. *Int. J. Comput. Vis.* **2015**, *115*, 211–252. [CrossRef]
22. Howard, J.; Gugger, S. Fastai: A layered API for deep learning. *Information* **2020**, *11*, 108. [CrossRef]
23. Esteva, A.; Kuprel, B.; Novoa, R.A.; Ko, J.; Swetter, S.M.; Blau, H.M.; Thrun, S. Dermatologist-level classification of skin cancer with deep neural networks. *Nature* **2017**, *542*, 115–118. [CrossRef] [PubMed]
24. Cheng, C.-T.; Wang, Y.; Chen, H.-W.; Hsiao, P.-M.; Yeh, C.-N.; Hsieh, C.-H.; Miao, S.; Xiao, J.; Liao, C.-H.; Lu, L. A scalable physician-level deep learning algorithm detects universal trauma on pelvic radiographs. *Nat. Commun.* **2021**, *12*, 1066. [CrossRef]
25. Gulshan, V.; Peng, L.; Coram, M.; Stumpe, M.C.; Wu, D.; Narayanaswamy, A.; Venugopalan, S.; Widner, K.; Madams, T.; Cuadros, J.; et al. Development and validation of a deep learning algorithm for detection of diabetic retinopathy in retinal fundus photographs. *JAMA* **2016**, *316*, 2402–2410. [CrossRef]
26. Tobore, I.; Li, J.; Yuhang, L.; Al-Handarish, Y.; Kandwal, A.; Nie, Z.; Wang, L. Deep learning intervention for health care challenges: Some biomedical domain considerations. *JMIR Mhealth Uhealth* **2019**, *7*, e11966. [CrossRef] [PubMed]
27. Meermans, G.; Malik, K.; Witt, J.; Haddad, F. Preoperative radiographic assessment of limb-length discrepancy in total hip arthroplasty. *Clin. Orthop. Relat. Res.* **2011**, *469*, 1677–1682. [CrossRef] [PubMed]
28. Schröter, S.; Ihle, C.; Mueller, J.; Lobenhoffer, P.; Stöckle, U.; van Heerwaarden, R. Digital planning of high tibial osteotomy. Interrater reliability by using two different software. *Knee Surgery Sports Traumatol. Arthrosc.* **2013**, *21*, 189–196. [CrossRef] [PubMed]

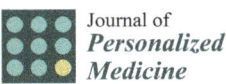 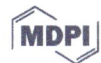

Article

Restoring the Patient's Pre-Arthritic Posterior Slope Is the Correct Target for Maximizing Internal Tibial Rotation When Implanting a PCL Retaining TKA with Calipered Kinematic Alignment

Alexander J. Nedopil [1,2,*], Connor Delman [3], Stephen M. Howell [2] and Maury L. Hull [2,3]

1. Orthopädische Klinik König-Ludwig-Haus, Lehrstuhl für Orthopädie der Universität Würzburg, 97074 Würzburg, Germany
2. Department of Biomedical Engineering, University of California, Davis, CA 95616, USA; sebhowell@mac.com (S.M.H.); mlhull@ucdavis.edu (M.L.H.)
3. Department of Orthopedic Surgery, University of California, Davis, CA 95817, USA; cdelman@ucdavis.edu
* Correspondence: nedopil@me.com

Abstract: Introduction: The calipered kinematically-aligned (KA) total knee arthroplasty (TKA) strives to restore the patient's individual pre-arthritic (i.e., native) posterior tibial slope when retaining the posterior cruciate ligament (PCL). Deviations from the patient's individual pre-arthritic posterior slope tighten and slacken the PCL in flexion that drives tibial rotation, and such a change might compromise passive internal tibial rotation and coupled patellofemoral kinematics. Methods: Twenty-one patients were treated with a calipered KA TKA and a PCL retaining implant with a medial ball-in-socket and a lateral flat articular insert conformity that mimics the native (i.e., healthy) knee. The slope of the tibial resection was set parallel to the medial joint line by adjusting the plane of an angel wing inserted in the tibial guide. Three trial inserts that matched and deviated 2°> and 2°< from the patient's pre-arthritic slope were 3D printed with goniometric markings. The goniometer measured the orientation of the tibia (i.e., trial insert) relative to the femoral component. Results: There was no difference between the radiographic preoperative and postoperative tibial slope (0.7 ± 3.2°, NS). From extension to 90° flexion, the mean passive internal tibial rotation with the pre-arthritic slope insert of 19° was greater than the 15° for the 2°> slope ($p < 0.000$), and 15° for the 2°< slope ($p < 0.000$). Discussion: When performing a calipered KA TKA with PCL retention, the correct target for setting the tibial component is the patient's individual pre-arthritic slope within a tolerance of ±2°, as this target resulted in a 15–19° range of internal tibial rotation that is comparable to the 15–18° range reported for the native knee from extension to 90° flexion.

Keywords: total knee replacement; total knee arthroplasty; kinematic alignment; slope; rotation

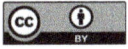

1. Introduction

Total knee arthroplasty (TKA) should restore the native, or healthy, knee's resting length of the posterior cruciate ligament (PCL) throughout the range of motion to provide stability and to not over or under constrain the knee [1]. A tibial component set in a posterior slope that tightens or slackens the PCL in flexion can decrease the range of motion, increase the risks of tibial component subsidence and polyethylene wear, cause anterior tibial subluxation, and anteroposterior instability which can lead to pain, effusion, and impaired function [1–7].

The correct target for setting the posterior slope with PCL retention is debatable and depends on the alignment method. A target recommended for mechanical alignment (MA) is 3–7° of the posterior slope [8]. However, a 3–7° range does not account for the 20° inter-individual range of the native posterior slope, and its use changes PCL tension in most knees [8–10]. Because the PCL tension in flexion drives tibial rotation, setting the tibial component to an incorrect slope might cause a loss of internal tibial rotation, thereby compromising the coupled reduction in the Q-angle throughout knee flexion, adversely affecting the retinacular ligaments' tension and patellofemoral tracking [11–14].

In contrast to MA, the recommended slope target for calipered kinematic alignment (KA) is to restore the patient's individual pre-arthritic posterior slope when retaining the PCL. The caliper technique, which does not release ligaments, sets the femoral and tibial components within 0 ± 0.5 mm of the patient's individual pre-arthritic distal and posterior femoral joint lines [15,16]. Intraoperatively, the tibial resection slope is set parallel to the medial joint line's posterior slope by adjusting the plane of an angel wing inserted in the tibial guide (Figure 1). Since the posterior slope on a lateral radiograph is minimally affected by arthrosis, as long as the medial and lateral tibial plateaus closely superimpose, the difference between the pre and postoperative slope can determine the angel wing technique's accuracy [7–9].

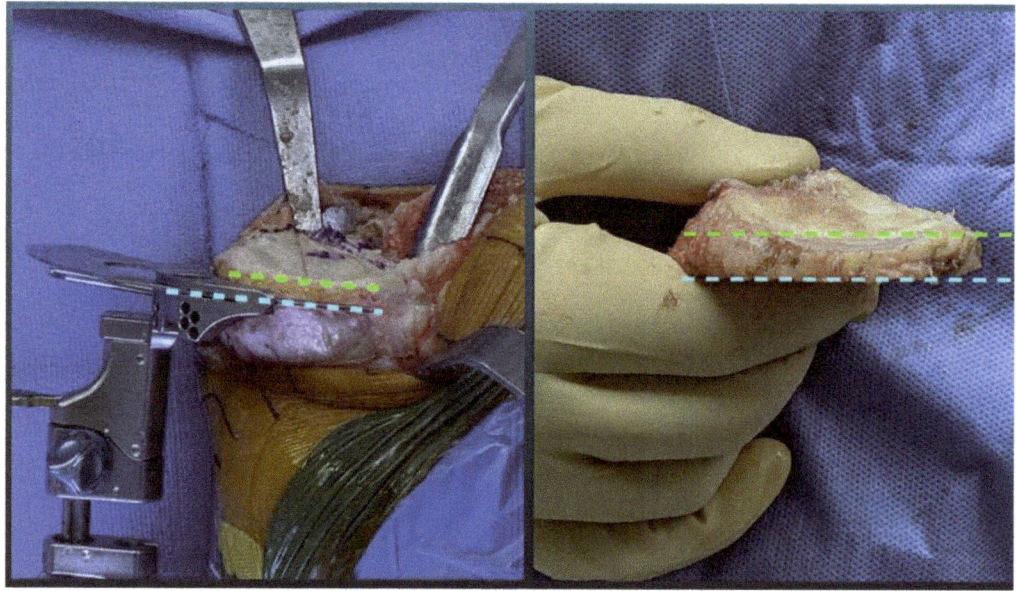

Figure 1. Intraoperative photographs of the medial side of a right knee show the method of setting the tibial resection (blue dotted line) parallel to the medial joint line (green dotted line) by adjusting the plane of an angel wing inserted in the tibial guide (**left**) and the visual verification check showing the tibial resection matches the patient's native slope (**right**).

There is a presumption that when a calipered KA retains the PCL and uses components that closely match the surface conformity of the native knee, the coupled internal rotation during passive flexion is also restored. Native knee dissections and image analysis by Freeman and Pinskerova showed that the medial femoral condyle behaves similarly to a ball-in-socket joint, and the lateral tibia and posteriorly mobile lateral meniscus form a flat articular surface, causing the tibia to internally rotate about the center of the medial compartment. The native knee's 15–18° range of internal tibial rotation from extension to 90° is a desirable arc of motion for TKA [11,17]. A trial insert with native knee conformity and a novel, built-in goniometer can intraoperatively measure the patient's specific tibial orientation and the degree of internal tibial rotation during flexion (Figure 2). It is unknown whether deviations from the patient's individual pre-arthritic posterior slope and the corresponding change in PCL tension adversely affect the tibial rotation.

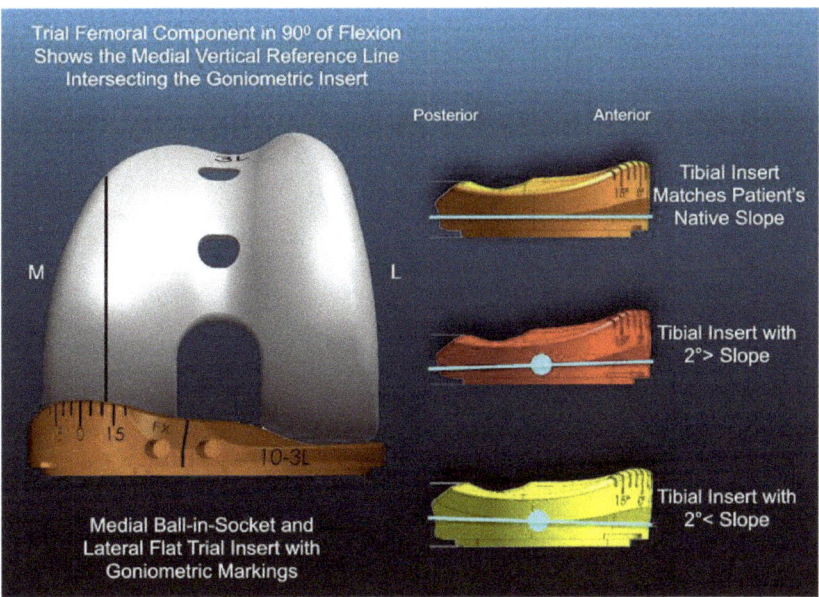

Figure 2. Schematics of a left TKA show the −12° of internal tibial orientation of the trial insert goniometer relative to the medial femoral condyle (left), and the method of creating the tibial inserts with a 2°> (=2° increased) and 2°< (=2° decreased) slope by pivoting the articular surface about the center (blue circle) of the insert that matched the patient's native slope.

Accordingly, the present study determined in 21 patients, using the insert with the novel built-in goniometer, whether there was a difference between the pre/postoperative posterior slope, and whether trial inserts that matched or deviated ±2° from the patient's individual pre-arthritic slope changed the patient's specific tibial orientation in extension and 90° flexion and internal tibial rotation in this range of flexion. The goal of the study was to test the hypotheses that (1) the visual method restores the patient's individual pre-arthritic slope with good reproducibility, and (2) the patient's individual pre-arthritic slope is the correct target within a tolerance of ±2° for a calipered KA TKA because it restores a 15–19° range of internal tibial rotation that is comparable to the native knee.

2. Materials and Methods

Our institutional review board approved the retrospective study (IRB 1632230-1). Between mid-May 2020 and early June 2020, two surgeons treated 36 consecutive patients with a primary TKA using a calipered KA, PCL retention, and patella resurfacing through a midvastus approach. Each patient fulfilled the Centers for Medicare and Medicaid Services guidelines for medical necessity for the TKA treatment, including: (1) radiographic evidence of Kellgren–Lawrence grade II to IV arthritic change or osteonecrosis; (2) any severity of clinical varus or valgus deformity; (3) and any severity of flexion contracture. Patients were treated with an implant designed by Freeman and Pinskerova, which featured a spherical medial femoral condyle and an insert with a medial ball-in-socket and a lateral flat articular surface (GMK Sphere, Medacta International, Available online: www.medacta.com (accessed on 31 May 2021)) (Figure 2). The implant manufacturer provided 3D printed one-time use trial goniometric inserts in three different slopes (i.e., matching patient's pre-arthritic slope, 2°> slope, 2°< slope). The three slopes were sterilized and packed for surgical use in 10-, 11- and 12-mm thicknesses and sizes 3, 4, and 5 left and right tibial baseplates (Figure 2) [18,19]. The implant manufacturer provided 3D printed one-time use trial goniometric inserts in three different slopes (i.e., matching patient's slope,

2°> slope, 2°< slope) in 10, 11, and 12 mm thicknesses for sizes 3, 4, and 5 left and right tibial baseplates (Figure 2). A total of thirty-six consecutive primary calipered KA TKAs were performed to assess 21 knees with the novel insert goniometer because some patients used implant sizes other than those available (i.e., sizes 14 and 17 inserts, and sizes 1, 2, and 6 tibial baseplates), and because some sizes of insert goniometers had been used and were no longer available. The tibial baseplate has an anatomically shaped footprint and a posterior cut-out for retention of the PCL that, when best fit to the tibial resection, sets the internal–external rotation so that the anterior–posterior (AP) axis is parallel to the flexion–extension (FE) plane of the native knee [20]. The first TKAs with an insert thickness and size selected for implantation that matched an available sterile triplet of trial goniometric inserts were studied.

The sample size calculation used the effect of deviating the slope by 2 degrees from the patient's pre-arthritic slope on passive internal rotation. Assuming a Type I error (alpha) of 0.05, a power (1-beta) of 80%, a minimum difference to detect a 3° change in rotation, and a standard deviation of ±6°, the sample size was 18 patients trialed with three different inserts. Twenty-one patients were included in the study consisting of 67% females with a mean age at the time of surgery of 70 ± 8 years (56 to 81) and a mean BMI of 29 ± 5 kg/m^2. Descriptive statistics of preoperative clinical characteristics, knee conditions, and function of included (n = 21) and not included (n = 15) patients are shown (Table 1). Preoperatively, there were no significant differences in age, proportion of women, body mass index, extension, flexion, varus or valgus deformities, Oxford Knee Score, Knee Society Score, or Knee Function Score between included and not included patients, which reduced the risk of a selection bias that could limit the generalization of the study's findings.

Table 1. Preoperative Patient Demographics and Clinical and Radiographic Characteristics of Included and Not-Included Patients.

Preoperative Demographics and Clinical and Radiographic Characteristics	Included Patients N = 21	Not-Included Patients N = 15	Significance
	DEMOGRAPHICS		
Age (years)	70 (±7.9)	68 (±8.8)	n.s.
Sex (male)	8 (38%)	7 (47%)	n.s.
Body Mass Index (kg/m^2)	29.2 (±5.3)	30.2 (±4.4)	n.s.
	PREOPERATIVE MOTION, DEFORMITY, ACL CONDITION, AND KELLGREN-LAWRENCE SCORE		
Extension (degrees)	7 (±5)	7 (±8)	n.s.
Flexion (degrees)	112 (±6.4)	110 (±8.7)	n.s.
Varus (+)/Valgus (−) Deformity (degrees)	−12.2 (±3.1)	−10.8 (±3.1)	n.s.
Kellgren- Lawrence Score	3.6 (±0.6)	3.4 (±0.5)	n.s.
	PREOPERATIVE FUNCTION		
Oxford Score (48 is best, 0 is worst)	21 (±8.4)	16 (±6.5)	n.s.
Knee Society Score	38 (±11.7)	38 (±16.4)	n.s.
Knee Function Score	55 (±21.5)	46 (±16.1)	n.s.

2.1. Overview of Unrestricted Calipered KA Technique and Accuracy Analysis of Component Placement

The following is an overview of the previously described unrestricted calipered KA technique performed through a midvastus approach using intraoperatively recorded verification checks and following a decision-tree [21]. For the femoral component, the varus–valgus (VV) and IE orientations and the AP and proximal–distal (PD) positions were set coincident with the patient's individual pre-arthritic distal and posterior joint lines by adjusting the calipered thicknesses of the distal and posterior femoral resections to within 0 ± 0.5 mm of those of the femoral component condyles after compensating for cartilage wear and the kerf of the saw blade. The basis for setting the distal and posterior femoral resection guide is knowing that the varus and valgus grade II to IV Kellgren–

Lawrence osteoarthritic knees have negligible bone wear at 0° and 90°, and that the mean full-thickness cartilage wear approximates 2 mm [22]. An accuracy analysis showed these steps restore the distal lateral femoral joint line of 97% of patients within the normal left to right symmetry and set the IE orientation of the femoral component with a deviation of 0.3° (external) ±1.1° from the KA target of the FE plane of the patient's knee [15,16,23,24].

The surgeon followed six options in a decision-tree to set the VV and posterior slope orientation of the tibial component to restore the patient's pre-arthritic tibial joint line and limb alignment and balance the knee by restoring the native tibial compartment forces [23–25]. The varus–valgus orientation of the proximal tibial resection was adjusted working in 1°–2° increments until there was negligible medial and lateral lift-off from the femoral component during a varus–valgus laxity assessment with the spacer block and trial tibial insert. An accuracy analysis showed these steps restore the proximal medial tibial joint line of 97% of patients within the normal left to right symmetry [16,24,26]. The method for visually selecting the posterior slope was to set an angel wing, inserted through the tibial guide's medial slot, parallel to the patient's pre-arthritic slope (Figure 2). A three-dimensional accuracy analysis in osteoarthritic varus knees reported a 0° mean difference between the patient's individual pre-arthritic and tibial component's posterior slope [27]. A best fit of the largest anatomically shaped trial tibial baseplate inside the cortical rim of the proximal tibial resection method set the IE orientation and AP and medial–lateral (ML) positions. An accuracy analysis showed a mean 2° (external) ± 5° deviation of the IE orientation of the tibial component from the KA target of the FE plane of the patient's knee [15,16,20,27–29].

The following steps determined the optimal insert thickness within a ±1 mm target. Place the knee in 90° flexion and palpate the PCL to verify that it is intact. Insert a goniometric tibial insert that matches the thickness of the spacer block. Place the knee in extension and verify that the knee hyperextends a few degrees, such as the pre-arthritic knee. When the knee has a flexion contracture, insert a thinner insert or release the posterior capsule. Verify that the VV laxity is negligible in full extension, the lateral compartment has a 3–4 mm gap and the medial compartment a negligible gap with the knee in 15°–30° flexion. When necessary, fine-tune the VV plane of the tibial resection. Place the knee in 90° flexion and determine whether passive IE rotation of the tibia approximates ±15°, such as the native knee [28].

2.2. Method for Radiographically Measuring the Preoperative Tibial Slope and Postoperative Tibial Component Slope

One author (A.J.N) measured the slope of the patient's tibia on a preoperative radiograph and the slope of the tibial component on a postoperative computer tomography scanogram using a previously described method with a 0.89 interobserver intraclass coefficient indicative of good interobserver agreement [4,26] (Figure 3).

2.3. Method of Measuring the Orientation of the Tibia with Trial Goniometric Insert

A goniometric trial insert that matched or deviated 2°> (=2° increased slope) and 2°< (=2° decreased slope) from the patient's individual pre-arthritic slope was randomly selected and inserted (Figure 2). The surgeon reduced the patella, placed the patient's heel on the back of the wrist, and lifted the leg to passively extend the knee without applying an IE moment to the ankle. The trial insert goniometer measured the IE tibial orientation relative to the femoral component (+external/−internal) with the knee in extension (Figure 4). The surgeon flexed the knee to 90° and rested the foot on the operating table, and the goniometer measured the tibial orientation (Figure 5). In random order, the surgeon inserted the two remaining inserts and repeated the tibial orientation measurements.

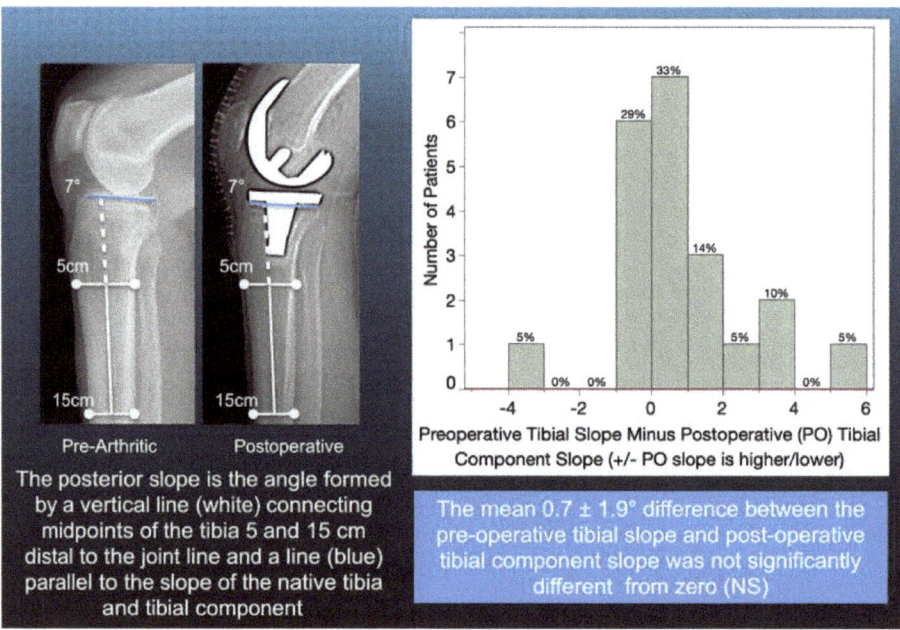

Figure 3. The figure shows the radiographic method for measuring the posterior slope of the preoperative tibia and postoperative tibial component (**left**) and the distribution of the difference in slope for the 21 patients as a measure of the reproducibility in setting the tibial component to the patient's native slope using the angel wing (**right**).

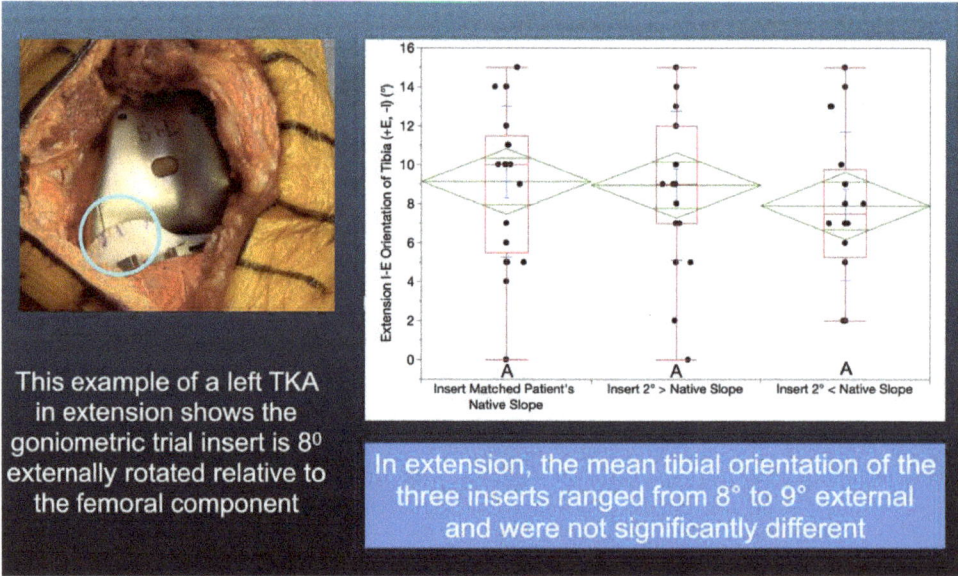

Figure 4. The figure shows an intraoperative photograph of the insert goniometer of a left TKA in extension reading 8° of external tibial orientation (**left**) and box plots of 21 patients that show the mean external tibial orientation was not significantly different between the three inserts (**right**). The top and bottom edges of the green diamond indicate the 95% confidence interval limits.

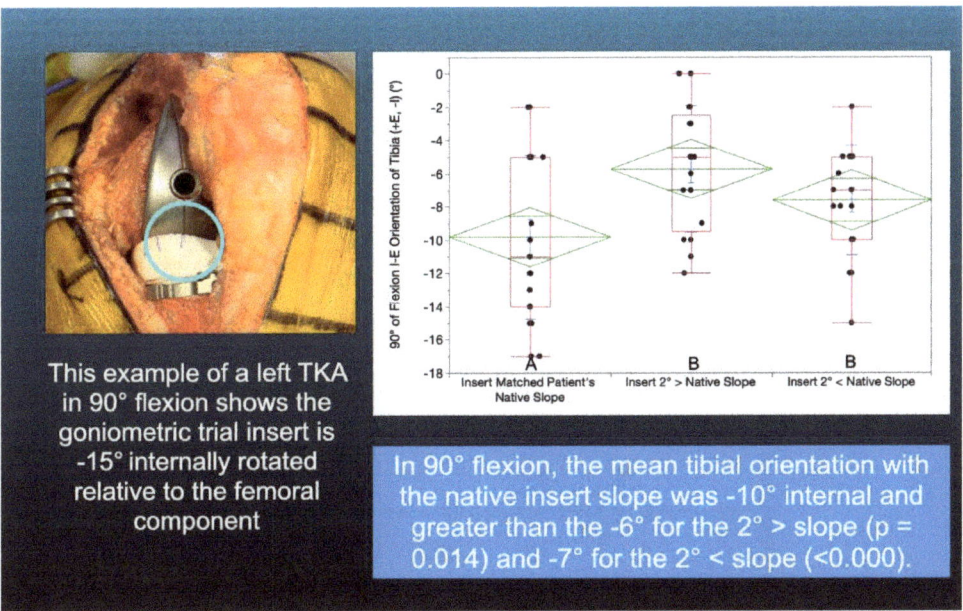

Figure 5. The figure shows an intraoperative photograph of the insert goniometer of a left TKA in 90° flexion reading −15° of internal tibial orientation (**left**) and the box plots show the internal tibial orientation for 21 patients and the insert slopes with different letters are significantly different (**right**).

2.4. Statistical Analysis

Data were analyzed using statistical software (JMP® Pro 15.2.1, Available online: www.jmp.com (accessed on 31 May 2021), SAS, Cary, NC, USA). The mean and standard deviation described the continuous variables. A Student's paired t-test determined whether the pre-arthritic and postoperative posterior tibial slope was radiographically different. A mixed-model repeated measured analysis with three fixed effects (i.e., trial goniometer insert that matched and deviated 2°> and 2°< from the patient's pre-arthritic slope) determined whether there was a difference in mean tibial orientation in extension and at 90° flexion and an internal tibial rotation from extension to 90° between the three insert slopes. For each analysis, a Tukey's Honest Significant Difference (HSD) post hoc test determined differences between all pairs of insert slopes. Significance was $p < 0.05$.

To quantify reproducibility, two observers (SMH and AJN) measured the slope of the tibia in seven knees. A two-factor mixed-model analysis of variance (ANOVA) with random effects computed the intraclass correlation coefficient (ICC). The first factor was the observer (2 levels), and the second was the patient (7 levels). ICC value of 0.89 indicated good reproducibility for the measurement of tibial slope.

3. Results

There was no difference between the radiographic preoperative and postoperative slope (0.7 ± 3.2°, NS), and 75% (16/21) of patients had a <2° difference (Figure 3). In extension, the tibial orientation of the three inserts with different slopes was comparable and ranged from 8° to 9° external (NS) (Figure 4). At 90°, the tibial orientation with the pre-arthritic slope insert was −10° internal and greater than the −6° for the 2°> slope ($p = 0.014$) and −7° for the 2°< slope (<0.000) (Figure 5). From extension to 90° flexion, the passive internal tibial rotation with the pre-arthritic slope insert was 19° and greater than the 15° for the 2°< slope ($p < 0.000$), and 15° for the 2°> slope ($p < 0.000$) (Figure 6).

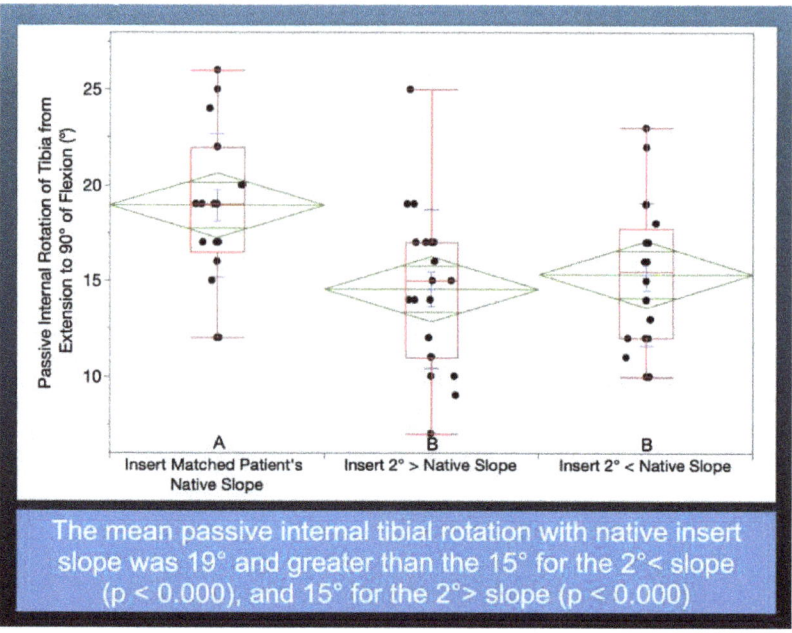

Figure 6. The box plots show the internal tibial rotation from extension to 90° flexion for 21 patients, and the insert slopes with different letters are significantly different.

4. Discussion

Knowing the target for setting the posterior slope when performing a calipered KA with PCL retention is necessary to restore internal tibial rotation and the coupled reduction in the Q-angle of the native knee throughout knee flexion and optimize the retinacular ligaments' tension and patellofemoral tracking. The most important findings of the present study of 21 patients were that (1) the visual method restored the patient's individual pre-arthritic slope with good reproducibility, and (2) the pre-arthritic slope is the correct target within a tolerance of ±2° for a calipered KA TKA because it restored a 15–19° range of internal tibial rotation that is comparable to the pre-arthritic knee [11,29].

The radiographic reproducibility of the visual method that set the tibial resection plane by aligning an angel wing in the tibial resection guide parallel to the patient's pre-arthritic joint line was comparable to a three-dimensional shape registration analysis between arthritic surface models segmented from preoperative magnetic resonance imaging scans and resected surface models segmented from postoperative computed tomography scans [27] (Figure 3). Setting the tibial resection to the patient's pre-arthritic slope is necessary to reduce the risks of tibial component subsidence and posterior polyethylene wear from not restoring the native PCL tension in flexion [4,6]. A study of thirty-three cemented MA TKA with PCL retention using instrumentation designed to cut the tibia with 0° posterior slope reported that ten tibial components had at least 2 mm of subsidence. The subsided tibial components had an 8° mean difference from the patient's pre-arthritic (i.e., preoperative) posterior slope. The non-subsided tibial components were within ±2° of their individual pre-arthritic slope [6]. A study of cemented calipered KA TKA with PCL retention reported 7 out of 2725 patients with tibial component failure from posterior subsidence or polyethylene wear with a 7° greater slope than the pre-arthritic slope [4]. A varus mechanism was not found to be associated with early tibial component failure after KA, whereas varus overload causing medial bone collapse and varus subsidence of the tibial component is responsible for a comparable—if not higher—incidence of 0.7% revisions after MA. Posterior subsidence generates cement debris, which leads to osteolysis of the tibia and accelerates the subsidence of the baseplate [30]. Hence, cutting the tibia to restore the patient's pre-arthritic slope is the correct target for reducing the risk of tibial component failure when performing a calipered KA and MA TKA with PCL retention.

The inserts with a 2°> and 2°< deviation from the patient's pre-arthritic slope in the present study, that slacken and tighten the PCL in flexion, caused a loss of internal tibial orientation only at 90° and not in extension, confirming the results of in vivo and in vitro studies that PCL tension, which progressively increases with flexion, drives internal tibial rotation (Figures 4 and 5) [12,13]. The PCL's resection in the cadaveric knee reduced internal tibial rotation at high flexion angles beginning at 60° [12]. A three-dimensional fluoroscopic analysis of a deep knee bend in patients with a PCL injury in one knee and the other intact showed a decreased internal tibial rotation throughout the range of flexion in the PCL-deficient knee, which correlated with patellar tilt ($R^2 = 0.73$) and medial–lateral patellar translation ($R^2 = 0.63$) [13,31]. Hence, surgeons and bioengineers should consider restoring the native knee's kinematic coupling between internal tibial rotation and patellofemoral tracking and loading when developing surgical techniques such as TKA [31].

The present study suggests that the correct target for setting the tibial component with a calipered KA TKA and PCL retention is the patient's individual pre-arthritic slope within a tolerance of ±2° because the 15–19° range of internal tibial rotation was comparable to the native knee and more significant deviations increase the risk of tibial component failure [4,6,11,17]. The fixed 3–7° slope range recommended for MA does not account for the 20° inter-individual range of the pre-arthritic posterior slope and should not be used with a calipered KA as only 33% (7 of 21) of the tibial components in the present study fit within this range [8–10,17]. MA surgeons commonly use techniques such as increasing the posterior slope and PCL recession and release to increase knee flexion; however, they cause a loss of internal tibial rotation and risk tibial component failure [3,5]. A Calipered KA that sets the components patient-specific to restore the patient's individual pre-arthritic joint lines within ±0.5 mm has the biomechanical advantage of retaining the PCL and restoring native knee tibial compartment forces and laxities during passive flexion without ligament release [23–25,32–34].

The present study has several limitations. These results are from a case series of two surgeons who require confirmation by others. The evaluation of the insert goniometer was with a medial ball-in-socket and a flat lateral insert designed to replicate the dynamic conformity of the native knee described by Freeman and Pinskerova [11,35–37]. It might function differently with posterior-stabilized, PCL-retaining, and ultra-congruent insert geometries that are less-conforming medially and more-constrained laterally with a posterior rim that stops internal rotation, such as a chock block. A medial concavity shallower than the ball-in-socket conformity enables the femur to translate anteriorly and posteriorly, thereby lowering the PCL's tension in flexion which drives internal tibial rotation. The internal tibial rotation might be less for implants placed with MA since the components commonly deviate from the patient-specific native joint lines, and ligaments are released to slacken an over-tensioned TKA [38–40].

5. Conclusions

The present study measured the passive internal tibial rotation with a novel goniometric insert between full extension and 90 degrees of flexion with the tibial component set to restore and deviate 2°> and 2°< from the patient's individual pre-arthritic slope in 21 patients treated with a calipered KA TKA and PCL retention, and showed that the pre-arthritic slope is the correct target as this resulted in a 15–19° range of internal tibial rotation, comparable to the 15–18° range reported for the native knee, whereas 2° deviations in slope caused a loss of tibial rotation.

Author Contributions: Conceptualization, A.J.N., S.M.H. and M.L.H.; methodology, A.J.N., S.M.H. and M.L.H.; software, A.J.N. and C.D.; validation, A.J.N., S.M.H. and M.L.H.; formal analysis, A.J.N., S.M.H. and M.L.H.; investigation, A.J.N., S.M.H. and M.L.H.; data curation, A.J.N. and S.M.H.; writing—original draft preparation, A.J.N. and S.M.H.; writing—review and editing, A.J.N., S.M.H. and M.L.H.; visualization, A.J.N. and S.M.H.; supervision, M.L.H. All authors have read and agreed to the published version of the manuscript.

Funding: Support for open access publication was provided by UC Davis and BaCaTeC.

Institutional Review Board Statement: The study was conducted according to the guidelines of the Declaration of Helsinki and approved by the Institutional Review Board of University California Davis (protocol code 1632230-1 and approved on 22 October 2020).

Informed Consent Statement: Patient consent was waived because the study is a retrospective review of de-identified preexisting patient data.

Acknowledgments: The authors thank Medacta International for providing the surgical instruments and trial implants to perform the study and BaCaTec for funding the open access publication fee.

Conflicts of Interest: The authors declare no conflict of interest.

References

1. Peters, C.L.; Jimenez, C.; Erickson, J.; Anderson, M.B.; Pelt, C.E. Lessons learned from selective soft-tissue release for gap balancing in primary total knee arthroplasty: An analysis of 1216 consecutive total knee arthroplasties: AAOS exhibit selection. *J. Bone Jt. Surg. Am.* **2013**, *95*, e152. [CrossRef] [PubMed]
2. Heesterbeek, P.J.; Wymenga, A.B. PCL balancing, an example of the need to couple detailed biomechanical parameters with clinical functional outcome. *Knee Surg. Sports Traumatol. Arthrosc.* **2010**, *18*, 1301–1303. [CrossRef] [PubMed]
3. Bellemans, J.; Robijns, F.; Duerinckx, J.; Banks, S.; Vandenneucker, H. The influence of tibial slope on maximal flexion after total knee arthroplasty. *Knee Surg. Sports Traumatol. Arthrosc.* **2005**, *13*, 193–196. [CrossRef] [PubMed]
4. Nedopil, A.J.; Howell, S.M.; Hull, M.L. What mechanisms are associated with tibial component failure after kinematically-aligned total knee arthroplasty? *Int. Orthop.* **2017**, *41*, 1561–1569. [CrossRef] [PubMed]
5. Scott, R.D.; Chmell, M.J. Balancing the posterior cruciate ligament during cruciate-retaining fixed and mobile-bearing total knee arthroplasty: Description of the pull-out lift-off and slide-back tests. *J. Arthroplast.* **2008**, *23*, 605–608. [CrossRef]
6. Hofmann, A.A.; Bachus, K.N.; Wyatt, R.W. Effect of the tibial cut on subsidence following total knee arthroplasty. *Clin. Orthop. Relat. Res.* **1991**, 63–69. [CrossRef]
7. Ahmad, R.; Patel, A.; Mandalia, V.; Toms, A. Posterior Tibial Slope: Effect on, and Interaction with, Knee Kinematics. *JBJS Rev.* **2016**, *4*, e3. [CrossRef]
8. Calek, A.K.; Hochreiter, B.; Hess, S.; Amsler, F.; Leclerq, V.; Hirschmann, M.T.; Behrend, H. High inter- and intraindividual differences in medial and lateral posterior tibial slope are not reproduced accurately by conventional TKA alignment techniques. *Knee Surg. Sports Traumatol. Arthrosc.* **2021**. [CrossRef]
9. Meier, M.; Janssen, D.; Koeck, F.X.; Thienpont, E.; Beckmann, J.; Best, R. Variations in medial and lateral slope and medial proximal tibial angle. *Knee Surg. Sports Traumatol. Arthrosc.* **2021**, *29*, 939–946. [CrossRef]
10. Nunley, R.M.; Nam, D.; Johnson, S.R.; Barnes, C.L. Extreme variability in posterior slope of the proximal tibia: Measurements on 2395 CT scans of patients undergoing UKA? *J. Arthroplast.* **2014**, *29*, 1677–1680. [CrossRef]
11. Freeman, M.A.; Pinskerova, V. The movement of the knee studied by magnetic resonance imaging. *Clin. Orthop. Relat. Res.* **2003**, *410*, 35–43. [CrossRef] [PubMed]
12. Li, G.; Gill, T.J.; DeFrate, L.E.; Zayontz, S.; Glatt, V.; Zarins, B. Biomechanical consequences of PCL deficiency in the knee under simulated muscle loads—An in vitro experimental study. *J. Orthop. Res.* **2002**, *20*, 887–892. [CrossRef]
13. Li, G.; Papannagari, R.; Li, M.; Bingham, J.; Nha, K.W.; Allred, D.; Gill, T. Effect of posterior cruciate ligament deficiency on in vivo translation and rotation of the knee during weightbearing flexion. *Am. J. Sports Med.* **2008**, *36*, 474–479. [CrossRef] [PubMed]
14. Fukubayashi, T.; Torzilli, P.A.; Sherman, M.F.; Warren, R.F. An in vitro biomechanical evaluation of anterior-posterior motion of the knee. Tibial displacement, rotation, and torque. *J. Bone Jt. Surg. Am.* **1982**, *64*, 258–264. [CrossRef]
15. Nedopil, A.J.; Howell, S.M.; Hull, M.L. Deviations in femoral joint lines using calipered kinematically aligned TKA from virtually planned joint lines are small and do not affect clinical outcomes. *Knee Surg. Sports Traumatol. Arthrosc.* **2020**, *28*, 3118–3127. [CrossRef]
16. Nedopil, A.J.; Singh, A.K.; Howell, S.M.; Hull, M.L. Does Calipered Kinematically Aligned TKA Restore Native Left to Right Symmetry of the Lower Limb and Improve Function? *J. Arthroplast.* **2018**, *33*, 398–406. [CrossRef]
17. Dennis, D.A.; Mahfouz, M.R.; Komistek, R.D.; Hoff, W. In vivo determination of normal and anterior cruciate ligament-deficient knee kinematics. *J. Biomech.* **2005**, *38*, 241–253. [CrossRef] [PubMed]

18. Schutz, P.; Taylor, W.R.; Postolka, B.; Fucentese, S.F.; Koch, P.P.; Freeman, M.A.R.; Pinskerova, V.; List, R. Kinematic Evaluation of the GMK Sphere Implant During Gait Activities: A Dynamic Videofluoroscopy Study. *J. Orthop. Res.* **2019**, *37*, 2337–2347. [CrossRef]
19. Gray, H.A.; Guan, S.; Young, T.J.; Dowsey, M.M.; Choong, P.F.; Pandy, M.G. Comparison of posterior-stabilized, cruciate-retaining, and medial-stabilized knee implant motion during gait. *J. Orthop. Res.* **2020**, *38*, 1753–1768. [CrossRef] [PubMed]
20. Nedopil, A.J.; Zamora, T.; Shelton, T.; Howell, S.M.; Hull, M. A Best-Fit of an Anatomic Tibial Baseplate Closely Parallels the Flexion-Extension Plane and Covers a High Percentage of the Proximal Tibia. *J. Knee Surg.* **2020**. [CrossRef]
21. Howell, S.M.; Shelton, T.J.; Gill, M.; Hull, M.L. A cruciate-retaining implant can treat both knees of most windswept deformities when performed with calipered kinematically aligned TKA. *Knee Surg. Sports Traumatol. Arthrosc.* **2021**, *29*, 437–445. [CrossRef]
22. Nam, D.; Lin, K.M.; Howell, S.M.; Hull, M.L. Femoral bone and cartilage wear is predictable at 0 degrees and 90 degrees in the osteoarthritic knee treated with total knee arthroplasty. *Knee Surg. Sports Traumatol. Arthrosc.* **2014**, *22*, 2975–2981. [CrossRef]
23. Nedopil, A.J.; Howell, S.M.; Hull, M.L. Does Malrotation of the Tibial and Femoral Components Compromise Function in Kinematically Aligned Total Knee Arthroplasty? *Orthop. Clin. N. Am.* **2016**, *47*, 41–50. [CrossRef]
24. Howell, S.M.; Gill, M.; Shelton, T.J.; Nedopil, A.J. Reoperations are few and confined to the most valgus phenotypes 4 years after unrestricted calipered kinematically aligned TKA. *Knee Surg. Sports Traumatol. Arthrosc.* **2021**. [CrossRef]
25. Roth, J.D.; Howell, S.M.; Hull, M.L. Kinematically aligned total knee arthroplasty limits high tibial forces, differences in tibial forces between compartments, and abnormal tibial contact kinematics during passive flexion. *Knee Surg. Sports Traumatol. Arthrosc.* **2018**, *26*, 1589–1601. [CrossRef]
26. Johnson, J.M.; Mahfouz, M.R.; Midillioglu, M.R.; Nedopil, A.J.; Howell, S.M. Three-dimensional analysis of the tibial resection plane relative to the arthritic tibial plateau in total knee arthroplasty. *J. Exp. Orthop.* **2017**, *4*, 27. [CrossRef] [PubMed]
27. Shelton, T.J.; Howell, S.M.; Hull, M.L. Is There a Force Target That Predicts Early Patient-reported Outcomes After Kinematically Aligned TKA? *Clin. Orthop. Relat. Res.* **2019**, *477*, 1200–1207. [CrossRef]
28. Shelton, T.J.; Nedopil, A.J.; Howell, S.M.; Hull, M.L. Do varus or valgus outliers have higher forces in the medial or lateral compartments than those which are in-range after a kinematically aligned total knee arthroplasty? limb and joint line alignment after kinematically aligned total knee arthroplasty. *Bone Jt. J.* **2017**, *99-B*, 1319–1328. [CrossRef] [PubMed]
29. Roth, J.D.; Howell, S.M.; Hull, M.L. Analysis of differences in laxities and neutral positions from native after kinematically aligned TKA using cruciate retaining implants. *J. Orthop. Res.* **2019**, *37*, 358–369. [CrossRef]
30. Roth, J.D.; Howell, S.M.; Hull, M.L. Native Knee Laxities at 0 degrees, 45 degrees, and 90 degrees of Flexion and Their Relationship to the Goal of the Gap-Balancing Alignment Method of Total Knee Arthroplasty. *J. Bone Jt. Surg. Am.* **2015**, *97*, 1678–1684. [CrossRef] [PubMed]
31. Dean, R.S.; DePhillipo, N.N.; Chahla, J.; Larson, C.M.; LaPrade, R.F. Posterior Tibial Slope Measurements Using the Anatomic Axis Are Significantly Increased Compared With Those That Use the Mechanical Axis. *Arthroscopy* **2021**, *37*, 243–249. [CrossRef] [PubMed]
32. Hozan, C.T.; Cavalu, S.; Cinta Pinzaru, S.; Mohan, A.G.; Beteg, F.; Murvai, G. Rapid Screening of Retrieved Knee Prosthesis Components by Confocal Raman Micro-Spectroscopy. *Appl. Sci.* **2020**, *10*, 5343. [CrossRef]
33. Li, G.; Papannagari, R.; Nha, K.W.; Defrate, L.E.; Gill, T.J.; Rubash, H.E. The coupled motion of the femur and patella during in vivo weightbearing knee flexion. *J. Biomech. Eng.* **2007**, *129*, 937–943. [CrossRef] [PubMed]
34. Jiang, C.C.; Yip, K.M.; Liu, T.K. Posterior slope angle of the medial tibial plateau. *J. Formos. Med. Assoc.* **1994**, *93*, 509–512.
35. Freeman, M.A.; Pinskerova, V. The movement of the normal tibio-femoral joint. *J. Biomech.* **2005**, *38*, 197–208. [CrossRef]
36. Pinskerova, V.; Samuelson, K.M.; Stammers, J.; Maruthainar, K.; Sosna, A.; Freeman, M.A. The knee in full flexion: An anatomical study. *J. Bone Jt. Surg. Br.* **2009**, *91*, 830–834. [CrossRef] [PubMed]
37. Hirschmann, M.T.; Moser, L.B.; Amsler, F.; Behrend, H.; Leclerq, V.; Hess, S. Functional knee phenotypes: A novel classification for phenotyping the coronal lower limb alignment based on the native alignment in young non-osteoarthritic patients. *Knee Surg. Sports Traumatol. Arthrosc.* **2019**, *27*, 1394–1402. [CrossRef] [PubMed]
38. Riley, J.; Roth, J.D.; Howell, S.M.; Hull, M.L. Increases in tibial force imbalance but not changes in tibiofemoral laxities are caused by varus-valgus malalignment of the femoral component in kinematically aligned TKA. *Knee Surg. Sports Traumatol. Arthrosc.* **2018**, *26*, 3238–3248. [CrossRef]
39. Riley, J.; Roth, J.D.; Howell, S.M.; Hull, M.L. Internal-external malalignment of the femoral component in kinematically aligned total knee arthroplasty increases tibial force imbalance but does not change laxities of the tibiofemoral joint. *Knee Surg. Sports Traumatol. Arthrosc.* **2018**, *26*, 1618–1628. [CrossRef]
40. Roth, J.D.; Howell, S.M.; Hull, M.L. Measuring Tibial Forces is More Useful than Varus-Valgus Laxities for Identifying and Correcting Overstuffing in Kinematically Aligned Total Knee Arthroplasty. *J. Orthop. Res.* **2020**. [CrossRef]

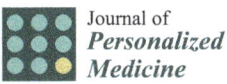 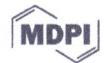

Review

Complex Bone Tumors of the Trunk—The Role of 3D Printing and Navigation in Tumor Orthopedics: A Case Series and Review of the Literature

Martin Schulze [1,*], Georg Gosheger [1], Sebastian Bockholt [1], Marieke De Vaal [1], Tymo Budny [1], Max Tönnemann [1], Jan Pützler [1], Albert Schulze Bövingloh [1], Robert Rischen [2], Vincent Hofbauer [1], Timo Lübben [1], Niklas Deventer [1] and Helmut Ahrens [1]

[1] Department of Orthopedics and Tumor Orthopedics, Muenster University Hospital, Albert-Schweitzer-Campus 1, 48149 Münster, Germany; georg.gosheger@ukmuenster.de (G.G.); sebastian.bockholt@ukmuenster.de (S.B.); mariekemathilda.devaal@ukmuenster.de (M.D.V.); Tymoteusz.budny@ukmuenster.de (T.B.); m.toennemann@uni-muenster.de (M.T.); jan.puetzler@uni-muenster.de (J.P.); albert.schulzeboevingloh@ukmuenster.de (A.S.B.); Vincent.hofbauer@ukmuenster.de (V.H.); dr.luebben@gmail.com (T.L.); niklas.deventer@ukmuenster.de (N.D.); helmut.ahrens@ukmuenster.de (H.A.)

[2] Clinic for Radiology, Muenster University Hospital, Albert-Schweitzer-Campus 1, 48149 Muenster, Germany; robert.rischen@ukmuenster.de

* Correspondence: schulze.martin@uni-muenster.de

Abstract: The combination of 3D printing and navigation promises improvements in surgical procedures and outcomes for complex bone tumor resection of the trunk, but its features have rarely been described in the literature. Five patients with trunk tumors were surgically treated in our institution using a combination of 3D printing and navigation. The main process includes segmentation, virtual modeling and build preparation, as well as quality assessment. Tumor resection was performed with navigated instruments. Preoperative planning supported clear margin multiplanar resections with intraoperatively adaptable real-time visualization of navigated instruments. The follow-up ranged from 2–15 months with a good functional result. The present results and the review of the current literature reflect the trend and the diverse applications of 3D printing in the medical field. 3D printing at hospital sites is often not standardized, but regulatory aspects may serve as disincentives. However, 3D printing has an increasing impact on precision medicine, and we are convinced that our process represents a valuable contribution in the context of patient-centered individual care.

Keywords: 3D printing; navigation-assisted surgery; tumor orthopedics; oncologic orthopedics; patient specific; tumor surgery; bone defects

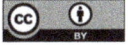

1. Introduction

Bone tumors are rare and account for less than 0.2% of primary malignant neoplasms registered in the database for the European Cancer Registry-based study on the survival and care of cancer patients (EUROCARE) [1].

The classification system for surgical treatment of malignant bone and soft tissue tumors was defined by Enneking [2]. The main objective of surgical treatment is wide tumor resection with sufficient safety margins free of tumor cells [3]. Resection is followed by reconstruction in a subsequent procedure. Tumors close to the trunk, e.g., in the thorax/spine, sacrum and pelvis, involve highly challenging surgical resection techniques compared to tumors of the extremities. Critical aspects are acceptable postoperative function, the preservation of critical neurovascular structures and low perioperative morbidity, mortality and recurrence rates [4,5].

For pelvic tumors, resection defects are classified according to the Dunham system (P1–P4). Functional limitations due to the loss of at least one hip joint component (P2)

in combination with very limited reconstruction possibilities make convalescence and mobilization of patients more difficult [6–8].

To improve the surgical procedure and outcome, two approaches may be considered. First, navigation-assisted surgical oncology has already proven its potential to reduce operation time, blood loss and the risk of intralesional resections in pelvic and sacral tumors [5,9]. Second, additive manufacturing (AM) processes are advancing in everyday clinical practice and are increasingly being used in trauma surgery, revision endoprosthetics and tumor orthopedics. In tumor orthopedics, in addition to the application of cutting guides for resection, reconstruction using individual implants is particularly notable [10–15].

The first and indispensable steps are the preparation of cross-sectional images and 3D modeling. Often, there is special interest in the early initiation of therapy, especially if the tumor progresses rapidly. Depending on the further processing of the 3D model, subsequent work steps may represent limiting factors to the aforementioned model.

By combining established intraoperative navigation with preoperative planning and creation of a patient-specific, full-size 3D-printed model, resection planes can be planned more precisely, healthy tissue and bone substances can be spared, biomechanics can be preserved and, if necessary, findings conventionally classified as inoperable can be surgically treated. Since there is no time required for design and production, therapy can be started almost immediately.

The aims of the present manuscript are to describe the combination of navigation and AM based on a retrospective analysis of a series of five cases and to review the current application of AM in tumor orthopedics.

Achievable advantages of combining navigation and AM include preservation of functional structures and joints, reduction of the risk of injury to internal organs, and planning of the operation using models true to the original to determine the most reasonable alternative for the patient without significant delay. A particular advantage is the opportunity to simulate functions and reconstruction of joint partners in advance in the 3D-printed model.

2. Materials and Methods

Five patients (aged 22 to 63 years) with malignancies close to the trunk were surgically treated in our institution between August 2019 and September 2020 using the combination of 3D printing and navigation. Admission of the patients to the combination of 3D printing and navigation was decided by the senior surgeons. In particular, the decision was based on the extent of the tumor and the expected complexity of the procedure, as well as potentially compromised anatomical structures in close spatial relationship to the tumor. Since this is of special relevance for tumors in the trunk region, different clinical entities were grouped as tumors close to the trunk for the present case series. All cases were histopathologically confirmed, staged, and presented to our interdisciplinary tumor board prior to surgery. All patients provided written informed consent for 3D print-assisted planning and navigation. Ethics committee permission was obtained for the present study (Ethics Committee of Medical Association of Westphalia-Lippe and the Medical Faculty of WWU Münster protocol code 2020-282-f-S, date of approval 30 April 2020).

Preoperative planning was based on diagnostic cross-sectional imaging. This requires both computed tomography (CT) with a maximum slice thickness of 1 mm [16] and contrast-enhanced magnetic resonance (MR) tomography with 1.5-Tesla field strength and multiaxial reconstruction in the T1/T2 sequences. The subsequent main process includes segmentation, virtual modeling and build preparation, as well as quality assessment, as depicted in Figure 1.

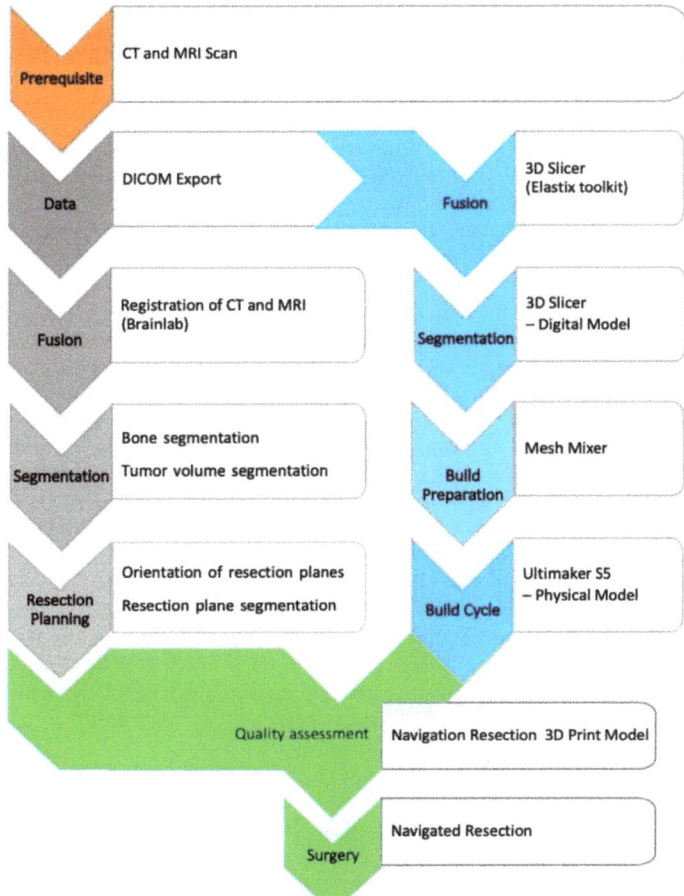

Figure 1. Flow chart for model processing.

The digital imaging and communications in medicine (DICOM) image data are transferred to software for further processing, segmentation, and model creation. Commercial software is available (for example, the approved medical device from *Materialise*; Leuven, Belgium). However, not every clinic has the resources to use this software, so experimental alternatives are being considered. One of these alternatives is the free open-source software *3D-Slicer* (release 4.10.2 from www.slicer.org (accessed on 27 October 2020)), which has been an established imaging tool in the biomedical sciences [17].

Segmentation is an essential part of model creation. Segmentation is the process of marking image elements layer by layer (2D) in a data set to allow grouping of similar elements into regions or volumes (3D). The tools used were thresholding, region growing, and manual sculpting. CT data can be used to mark anatomical bony structures particularly well, allowing a semi-automated approach. Soft tissue structures may be better segmented using magnetic resonance imaging (MRI) data. Databases of anatomical atlases are steadily improving and increasingly facilitate detection and segmentation [18–20]. However, tumors represent a special challenge, as they may contain both bony and soft tissue components and are individually distinct in terms of their geometry and spatial extent. We determined the tumor margin by looking at the transition of the marrow signal from abnormal to normal in T1-weighted MR images [21] (p. 2534).

The 3D model was exported as a mesh surface from planar triangles in a special format as standard tessellation language (STL) and prepared for 3D printing. A wide variety of processes can be suitable for model printing. Essential criteria are sufficient build space, speed, cost, and resolution of the print. We used an *Ultimaker-S5* printer (Ultimaker B.V., Utrecht, The Netherlands) with two print heads for printing with polylactide acid (PLA) polymer. This allows separate printing of support structures or the tumor component for visualization. The free software *Meshmixer* (Autodesk Inc., Dublin, Ireland) was used for preparation. Among other things, it can be used to optimize support structures. Furthermore, the software provides an inspection and repair tool to verify the mesh integrity and avoid print errors. Since the printing process can be fully simulated, material- and time-oriented optimization is possible. Printing is performed in a one-to-one model.

In the next essential step, the model was validated against the navigation system (*Kick—Brainlab*, Munich, Germany) in terms of its correspondence to the CT/MR image data. This can be done by region registration based on the acquisition of landmarks. Alternatively, registration using X-ray in two planes and subsequent matching for cross-sectional imaging is possible. The latter requires an additional contrast for X-rays, e.g., by means of zinc-containing coating. If there is sufficient accuracy within the error specified by the navigation manufacturer, it is possible for the surgical team to comprehensively evaluate the subsequent surgical steps and resection planes, as well as reconstruction options.

A systematic literature search was conducted via PubMed and Scopus plus Medical Subject Headings (MeSH) terms. After screening for duplicates, all titles and abstracts were reviewed. To maintain a broad perspective and include relevant articles, the references of the eligible articles were included in the search and added to the review where appropriate.

Articles that met the following exclusion criteria were not considered: studies on maxillofacial, cranium, or extremity tumors; studies in languages other than English or German; conference proceedings; studies solely for patient education; and studies solely on the printing of biomaterials.

3. Results

All surgeries were conducted as conventional operations, except the osteotomies and the speed burring, for which the navigation system was used. Image-to-patient registration was performed using one of the following three methods: paired points, surface matching or matching radiographs in two planes (*Xspot*, *Brainlab*, Munich, Germany).

3.1. Case 1

Case 1 involved a 22-year-old female patient suffering from a multiple cartilaginous exostosis disease with a secondary peripheral chondrosarcoma G3 of the right ilium without metastasis. The resection was performed as navigated internal hemipelvectomy (P1a), followed by augmentation of the right ileum with a standard screw-rod system (*Expedium, DePuy Synthes Spine Inc.*, Raynham, MA, USA) and revision cement (COPAL® G+C, Heraeus, Wehrheim, Germany) (Figure 2). This procedure allowed preservation of the hip joint. Trochanter resection was followed by reconstruction of the ventral hip joint capsule and reinsertion of the musculature using an attachment tube (*Implantcast*, Buxtehude, Germany). During treatment, superficial dry skin necrosis at the Enneking approach site occurred without signs of infection and eventually healed. The first follow-up 3 months after surgery showed a stable and increasingly fluid gait pattern with a positive Trendelenburg sign. The range of motion of the right hip joint was fully preserved. At the 15-month follow-up, the patient was free of pain and was able to walk a three-kilometer distance. The native X-ray and MRI of the pelvis showed no signs of tumor recurrence.

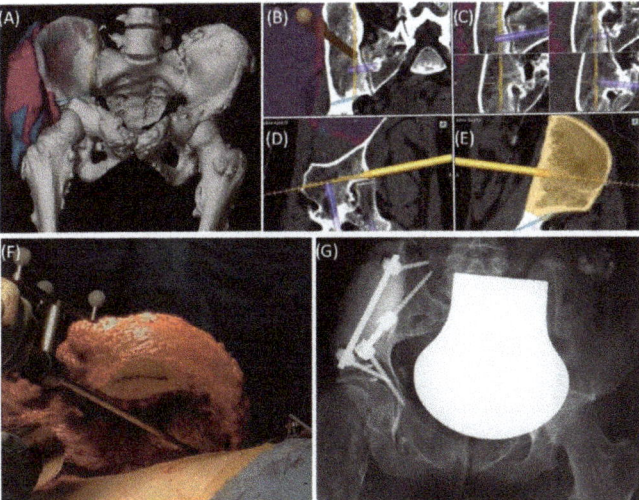

Figure 2. Case 1: Preoperative planning and segmentation of tumor volume components [bony (pink) and soft tissue (teal)] (**A**); resection planes [transverse (orange) and axial (blue)] during surgery with navigated chisel (orange) (**B–E**) intraoperative situs during resection (**F**); postoperative radiograph with reconstructed iliac defect (**G**).

3.2. Case 2

A 59-year-old female patient was diagnosed with bone metastasis of endometrial carcinoma of the sacrum with increasing and immobilizing pain. Primary radiation was discussed, but primary surgery and adjuvant radiation were preferred. Preoperatively, bladder/rectum dysfunction and a bladder-vaginal fistula were already present due to significant metastatic progression. The goal of 3D model-based planning and navigation was marginal resection of the metastasis in terms of a partial sacrectomy below S2 with ligation of the dural tube and the descending nerve roots below S2 (Figures 3 and 4). Repeated revision surgery and systemic antibiotic treatment after wound infection were necessary. At the two-month follow-up, further metastases with pulmonary foci, which did not exist preoperatively, were found. Palliative treatment and radiation followed.

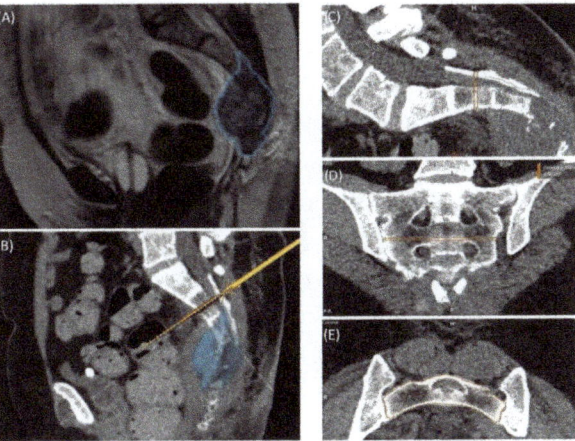

Figure 3. Case 2: Tumor segmentation (**A**) and resection plane planning (**B**), as well as preoperative validation of model accuracy with a navigated chisel resection of the 3D-printed model (**B–E**).

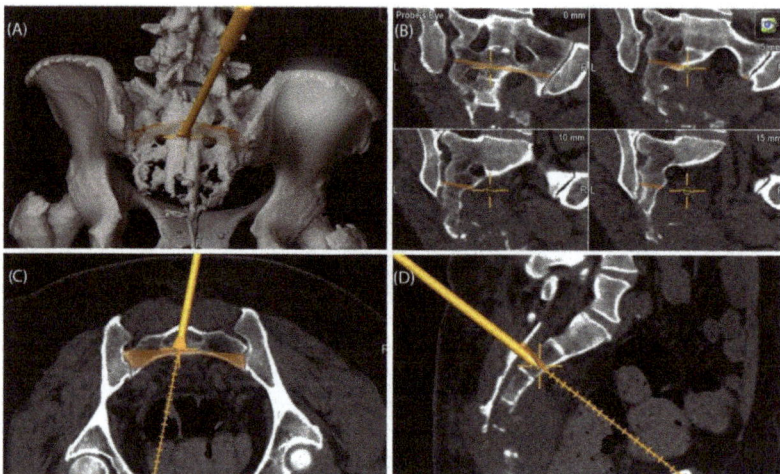

Figure 4. Case 2: 3D model of navigated chisel resection (**A**); resection planes in the axial and transversal planes (**C,D**); intraoperative view of the navigated chisel with crosshairs showing the location of the tip (**B**).

3.3. Case 3

Case 3 involved a 63-year-old female patient with a diagnosed inner thoracic chondrosarcoma (G2) of the 9th left rib. The soft tissue component extended from the 7th to the 11th rib next to the aorta and lungs (Figure 5). After CT-MRI fusion and planning, marginal resection was possible by combining a partial corpectomy T7–T11 with laminectomy T7–T11 and partial resection of ribs 7–11 on the left side. Reconstruction was carried out by instrumentation spondylodesis with a screw-rod system from T5-T11 and extensive coverage with bovine pericardium (Baxter, Deerfield, IL USA) (Figure 6). The postoperative histopathological examinations confirmed tumor-free resection margins and revealed a high-grade tumor (G3). After adjuvant radiation and a four-month postoperative follow-up, there was no sign of local recurrence. The patient returned to daily life without any sensomotoric deficit.

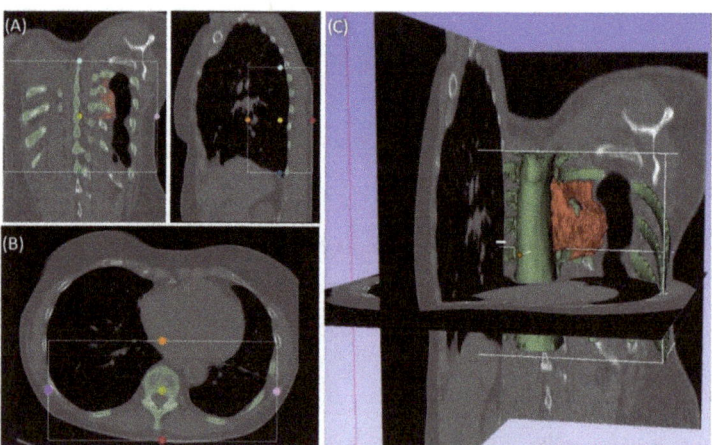

Figure 5. Segmentation of a thoracic chondrosarcoma and preparation for 3D model printing; cross-sectional segmentation (**A,B**) and 3D model with tumor volume (red) (**C**).

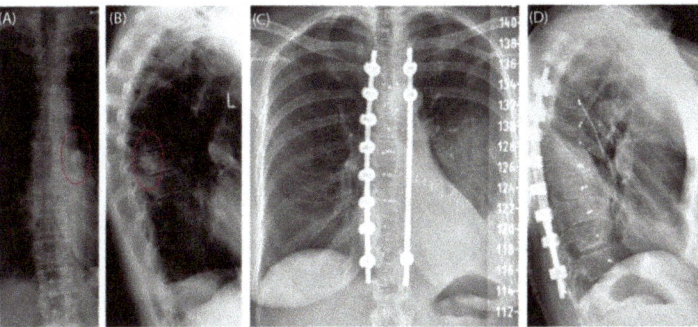

Figure 6. Case 3: Preoperative radiographs in frontal (**A**) and lateral (**B**) views, red circles indicate the bony tumor mass; postoperative radiographs in frontal (**C**) and lateral (**D**) views.

3.4. Case 4

A 49-year-old female patient was diagnosed with an unclear sacral/coccygeal mass that was painful on palpation. The patient reported load-dependent coccydynia for 6–7 months with no typical radiculopathy, intact sensorimotor function, and regular fecal/urinary continence. After biopsy, high-grade osteoblastic osteosarcoma was diagnosed, and four cycles of neoadjuvant chemotherapy were administered according to the EURO-BOSS protocol. Navigated resection of the sacral region S2/S3 to S5, including the coccyx (Figure 7), reconstruction of the defect of the rectal intestinal wall and reconstruction using a Vicryl mesh loaded with gentamycin chains, were conducted. Histopathologically, a R0 resection with a regression degree of 4 according to Salzer–Kuntschik was confirmed. Incontinence remained due to the resection of the sacral nerve roots. Because of reduced physical status, chemotherapy was not continued postoperatively.

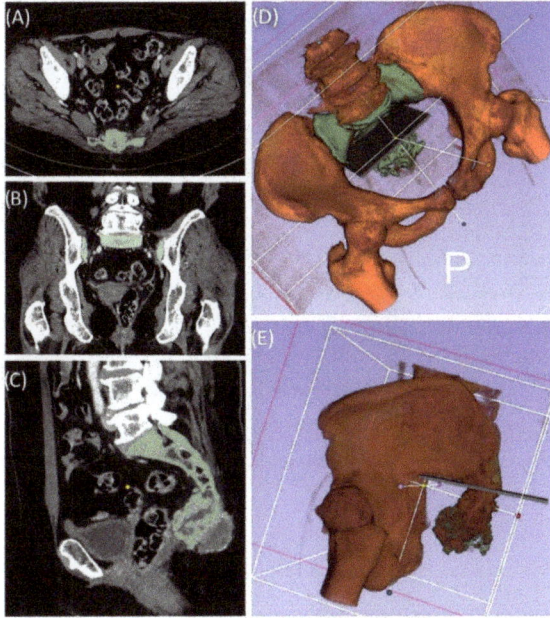

Figure 7. Case 4: Segmentation and resection plane planning of a high-grade osteoblastic osteosarcoma of the sacrum; cross-sectional segmentation (**A–C**) and 3D model with the resection plane as the volume (gray) (**D**,**E**).

3.5. Case 5

A 58-year-old male patient was diagnosed with a giant cell tumor of the left pelvis in 2013. After five years of conservative treatment with denosumab, he developed recurrent jawbone osteonecrosis. Therefore, the treatment was stopped in 2018. Consequently, tumor progression with increasing symptoms occurred, and surgical resection was indicated after rebiopsy and histopathological confirmation. Intralesional resection was performed via high-speed burr curettage followed by adjuvant polymethyl methacrylate filling (Figures 8 and 9). This approach allowed preservation of the hip joint. Foot drop on the left side was noted postoperatively, and hip flexion was restricted to 60° for 4 weeks postoperatively to avoid luxation. At the 6-month follow-up, the patient had free range of motion of the hip in all directions except for a maximum of 10° external rotation. The foot drop increasingly improved, and orthosis was no longer necessary at this point.

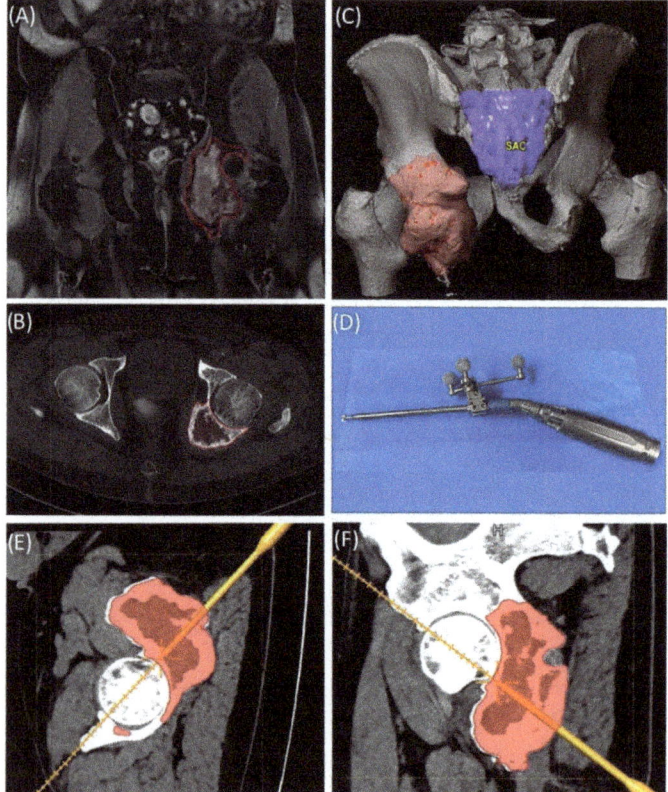

Figure 8. Case 5: Segmentation of the giant cell tumor in magnetic resonance imagining (MRI) (**A**) and computed tomography (CT) (**B**) scans, segmented tumor volume (**C**), high-speed burr navigation (**D**), intraoperative navigation of the tumor volume with the high-speed burr tool tip (**E,F**).

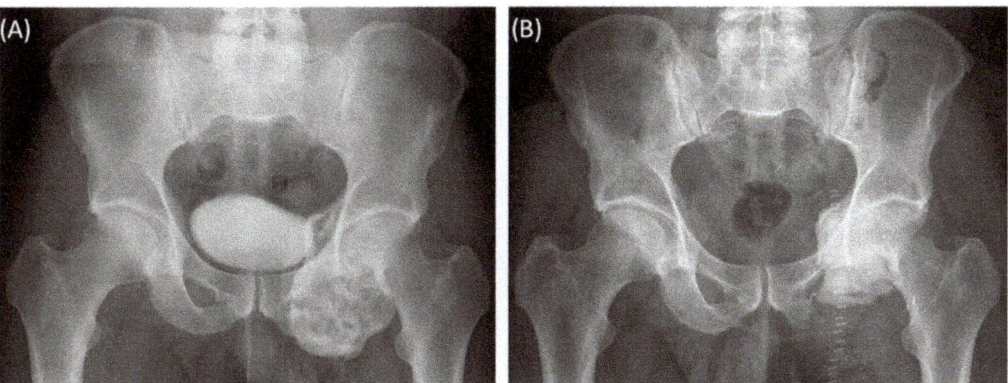

Figure 9. Case 5: Preoperative plain radiograph of the acetabular giant cell tumor (**A**) and postoperative result after resection of the dorsal parts and intralesional curettage with a navigated burr and augmentation with polymethyl methacrylate (**B**).

3.6. Review of Literature

The initial search with "bone tumor AND 3D printing" resulted in 254 PubMed and 205 Scopus matches up to 27 October 2020. Of these, the majority were articles and case reports; some were reviews (21 in PubMed and 22 in Scopus), and only one was a systematic review.

The results for "(printing, three-dimensional [MeSH Terms]) AND (surgery, computer-assisted [MeSH Terms]) AND (bone and bones)" included 138 articles but decreased to seven when excluding the terms "cranio", "maxilla" and "facial" (Figure 10).

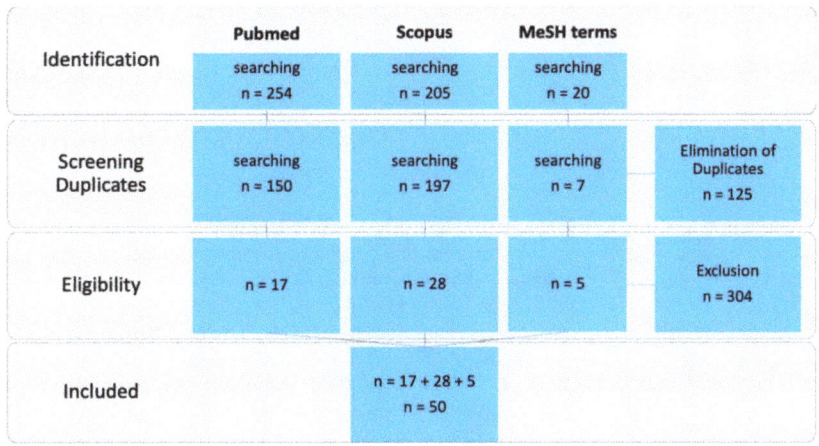

Figure 10. PRISMA (Preferred Reporting Items for Systematic Reviews and Meta-Analyses) flow chart with 50 articles included.

4. Discussion

In our case series, we combined navigated tumor resection with preoperative planning by 3D modeling and printing and successfully evaluated the navigation steps from the printed model for complex bone tumor resection of the trunk. From our process and clinical follow-up, we are encouraged and convinced of its safety. However, this study involves the development and testing of an experimental approach. The development of an in-house standard with further quality assessment is a future task. For this reason, a review of the current literature was conducted, and key aspects were identified that could help with in-house validation.

The overall 5-year survival of pelvic sarcomas is reported to be less than 28% [22]. Oncological and functional outcomes depend on several factors. One factor is a tumor-free margin which can compete with the wish of a good functional outcome. Without any technical assistance, e.g., navigation, even an experienced surgeon is challenged to consequently achieve a clearly defined margin with the complex anatomy of the pelvis [23]. Clinical findings of conventional resections report an incidence of intralesional resection at the pelvis of 29% and a recurrence rate of 27% [24]. Therefore, the request for improvement is justified.

In a case series of 13 patients (seven with pelvic tumors, six with upper extremity tumors), individual implants for reconstruction were presented by Angelini et al. in 2019. At the two-year follow-up, at least good functional results were reported, with a complication rate of 38.5%. The authors suggested an experience-based decision-making algorithm for deciding on reconstruction of the pelvis rather than modular prosthesis for individual implant construction depending on the resection level [25]. No information on the time span for planning, construction and manufacturing until surgery was given.

The indirect effects of 3D printing on surgical procedures, including reduced surgery time, reduced blood loss or radiation time, are reported in the literature [26,27]. This may contribute to a reduced complication rate of wound infections and wound healing disorders [6–8] and therefore enable earlier adjuvant therapy initiation.

As another result of these observations, it is clear that 3D printing in the context of preoperative planning helps to avoid wasting resources, e.g., by not having to try out appropriate instruments in the operating room first, thus avoiding unnecessary reserialization or disposal [28].

As early as 2018, the 3D printing Special Interest Group (SIG) unveiled a rating system that highlighted the suitability of medical 3D printing for clinical use, research, scientific, and informative purposes [28]. According to this evaluation system, four particularly suitable main groups were identified: craniomaxillofacial trauma, congenital malformations, acquired/developmental deformities, and neoplasms. In particular, the last group applies to the cases presented here. While Chepelev et al. mainly focused on technical aspects, from a tumor orthopedic point of view, there are additional aspects to be considered regarding disease progression, therapy stages, and surgical safety.

In the course of this review, we would like to take a closer look at further aspects and perspectives of recent findings from research.

4.1. 3D Printing for the Treatment of Tumors

Future trends in the treatment of bone metastasis aim to improve local recurrence control and to overcome systemic side effects by local solutions using therapeutic osteoinductive and osteoconductive adjuvants in 3D-printed biodegradable spacers with structural support. In their review on advances in personalized metastatic therapy, Ahangar et al. mentioned their promising results from an in vitro study on drug-eluting nanoporous 3D-printed scaffolds [29]. They concluded that tissue-engineered bone substitutes have high potential to circumvent the limitations of conventional therapy strategies, e.g., donor site morbidity of bone grafts. Despite these encouraging innovations, clinical data and experience are still limited.

Haleem et al. 2020 conducted a literature review on the basic applications of 3D printing to improve tumor therapy. In their article, the authors grouped the applications of 3D printing as follows: replicas of cancerous parts, 3D phantoms of tumors and organs, treatment of tumor tissue, study cancer growth, monitoring of cancer treatment, teaching tools, etc. With their concise look at 3D printing on bioprintables, they shed light on the potential of this manufacturing technology for cancer therapy. However, this has to be distinguished from classical AM methods using plastics, ceramics, or metals due to the effects on active cells and metabolic activity.

Consequently, there is no reference in their work to an application using or combining 3D printing with intraoperative navigation or custom endoprosthetics [30].

4.2. Patient-Specific Devices—Personal Surgical Instruments (PSIs)

Patient-specific devices are increasingly used and include any anatomy-fitted jigs, cutting guides, templates for implant positioning and implants [12–14,27,31–34]. Numerous case reports illustrate and complement the versatility of using personal surgical instruments (PSIs) [35].

Although software and development are steadily improving, technical demands for accurate automatic algorithms for medical image processing, especially in the field of image segmentation and registration, are unabated. The user friendliness of powerful software tools is only one factor, among others, to provide access to a patient-specific design of instruments and implants [36]. Aside from the technical aspects, the use of these individual solutions also raises several questions in clinical practice.

The use of custom instruments has raised the question of possible effects on wound healing. For pelvic tumor surgery, complications such as wound infections can occur, e.g., after a longer operation time and extended resection, including custom implants [37]. In a retrospective analysis, Shea et al. presented a large cohort of more than 100 patients who received patient-specific devices or intraoperatively used anatomical models within a 4-year period. In their study, they presented a detailed workflow and examined the infection rate associated with the intraoperative patient-specific models used after hydrogen peroxide plasma sterilization. In the published results, the infection rate of 7% was not significantly different from that with standard surgical procedures. Shea et al. concluded that their process is safe for continuation and implementation elsewhere [38].

Another significant aspect from the orthopedic tumor point of view is the recurrence rate. In a prospective study of nine cases in comparison to a historical control group of 19 cases, Robin et al. reported a reduction in the local recurrence rate to zero with the use of 3D-printed patient-specific instruments [39].

The use of customized 3D-printed implants has introduced a wide range of possibilities [40]. However, outcome and function depend largely on correct positioning and the quality of the implant-bone interface in terms of primary and secondary stability [33,41]. In particular, the design of porous implant structures has an important influence on osteointegration, osteoconduction and osteoinduction and should match the patients' needs [42,43]. The choice of optimal design parameters is only one of many factors that still require close collaboration between clinicians and engineers. The articles by Kwok et al. 2016 [33] or Mitsouras et al. 2015 already illustrated this clearly [44].

Since the cutting templates and individual implants, or at least the manufacturing process itself, require approval as medical devices, the application may be limited to a small circle of users; in our experience, this type of approach cannot feasibly be made available to all users in a timely manner at present.

4.3. Navigation-Assisted Surgery

Cho et al. investigated the long-term outcomes of navigation-assisted bone tumor surgery in 18 cases and used software-based preoperative resection planning. The described MRI to CT image-to-image registration was performed using K-wire or resorbable pin placement before imaging. The author's defined acceptable error was <2 mm. Comparison of the histopathological margins to the preoperative plan showed a maximum error of 3 mm. The time for navigation setup was reported to be less than 30 min [9]. The average intraoperative navigation time during surgery was reported by Wong et al. to be less than 25 min [21].

In another retrospective analysis of pelvic and sacral primary tumors of navigation-assisted resections, Jeys et al. demonstrated that navigation helped to preserve sacral nerve roots, convert inoperable findings into operable ones, and avoid hindquarter amputations. The authors concluded that the risk of intralesional resection and, at least in an over short observation period, the local recurrence rate can be positively influenced by navigation [24].

A direct comparison of standard versus navigation-assisted resection was performed by Laitinen et al. in a retrospective study. They confirmed the aforementioned findings and additionally reported significantly reduced blood loss and a non-significantly reduced operation time. Based on these results and with reference to other authors, the authors concluded that navigation allows accurate visualization of the tumor, predictable alignment of osteotomies, and accurate placement of custom prostheses. Accordingly, more accurate resection may allow preservation of articular surfaces, which is unlikely without navigation [5].

Consistently, the authors concluded that computer-assisted navigation reduces the risk of intralesional resections and recurrence rates and furthermore improves functional outcomes.

Image-to-patient registration errors less than 2 mm seem to be a minimum requirement [9], but less than 1 mm is considered acceptable [5,24,45].

For spinal screw insertion, a surface registration accuracy of 0.5 mm is advised in CT-guided navigation as the clinical threshold [46]. Thus, CT scan data should provide similar accuracy, depending on the anatomic region and surgical needs, with commonly reported slice thicknesses between 0.5 for fine bone structures and 2.0 mm for larger structures, such as the pelvis and sacrum [47,48]. In line with these requirements, our scan parameters ranged from 0.6–1.5 mm. The detailed scan parameters are presented in Table A1 in Appendix A.

Cartiaux et al. demonstrated improved accuracy with navigation in simulated bone tumor surgery compared to freehand resection and concluded a possible benefit for pelvic tumor surgery by achieving clinically acceptable margins [49].

4.4. Navigation and Anatomic Modeling

The use of 3D anatomical models in combination with intraoperative navigation for pelvic tumors has been reported in the past. Zhang et al. described a case of hemipelvectomy and concluded that the combination allows a more targeted approach and safe osteotomies. However, in their study, the 3D model based on CT data was used only for spatial orientation. Navigation of the model for preoperative preparation did not occur. Accordingly, it is not clear whether a control of the dimensions and thus an actual 1:1 model was used [50].

Another case report by Heunis et al. describes a similar approach. The model was created by an external company, and intraoperative navigation was performed, in which the model only served as a visual guide and supplementary physical orientation aid [51].

Considering these rare literature results, our case series represents the first comprehensively described combination of preoperative planning and navigation on individual 3D models.

4.5. Accuracy of PSIs and Individual Implants vs. Navigation

The resection error ranges from 1 to 4 mm from planned resection to implant position with PSIs [52].

In a subsequent study, Cartiaux et al. compared the osteotomy results from three different modalities with their pelvic bone model: free hand, PSI and navigation assisted. They evaluated the location accuracy of defined osteotomy planes at the pelvis with a PSI in a saw bone model with the aim of a 10 mm safe margin to a virtual tumor volume. Compared to free-hand osteotomy, this approach yielded a significantly higher average accuracy of 1.0 to 3.7 mm and a lower difference of 3.1 to 5.1 mm from the targeted safe margin. The navigation-assisted osteotomy results were comparable, suggesting an equivalence to the PSI. In this model, the PSI was superior to navigation in terms of time consumption, which they explained by the predefined best-fit position of the PSI on the bony surface [53]. While these results are from an ideal in vitro setup without soft tissue and vulnerable in situ structures, the reported time consumption for the setup of the navigation system and patient registration are routine and system dependent.

In a prospective cohort of 11 patients, Gouin et al. resected pelvic bone tumors using PSIs. The authors defined different distances (from 3 to 15 mm) as desired safe margins. The location accuracy of the PSIs was reported to range from 1.5 to 4.4 mm. Deviations from the desired margins were within the acceptable range. One instance of local recurrence after

18 months of follow-up was reported. These results are comparable to those of a cadaver study from Sallent et al., which showed that a mean improvement of the accuracy up to 9.6 mm in sacroiliac osteotomies could be achieved by using PSIs [54]. The authors concluded that PSI-assisted surgeries can be performed safely with an accuracy that is clinically relevant for pelvic bone tumor surgery. The limitations of the study included the lack of a control group and randomization. Nevertheless, this study shows that multiplanar resection of tumors benefits from comprehensive preoperative planning and that the presented approach has the potential to improve patient safety and thus recurrence-free survival under certain conditions.

Depending on the rapid prototyping technology, PSIs are provided with a dimensional tolerance, e.g., 0.2 mm. These instruments are often made of plastics and carry a risk of unintentional material removal during drilling or osteotomy. The possible unintentional retention of the fine particles in situ must be viewed extremely critically.

One possible critical aspect of individual surgical instruments and implants is the time-consuming design and verification process, including biomechanical considerations. Even in a print-on-demand setup with professional engineer support in a standardized process, this may take several months, excluding analysis with the finite element method (FEM) [52,55].

4.6. Biomechanical Considerations

The FEM supports the mathematical consideration of complex relationships of material properties, such as stresses, reactions in the implant bearing with bearing forces and deformations. The models are often validated empirically. As early as the 1990s, Dalstra and Huiskes used the FEM to investigate the main loading zones of the pelvis. With their results, they were able to show that despite considerable variance in the force applied to the hip joint, the resulting vector affects the anterior and superior portions of the acetabulum. Accordingly, the most important load-bearing portions of the pelvic bone are the sacroiliac joint and pubic symphysis, with load transfer through the superior acetabular rim, the incisura ischiadicae, and, to a lesser extent, the pubic bone [56].

The importance of the biomechanics of the pelvis and hip joints was revealed by several preliminary works and different parameters [57,58]. Lee et al. showed with an FEM investigation of a case of periacetabular osteotomy that by changing the joint angles by a few degrees, the contact area of the joint partners could be increased by a factor of 10, and surface pressure in the joint could be halved [57].

Simulation using an FEM approach can help to make the decision between several reconstruction and anchorage alternatives [52,59,60]. The anatomical variability of different individuals is difficult to account for in models based on image data of one patient. Sophisticated models are often based on extensive validation with numerous material parameters. These are typically limited to passive structures such as bone, cartilage, and ligaments [59]. Consideration of active muscle forces is the subject of current research, and to date, metabolic processes for prognosis can hardly be represented in an individual model.

For a realistic biomechanical assessment, surgical planning and, if necessary, an individual endoprosthesis, the open source database OrtohLoad.com (accessed on 28 October 2020) offers additional comprehensive in vivo data samples of joint contact forces and moments, whole body kinematics and ground reaction forces [61].

This existing knowledge should be considered when planning resection levels and individual reconstructions, and recent developments in simulation should be carefully implemented and included in considerations when possible. This can help to identify unfavorable loading situations of implants to optimize implant positioning and thus effectively reduce risks such as loosening or material failure.

Beyond that, however, in a clinical setting, it is questionable whether the time required for an individual FEM approach justifies planning for tumor resection and reconstruction.

4.7. Regulatory and Technical Considerations

As already stated by Chepelev et al., "The United States Food and Drug Administration (FDA) classifies medical 3D printing software into design manipulation software that enables medical device design and modification and build preparation software that enables the conversion of the digital design into a file format that is 3D printable [. . .]" [62]. The FDA expert group identified various critical aspects in the AM process. In their non-binding recommendation, they describe these considerations, e.g., the effects of medical imaging: quality and resolution for matching, smoothing or image processing algorithms that could influence the dimensions compared to the referenced anatomy, effects from soft and bony tissue structures and uniqueness of anatomic landmarks. As an example, the geometry and volume of a tumor could not be consistent over time or may have been influenced by patient movement during examination, leading to a mismatch of imaging and patient features. Therefore, a risk-based approach for process validation is recommended to prevent these effects/meet these constraints. This also includes but is not limited to a validation of [63]:

1. File format conversions, for example, when changing the applied software.
2. Digital device design in a general four-step process: 1. The placement of the model in the build volume, 2. the addition of support structures, 3. slicing and 4. build path generation. For example, support structures can influence surface quality or geometry, or warping can occur.
3. Machine parameters and environment: preventive maintenance intervals, calibration, environmental conditions in the build volume (temperature, atmospheric composition) and adjustable machine parameters should be documented.
4. Material controls: the raw material should be provided with detailed data sheets by the manufacturer. The printing process can influence these parameters. Therefore, further tests may be required for the processed material.
5. Postprocessing: this may include, among other things, the finishing of surfaces to improve surface quality. However, the device performance must not be negatively affected and must be ensured by suitable methods, such as mechanical tests.
6. Process validation: a manufactured model or device must have clear and verifiable quality characteristics. The variability of input parameters and manufacturing steps has an influence on this. If the AM process result is not fully verified, process validation must be performed. Test coupons that are printed together with the model or device can help with process validation. These have defined geometries and surface structures and can be positioned appropriately to serve as a worst-case scenario and assure quality control for the actual AM print job.

However, there is often a lack of in-house expertise on implant design and the necessary on-site manufacturing technology with a corresponding comprehensive quality management system for the design and manufacture of medical devices, e.g., according to ISO 13485 [55].

Even if the result of the in-house process is an anatomical model and not a higher classified patient-specific device, compliance with regulatory requirements is mandatory. The European Union (EU) Medical Device Regulation (MDR) guidelines require that all processes for the design and manufacturing of a device for medical use be registered. A certain imprecision of the MDR guidelines remains with regard to segmentation of image data and software packages used. It should therefore be in the interest of every facility to comply as closely as possible with the MDR guidelines for anatomic models. Processes described in detail by various authors, such as Chepelev et al. 2018 and Willemsen et al. 2019, who have already worked out a procedural workflow in consideration of the regulatory framework, could serve as a blueprint [28,55].

4.8. Costs, Print Time and Quality

In the literature, 3D printing has been repeatedly evaluated for its effects on surgical procedures. Reduced surgery time and reduced blood loss are among them [27]. However, there is also a comprehensive financial analysis of operating room costs. In a review by

Ballard et al., the repeatedly observed reduced surgery time of approximately 20–60 min on average indicates a significant cost reduction of the equivalent of 1200–3200 euros in the operating room. However, this is counterbalanced by the resources and expertise required for 3D printing. According to this, a break-even point is already reached at 1.2 models/week [64].

The choice of the printing method determines the extent of the investment and operating costs for an on-site printing system in a hospital. Fused filament fabrication (FFF)/fused deposition modeling (FDM) filament printers have become accessible for lower four-digit amounts (in euros), while PolyJet (liquid photopolymer jet) printers and other processes, such as laser sintering (SLS) or stereolithography (SLA), easily cost high six-digit amounts. In addition to the initial purchase expense of a device, higher costs can quickly be incurred for maintenance and materials. It is undisputed that filament printing is currently the most cost-effective method. Beyond this, the choice for the printing method should also depend on the intended use of the printed result (anatomic model, PSI or PSI) [44].

Chen et al. tested different printing technologies with different settings, such as infill, layer height, and orientation on a model print bed, and assessed their effect on the estimated duration and cost of anatomical models. The FDM method proved to be the most cost-effective method, with a cost of less than 20 USD per printed model. While 5% changes in infill had no significant impact, different orientations in the print bed resulted in cost increases of 35% and print duration increases of 40%. While printing with other methods is significantly more cost-effective, the expected printing time is up to $\frac{3}{4}$ shorter with the PolyJet method. However, the actual time required for a print job can differ significantly from the estimate [65]. With their study, Chen et al. provided a comparison of different AM technologies and also considered the orientation of the print model. However, technology is developing rapidly in a fast-growing market, and their overview is a limited snapshot. Each technology has its benefits, and there is an increasing number of options for materials or even compounds in the field of AM. Therefore, the choice for the right printer should never be influenced solely by the purchase price.

The cost and effort of postprocessing or maintenance have not been specified in the literature as of the time of our review but should be considered when choosing the printing method and printer.

Due to the high resolution of the printers, the achievable quality of the print result usually exceeds the quality of the diagnostic imaging used for modeling, since slice thicknesses of several millimeters are often used here. However, numerous process variables must be considered for the print result.

Beyond this, print time and accuracy are dependent on essential parameters such as the resolution. There is a difference in printing resolution in the xy-direction, which represents the horizontal plane, and the z-resolution, which is given with the layer height of the print [66]. In the field of FFF/FDM printers, the normal resolution of the nozzle is 0.4 mm. The laser resolution of SLS Printers is normally 0.1 mm, and the resolution of PolyJet printers is approximately 600 PPI. You can easily change the nozzle of an FFF/FDM printer to 0.6 mm or 0.8 mm. In contrast to the layer height, a software setting, these are hardware settings that can only be modified by exchanging printer components. It should also be noted that not every manufacturer offers this option.

Consequently, the print-speed-accuracy matrix is not a 2D but a 3D function of layer height, object size and xy-resolution (Figure 11). A large object printed with a thin xy-resolution and a small layer height takes the longest print time. A small object printed with a thick xy-resolution and a large layer height can be printed faster. The accuracy correlates negatively with the print time. Furthermore, a large layer height may result in the loss of details in the z-direction. A higher xy-resolution allows a smaller radius at edges in the horizontal plane. This effect is comparable to industrial milling, where a small radius is the effect of a cutter with a small diameter.

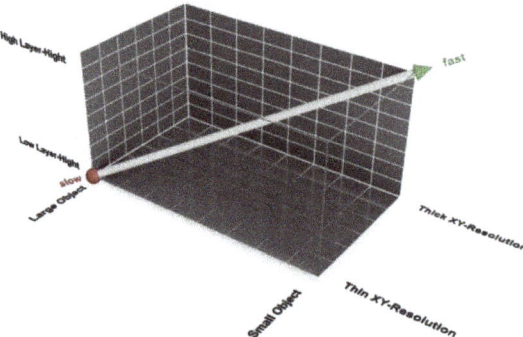

Figure 11. Print duration as a function of layer height, object size and xy-plane resolution for fused filament fabrication/fused deposition modeling (FFF/FDM) filament printing methods.

4.9. Special Considerations and Pitfalls

- Input image quality, slice thickness/step phenomenon, kernel [67], noise reduction, mesh quality and number of triangles [44] scaling errors in import/export processes and wrapping.
- Smoothing of relevant structures.
- Resection margins should not be reduced.
- Rapid tumor progression must be considered, so images must be up to date.

When considering the aforementioned aspects and perspectives on accuracy, time savings, and additional costs for the possible applications of AM, regulatory aspects also play a key role. Finally, the production processes and the large number of selectable input variables are determining factors for the printing result. Therefore, statements on comparisons in the literature that suggest general validity should be interpreted with caution. For an illustrative model for discussion with the patient or for teaching purposes, different requirements must certainly be met compared to a model that is directly associated with the treatment of the patient, especially if it is used for the design of patient-specific templates, implants, or the planning of planes for navigated resection. For clinicians aiming to design their first experimental models, a step-by-step guide with valuable hints would be helpful to get started in this exciting but also partially complex field of medical 3D printing [62,68].

4.10. Advantages of Our Approach

The presented procedure allows a clinical team of surgeons and radiologists to become familiar with the techniques and possibilities of AM technologies. The generation of a 3D model and validation of its accuracy were the first steps towards patient-centered treatment using 3D printing in our hospital. The experience gained enables the development of a process standard in one's own clinic, which can facilitate the step towards the development of individualized patient instruments and implants.

The benefits of our approach are as follows:

1. Replicates individual anatomy for preoperative planning, respecting critical structures.
2. Decreased surgical time and blood loss.
3. Preoperatively and intraoperatively adaptable with real-time visualization of multi-planar resections.
4. Variable navigated instruments (chisel, saw) for precise real-time visual control during resection.
5. Safe usability in simple and complex soft tissue situations.
6. Improved possibility for implant placement (without additional traumatic surgical preparation for drill holes or fixation pins for jigs and patient-specific instruments).

7. Decreased radiation exposure.
8. Supports tumor clear margin resection.

5. Conclusions

In our study, we presented a series of cases with complex bone tumor resection and described the combination of navigation and additively manufactured 3D models as an option for improved tumor resection planning.

The review of the current literature confirms the trend and diverse applications of 3D printing in the medical field. It also revealed that 3D printing in hospitals allows it to be used in a variety of applications and that processing is not standardized. Often, quality assurance standards are missing, partially because different perspectives and disciplines as well as regulatory aspects must be considered. For a safe procedure, the process should be transparently validated for patient-specific care at each hospital. For this purpose, it is recommended to have a clear process evaluation plan.

Like other authors, we are convinced that the increasing number of cases and presented evidence indicate that these methods can influence parameters in the treatment of complex musculoskeletal diseases. This includes patient and physician satisfaction, operation time, blood loss and various direct and indirect costs associated with shared decision making and patient-centered processes [28].

Three-dimensional (3D) printing has an increasing impact on precision medicine, and the presented case series represents a good alternative contributing to patient-centered individual care. It is expected that the future development of 3D printing will offer more solutions for patient-specific care in hospitals. It is our responsibility to take the next step and set up a framework in conformity with regulatory demands and to validate our approach to provide safety information and meet the highest medical standards.

Author Contributions: All authors substantially contributed throughout the study and approved the final submitted version of this manuscript. Individual contributions were as follows: conceptualization and methodology, G.G., V.H., R.R., H.A. and M.S.; software: segmentation and modeling, M.S., V.H., N.D., T.L. and T.B.; validation, T.L., N.D. and V.H.; formal Analysis, T.B. and R.R.; investigation, N.D., M.D.V., H.A. and M.S.; writing—original draft preparation, M.S., R.R., J.P. and T.L.; writing—review and editing, N.D., H.A., V.H., M.T., S.B., A.S.B., M.D.V., T.B., J.P. and R.R.; visualization, M.S. and M.T.; and supervision, G.G., N.D. and H.A. All authors have read the manuscript and concur with its content. The authors affirm that the material within this work has not been published or submitted for publication elsewhere. All authors have read and agreed to the published version of the manuscript.

Funding: This research received no external funding.

Institutional Review Board Statement: The study was conducted according to the guidelines of the Declaration of Helsinki and approved by the Ethics Committee of the Medical Association of Westphalia-Lippe and the Medical Faculty of WWU Münster (protocol code 2020-282-f-S, date of approval 30 April 2020).

Informed Consent Statement: Informed consent was obtained from all subjects involved in the study.

Conflicts of Interest: The authors declare no conflict of interest.

Appendix A

Table A1. Computed tomography (CT) scan parameters in cases 1–5, all in a matrix of 512 × 512.

Case	Device	Voltage (kV)	Electric Current (mAs)	Dose-Length Product (mGy*cm)	Slice Thickness (mm)	Pitch	Kernel
1	Siemens Somatom Definition Flash	100	2976	435	1.5	0.6	I26f
2	Siemens Somatom Definition Flash	120	1207	286	0.6	0.8	B20f
3	Siemens Somatom Definition Force	100	1145	233	0.75	0.8	Br69
4	Siemens Perspective	n/a	n/a	n/a	1.0	1.5	I80s
5	Siemens Somatom Definition Navigator S16	100	3862	313	1.0	0.9	B70F

References

1. Stiller, C.; Trama, A.; Serraino, D.; Rossi, S.; Navarro, C.; Chirlaque, M.; Casali, P.G. Descriptive epidemiology of sarcomas in Europe: Report from the RARECARE project. *Eur. J. Cancer* **2013**, *49*, 684–695. [CrossRef] [PubMed]
2. Enneking, W.F.; Dunham, W.K. Resection and reconstruction for primary neoplasms involving the innominate bone. *J. Bone Jt. Surg.* **1978**, *60*, 731–746. [CrossRef]
3. Casali, P.G.; Bielack, S.; Abecassis, N.; Aro, H.; Bauer, S.; Biagini, R.; Bonvalot, S.; Boukovinas, I.; Bovee, J.V.M.G.; Brennan, B.; et al. Bone sarcomas: ESMO–PaedCan–EURACAN Clinical Practice Guidelines for diagnosis, treatment and follow-up. *Ann. Oncol.* **2018**, *29*, iv79–iv95. [CrossRef] [PubMed]
4. Fiorenza, F.; Abudu, A.; Grimer, R.J.; Carter, S.R.; Tillman, R.M.; Ayoub, K.; Mangham, D.C.; Davies, A.M. Risk factors for survival and local control in chondrosarcoma of bone. *J. Bone Jt. Surg.* **2002**, *84*, 93–99. [CrossRef]
5. Laitinen, M.; Parry, M.C.; Albergo, J.I.; Grimer, R.J.; Jeys, L.M. Is computer navigation when used in the surgery of iliosacral pelvic bone tumours safer for the patient? *Bone Jt. J.* **2017**, *99-B*, 261–266. [CrossRef]
6. Ogura, K.; Boland, P.J.; Fabbri, N.; Healey, J. Rate and risk factors for wound complications after internal hemipelvectomy. *Bone Jt. J.* **2020**, *102-B*, 280–284. [CrossRef]
7. Senchenkov, A.; Moran, S.L.; Petty, P.M.; Knoetgen, J.; Clay, R.P.; Bite, U.; Barnes, S.A.; Sim, F.H. Predictors of Complications and Outcomes of External Hemipelvectomy Wounds: Account of 160 Consecutive Cases. *Ann. Surg. Oncol.* **2007**, *15*, 355–363. [CrossRef]
8. Rudert, M.; Holzapfel, B.; Pilge, H.; Rechl, H.; Gradinger, R. Beckenteilresektion (innere Hemipelvektomie) und endoprothetischer Ersatz bei hüftgelenksnahen Tumoren. *Oper. Orthop. Traumatol.* **2012**, *24*, 196–214. [CrossRef]
9. Cho, H.S.; Oh, J.H.; Han, I.; Kim, H.-S. The outcomes of navigation-assisted bone tumour surgery. *J. Bone Jt. Surg.* **2012**, *94*, 1414–1420. [CrossRef]
10. Fang, C.; Cai, H.; Kuong, E.; Chui, E.; Siu, Y.C.; Ji, T.; Drstvenšek, I. Surgical applications of three-dimensional printing in the pelvis and acetabulum: From models and tools to implants. *Der Unf.* **2019**, *122*, 278–285. [CrossRef]
11. Moreta-Martinez, R.; García-Mato, D.; García-Sevilla, M.; Pérez-Mañanes, R.; Calvo-Haro, J.; Pascau, J. Augmented reality in computer-assisted interventions based on patient-specific 3D printed reference. *Health Technol. Lett.* **2018**, *5*, 162–166. [CrossRef]
12. Gómez-Palomo, J.M.; Estades-Rubio, F.J.; Meschian-Coretti, S.; Montañez-Heredia, E.; Fuente, F.J.D.S.-D.L. Internal Hemipelvectomy and Reconstruction Assisted by 3D Printing Technology Using Premade Intraoperative Cutting and Placement Guides in a Patient With Pelvic Sarcoma. *JBJS Case Connect.* **2019**, *9*, e0060. [CrossRef]
13. Liu, X.; Liu, Y.; Lu, W.; Liao, S.; Du, Q.; Deng, Z.; Lu, W. Combined Application of Modified Three-Dimensional Printed Anatomic Templates and Customized Cutting Blocks in Pelvic Reconstruction after Pelvic Tumor Resection. *J. Arthroplast.* **2019**, *34*, 338–345.e1. [CrossRef]
14. Ma, L.; Zhou, Y.; Lin, Z.; Wang, Y.; Zhang, Y.; Xia, H.; Mao, C. 3D-printed guiding templates for improved osteosarcoma resection. *Sci. Rep.* **2016**, *6*, 23335. [CrossRef]
15. Lador, R.; Regev, G.; Salame, K.; Khashan, M.; Lidar, Z. Use of 3-Dimensional Printing Technology in Complex Spine Surgeries. *World Neurosurg.* **2020**, *133*, e327–e341. [CrossRef]
16. Dalrymple, N.C.; Prasad, S.R.; Freckleton, M.W.; Chintapalli, K.N. Introduction to the Language of Three-dimensional Imaging with Multidetector CT. *RadioGraphics* **2005**, *25*, 1409–1428. [CrossRef]
17. Kikinis, R.; Pieper, S.D.; Vosburgh, K.G. 3D Slicer: A Platform for Subject-Specific Image Analysis, Visualization, and Clinical Support. In *Intraoperative Imaging and Image-Guided Therapy*; Jólesz, F.A., Ed.; Springer: New York, NY, USA, 2014; pp. 277–289. ISBN 978-1-4614-7657-3.
18. Ehrhardt, J.; Handels, H.; Malina, T.; Strathmann, B.; Plötz, W.; Pöppl, S.J. Atlas-based segmentation of bone structures to support the virtual planning of hip operations. *Int. J. Med. Inform.* **2001**, *64*, 439–447. [CrossRef]
19. Kennedy, A.; Dowling, J.; Greer, P.B.; Holloway, L.; Jameson, M.G.; Roach, D.; Ghose, S.; Rivest-Hénault, D.; Marcello, M.; Ebert, M.A. Similarity clustering-based atlas selection for pelvic CT image segmentation. *Med. Phys.* **2019**, *46*, 2243–2250. [CrossRef]

20. Kikuchi, A.; Onoguchi, M.; Horikoshi, H.; Sjöstrand, K.; Edenbrandt, L. Automated segmentation of the skeleton in whole-body bone scans. *Nucl. Med. Commun.* **2012**, *33*, 947–953. [CrossRef]
21. Wong, K.C.; Kumta, S.M.; Antonio, G.E.; Tse, L.F. Image Fusion for Computer-assisted Bone Tumor Surgery. *Clin. Orthop. Relat. Res.* **2008**, *466*, 2533–2541. [CrossRef]
22. Parry, M.C.; Laitinen, M.; Albergo, J.; Jeys, L.; Carter, S.; Gaston, C.L.; Sumathi, V.; Grimer, R.J. Osteosarcoma of the pelvis. *Bone Jt. J.* **2016**, *98*, 555–563. [CrossRef] [PubMed]
23. Cartiaux, O.; Docquier, P.-L.; Paul, L.; Francq, B.G.; Cornu, O.; Delloye, C.; Raucent, B.; Dehez, B.; Banse, X. Surgical inaccuracy of tumor resection and reconstruction within the pelvis: An experimental study. *Acta Orthop.* **2008**, *79*, 695–702. [CrossRef] [PubMed]
24. Jeys, L.; Matharu, G.S.; Nandra, R.S.; Grimer, R.J. Can computer navigation-assisted surgery reduce the risk of an intralesional margin and reduce the rate of local recurrence in patients with a tumour of the pelvis or sacrum? *Bone Jt. J.* **2013**, *95*, 1417–1424. [CrossRef] [PubMed]
25. Angelini, A.; Trovarelli, G.; Berizzi, A.; Pala, E.; Breda, A.; Ruggieri, P. Three-dimension-printed custom-made prosthetic reconstructions: From revision surgery to oncologic reconstructions. *Int. Orthop.* **2019**, *43*, 123–132. [CrossRef]
26. Garg, B.; Gupta, M.; Singh, M.; Kalyanasundaram, D. Outcome and safety analysis of 3D-printed patient-specific pedicle screw jigs for complex spinal deformities: A comparative study. *Spine J.* **2019**, *19*, 56–64. [CrossRef]
27. Hung, C.-C.; Li, Y.-T.; Chou, Y.-C.; Chen, J.-E.; Wu, C.-C.; Shen, H.-C.; Yeh, T.-T. Conventional plate fixation method versus pre-operative virtual simulation and three-dimensional printing-assisted contoured plate fixation method in the treatment of anterior pelvic ring fracture. *Int. Orthop.* **2019**, *43*, 425–431. [CrossRef]
28. Chepelev, L.; Wake, N.; Ryan, J.; Althobaity, W.; Gupta, A.; Arribas, E.; Santiago, L.; Ballard, D.H.; Wang, K.C.; Weadock, W.; et al. Radiological Society of North America (RSNA) 3D printing Special Interest Group (SIG): Guidelines for medical 3D printing and appropriateness for clinical scenarios. *3D Print. Med.* **2018**, *4*, 1–38. [CrossRef]
29. Ahangar, P.; Aziz, M.; Rosenzweig, D.H.; Weber, M.H. Advances in personalized treatment of metastatic spine disease. *Ann. Transl. Med.* **2019**, *7*, 223. [CrossRef]
30. Haleem, A.; Javaid, M.; Vaishya, R. 3D printing applications for the treatment of cancer. *Clin. Epidemiol. Glob. Health* **2020**, *8*, 1072–1076. [CrossRef]
31. Park, J.W.; Kang, H.G.; Lim, K.M.; Park, D.W.; Kim, J.H.; Kim, H.S. Bone tumor resection guide using three-dimensional printing for limb salvage surgery. *J. Surg. Oncol.* **2018**, *118*, 898–905. [CrossRef]
32. Gouin, F.; Paul, L.; Odri, G.-A.; Cartiaux, O. Computer-Assisted Planning and Patient-Specific Instruments for Bone Tumor Resection within the Pelvis: A Series of 11 Patients. *Sarcoma* **2014**, *2014*, 1–9. [CrossRef]
33. Wong, K.C. 3D-printed patient-specific applications in orthopedics. *Orthop. Res. Rev.* **2016**, *8*, 57–66. [CrossRef]
34. Lin, C.-L.; Fang, J.-J.; Lin, R.-M. Resection of giant invasive sacral schwannoma using image-based customized osteotomy tools. *Eur. Spine J.* **2016**, *25*, 4103–4107. [CrossRef]
35. Mobbs, R.J.; Coughlan, M.; Thompson, R.; Sutterlin, C.E.; Phan, K. The utility of 3D printing for surgical planning and patient-specific implant design for complex spinal pathologies: Case report. *J. Neurosurg. Spine* **2017**, *26*, 513–518. [CrossRef]
36. Chen, X.; Xu, L.; Wang, W.; Li, X.; Sun, Y.; Politis, C. Computer-aided design and manufacturing of surgical templates and their clinical applications: A review. *Expert Rev. Med. Devices* **2016**, *13*, 853–864. [CrossRef]
37. Wang, J.; Min, L.; Lu, M.; Zhang, Y.; Wang, Y.; Luo, Y.; Zhou, Y.; Duan, H.; Tu, C. What are the Complications of Three-dimensionally Printed, Custom-made, Integrative Hemipelvic Endoprostheses in Patients with Primary Malignancies Involving the Acetabulum, and What is the Function of These Patients? *Clin. Orthop. Relat. Res.* **2020**, *478*, 2487–2501. [CrossRef]
38. Shea, G.K.-H.; Wu, K.L.-K.; Li, I.W.-S.; Leung, M.-F.; Ko, A.L.-P.; Tse, L.; Pang, S.S.-Y.; Kwan, K.Y.-H.; Wong, T.-M.; Leung, F.K.-L.; et al. A review of the manufacturing process and infection rate of 3D-printed models and guides sterilized by hydrogen peroxide plasma and utilized intra-operatively. *3D Print. Med.* **2020**, *6*, 1–11. [CrossRef]
39. Evrard, R.; Schubert, T.; Paul, L.; Docquier, P.-L. Resection margins obtained with patient-specific instruments for resecting primary pelvic bone sarcomas: A case-control study. *Orthop. Traumatol. Surg. Res.* **2019**, *105*, 781–787. [CrossRef]
40. Šimić Jovičić, M.; Vuletić, F.; Ribičić, T.; Šimunić, S.; Petrović, T.; Kolundžić, R. Implementation of the three-dimensional printing technology in treatment of bone tumours: A case series. *Int. Orthop.* **2021**, *45*, 1079–1085. [CrossRef]
41. Wong, K.-C.; Scheinemann, P. Additive manufactured metallic implants for orthopaedic applications. *Sci. China Mater.* **2018**, *61*, 440–454. [CrossRef]
42. Karageorgiou, V.; Kaplan, D. Porosity of 3D biomaterial scaffolds and osteogenesis. *Biomaterials* **2005**, *26*, 5474–5491. [CrossRef] [PubMed]
43. Kumar, A.; Nune, K.C.; Murr, L.; Misra, R.D.K. Biocompatibility and mechanical behaviour of three-dimensional scaffolds for biomedical devices: Process–structure–property paradigm. *Int. Mater. Rev.* **2016**, *61*, 20–45. [CrossRef]
44. Mitsouras, D.; Liacouras, P.; Imanzadeh, A.; Giannopoulos, A.A.; Cai, T.; Kumamaru, K.K.; George, E.; Wake, N.; Caterson, E.J.; Pomahac, B.; et al. Medical 3D Printing for the Radiologist. *Radiographics* **2015**, *35*, 1965–1988. [CrossRef]
45. Wong, K.C.; Kumta, S.M. Computer-assisted Tumor Surgery in Malignant Bone Tumors. *Clin. Orthop. Relat. Res.* **2013**, *471*, 750–761. [CrossRef] [PubMed]

46. Uehara, M.; Takahashi, J.; Ikegami, S.; Kuraishi, S.; Futatsugi, T.; Oba, H.; Takizawa, T.; Munakata, R.; Koseki, M.; Kato, H. How Much Surface Registration Accuracy is Required Using Ct-based Navigation System in Adolescent Idiopathic Scoliosis Surgery? *Clin. Spine Surg.* **2019**, *32*, E166–E170. [CrossRef] [PubMed]
47. Liang, B.; Chen, Q.; Liu, S.; Chen, S.; Yao, Q.; Wei, B.; Xu, Y.; Tang, C.; Wang, L. A feasibility study of individual 3D-printed navigation template for the deep external fixator pin position on the iliac crest. *BMC Musculoskelet. Disord.* **2020**, *21*, 1–10. [CrossRef] [PubMed]
48. Tetsunaga, T.; Yamada, K.; Tetsunaga, T.; Furumatsu, T.; Sanki, T.; Kawamura, Y.; Ozaki, T. Comparison of the accuracy of CT- and accelerometer-based navigation systems for cup orientation in total hip arthroplasty. *HIP Int.* **2020**, 1120700020904940. [CrossRef]
49. Cartiaux, O.; Banse, X.; Paul, L.; Francq, B.G.; Aubin, C.-E.; Docquier, P.-L. Computer-assisted planning and navigation improves cutting accuracy during simulated bone tumor surgery of the pelvis. *Comput. Aided Surg.* **2012**, *18*, 19–26. [CrossRef]
50. Zhang, Y.; Wen, L.; Zhang, J.; Yan, G.; Zhou, Y.; Huang, B. Three-dimensional printing and computer navigation assisted hemipelvectomy for en bloc resection of osteochondroma. *Medicine* **2017**, *96*, e6414. [CrossRef]
51. Heunis, J.C.; Cheah, J.W.; Sabnis, A.J.; Wustrack, R.L. Use of three-dimensional printing and intraoperative navigation in the surgical resection of metastatic acetabular osteosarcoma. *BMJ Case Rep.* **2019**, *12*, e230238. [CrossRef]
52. Wong, K.C.; Kumta, S.M.; Geel, N.V.; Demol, J. One-step reconstruction with a 3D-printed, biomechanically evaluated custom implant after complex pelvic tumor resection. *Comput. Aided Surg.* **2015**, *20*, 14–23. [CrossRef]
53. Cartiaux, O.; Paul, L.; Francq, B.G.; Banse, X.; Docquier, P.-L. Improved Accuracy with 3D Planning and Patient-Specific Instruments During Simulated Pelvic Bone Tumor Surgery. *Ann. Biomed. Eng.* **2014**, *42*, 205–213. [CrossRef] [PubMed]
54. Sallent, A.; Vicente, M.; Reverte-Vinaixa, M.M.; Lopez, A.; Rodríguez-Baeza, A.; Pérez-Domínguez, M.; Velez, R. How 3D patient-specific instruments improve accuracy of pelvic bone tumour resection in a cadaveric study. *Bone Jt. Res.* **2017**, *6*, 577–583. [CrossRef] [PubMed]
55. Willemsen, K.; Nizak, R.; Noordmans, H.J.; Castelein, R.M.; Weinans, H.; Kruyt, M.C. Challenges in the design and regulatory approval of 3D-printed surgical implants: A two-case series. *Lancet Digit. Health* **2019**, *1*, e163–e171. [CrossRef]
56. Dalstra, M.; Huiskes, R. Load transfer across the pelvic bone. *J. Biomech.* **1995**, *28*, 715–724. [CrossRef]
57. Lee, K.-J.; Park, S.-J.; Lee, S.-J.; Naito, M.; Kwon, S.-Y. Biomechanical study on the efficacy of the periacetabular osteotomy using Patient-specific finite element analysis. *Int. J. Precis. Eng. Manuf.* **2015**, *16*, 823–829. [CrossRef]
58. Park, D.W.; Lim, A.; Park, J.W.; Lim, K.M.; Kang, H.G. Biomechanical Evaluation of a New Fixation Type in 3D-Printed Periacetabular Implants using a Finite Element Simulation. *Appl. Sci.* **2019**, *9*, 820. [CrossRef]
59. Wang, B.; Sun, P.; Xie, X.; Wu, W.; Tu, J.; Ouyang, J.; Shen, J. A novel combined hemipelvic endoprosthesis for peri-acetabular tumours involving sacroiliac joint: A finite element study. *Int. Orthop.* **2015**, *39*, 2253–2259. [CrossRef]
60. Sohn, S.; Park, T.H.; Chung, C.K.; Kim, Y.J.; Jang, J.W.; Han, I.-B.; Lee, S.J. Biomechanical characterization of three iliac screw fixation techniques: A finite element study. *J. Clin. Neurosci.* **2018**, *52*, 109–114. [CrossRef]
61. Bergmann, G. OrthoLoad. Available online: https://orthoload.com/ (accessed on 12 February 2021).
62. Chepelev, L.; Hodgdon, T.; Gupta, A.; Wang, A.; Torres, C.; Krishna, S.; Akyuz, E.; Mitsouras, D.; Sheikh, A. Medical 3D printing for vascular interventions and surgical oncology: A primer for the 2016 radiological society of North America (RSNA) hands-on course in 3D printing. *3D Print. Med.* **2016**, *2*, 5. [CrossRef]
63. U.S. Food and Drug Administration. Technical Considerations for Additive Manufactured Medical Devices. December 2017. Available online: https://www.fda.gov/regulatory-information/search-fda-guidance-documents/technical-considerations-additive-manufactured-medical-devices (accessed on 19 January 2021).
64. Ballard, D.H.; Mills, P.; Duszak, R.; Weisman, J.A.; Rybicki, F.J.; Woodard, P.K. Medical 3D Printing Cost-Savings in Orthopedic and Maxillofacial Surgery: Cost Analysis of Operating Room Time Saved with 3D Printed Anatomic Models and Surgical Guides. *Acad. Radiol.* **2020**, *27*, 1103–1113. [CrossRef] [PubMed]
65. Chen, J.V.; Dang, A.B.C.; Dang, A. Comparing cost and print time estimates for six commercially-available 3D printers obtained through slicing software for clinically relevant anatomical models. *3D Print. Med.* **2021**, *7*, 1–14. [CrossRef] [PubMed]
66. George, E.; Barile, M.; Tang, A.; Wiesel, O.; Coppolino, A.; Giannopoulos, A.; Mentzer, S.; Jaklitsch, M.; Hunsaker, A.; Mitsouras, D. Utility and reproducibility of 3-dimensional printed models in pre-operative planning of complex thoracic tumors. *J. Surg. Oncol.* **2017**, *116*, 407–415. [CrossRef] [PubMed]
67. Leng, S.; McGee, K.; Morris, J.; Alexander, A.; Kuhlmann, J.; Vrieze, T.; McCollough, C.H.; Matsumoto, J. Anatomic modeling using 3D printing: Quality assurance and optimization. *3D Print. Med.* **2017**, *3*, 1–14. [CrossRef]
68. Giannopoulos, A.A.; Chepelev, L.; Sheikh, A.; Wang, A.; Dang, W.; Akyuz, E.; Hong, C.; Wake, N.; Pietila, T.; Dydynski, P.B.; et al. 3D printed ventricular septal defect patch: A primer for the 2015 Radiological Society of North America (RSNA) hands-on course in 3D printing. *3D Print. Med.* **2015**, *1*, 1–20. [CrossRef]

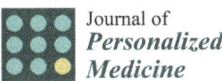 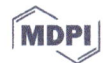

Opinion

Opinion Piece: Patient-Specific Implants May Be the Next Big Thing in Spinal Surgery

Tajrian Amin [1,2,3], William C.H. Parr [1,4,5] and Ralph J. Mobbs [1,2,3,*]

1. NeuroSpine Surgery Research Group (NSURG), Sydney 2000, Australia; tajamin1998@gmail.com (T.A.); parr.will@googlemail.com (W.C.H.P.)
2. Neuro Spine Clinic, Prince of Wales Private Hospital, Randwick 2031, Australia
3. Faculty of Medicine, University of New South Wales (UNSW), Sydney 2000, Australia
4. Surgical and Orthopaedic Research Laboratories (SORL), Prince of Wales Clinical School, Faculty of Medicine, University of New South Wales, Randwick 2031, Australia
5. 3DMorphic Pty Ltd., Matraville 2036, Australia
* Correspondence: r.mobbs@unsw.edu.au; Tel.: +61-(02)-9650-4766

Abstract: The emergence of 3D-Printing technologies and subsequent medical applications have allowed for the development of Patient-specific implants (PSIs). There have been increasing reports of PSI application to spinal surgery over the last 5 years, including throughout the spine and to a range of pathologies, though largely for complex cases. Through a number of potential benefits, including improvements to the implant–bone interface and surgical workflow, PSIs aim to improve patient and surgical outcomes, as well as potentially provide new avenues for combating challenges routinely faced by spinal surgeons. However, obstacles to widespread acceptance and routine application include the lack of quality long-term data, research challenges and the practicalities of production and navigating the regulatory environment. While recognition of the significant potential of Spinal PSIs is evident in the literature, it is clear a number of key questions must be answered to inform future clinical and research practices. The spinal surgical community must selectively and ethically continue to offer PSIs to patients, simultaneously allowing for the necessary larger, comparative studies to be conducted, as well as continuing to provide optimal patient care, thereby ultimately determining the exact role of this technology and potentially improving outcomes.

Keywords: Three-Dimensional Printing (3DP); custom implant; patient-specific implants (PSI); spinal surgery

1. Introduction

Three-Dimensional Printing (3DP) refers to the manufacturing method wherein 3D computer aided design (CAD) parts are physically realised through the sequential addition of fine cross-sectional (2D) layers of material. The technology has been widely influential and has seen significant medical application, including producing Patient-specific implants (PSIs) in orthopaedic surgery. PSIs refer to customised implants, tailored to the exact anatomical and surgical needs of each patient, with the key aims of minimising anatomical remodelling and improving implant–bone interface mechanics, osseointegration and surgical outcomes, as well as ultimately improving patient outcomes [1–3]. Since the early work of D'Urso et al. [4], 3DP has been extensively applied to spinal surgery, with multiple reports highlighting the utility of spinal biomodels, pedicle screw guides and PSIs [5]. PSIs in spinal surgery have become a particularly promising area, with an increasing number of case reports and small series, particularly of complex cases, emerging over the last 5 years [5–14]. Though the field is clearly at an early and formative stage, with more data required to validate this technology and its full potential likely yet to be realised, key questions about its future remain. What is the role of 3D-Printed PSIs in spinal surgery? Will every patient get a PSI in the future? Are they only for complex cases? Or will PSIs

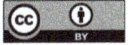

ultimately be left by the wayside? This article aims to outline the ongoing discussion on PSIs within the spinal surgical community, with particular attention toward current uses and trends.

2. Current State of PSI Use in Spinal Surgery

Since the early case reports of Xu et al. [15], Phan et al. [16] and Wei et al. [17] in 2016, there has been a rapid increase in reports of Spinal PSI use. An encouraging development has been the emergence of small case series over the last 3 years, namely the reports from Girolami et al. [6] and Wei et al. [7], indicating a growing acceptance by clinicians, the potential scalability of these technologies, and the transition to higher levels of research. PSIs have now been used to manage a range of pathologies, including infection [11], degeneration [18], malignancy [19] and deformity [9], throughout the spine at the cervical [7], thoracic [19], lumbar [6] and sacral [17] levels. These cases have generally involved highly complex patho-anatomies, with a PSI indicated following the assessment of the surgical team that no commercially available generic or Off-The-Shelf (OTS) implant would provide an acceptable surgical outcome. In these scenarios, OTS implants are often deemed unlikely to produce good outcomes due to a significant implant–bone shape mismatch. Generally, this mismatch will be compensated for through extensive remodelling of the bony anatomy to fit the implant, likely resulting in increased operative time and trauma due to high-speed bone burring, a weakened bony anatomy and possibly increased subsidence risk, as well as a likely suboptimal implant–bone contact area and suboptimal force distribution. Regarding the literature to date, implants have largely been high cervical spine, vertebrectomy, interbody and sacral devices, generally manufactured from Titanium alloy. Figures 1–3 illustrate a range of PSI types used in our own practice.

A large suite of custom features have been described, including endplate matching, integral fixation, planned screw trajectories, windows for bone growth and radiographic assessment, variable surface porosity, biomimetic structures and integration with posterior hardware [5,6,11,20]. While authors have frequently emphasised the need for further research, with larger samples and comparative methodologies, as well as the limitations associated with 3DP and PSIs, these early reports have been largely favourabe, and a general appreciation of the promise of this technology is apparent [1,5]. However, the current evidence, at best, may be used to support PSI use only by highly experienced surgical teams in highly selected cases, namely patients with complex patho-anatomies, where the use of an OTS implant is unlikely to produce acceptable outcomes, and who provide informed consent after a comprehensive education, including the overall early stage, unproven and, sometimes, experimental nature of this emerging technology.

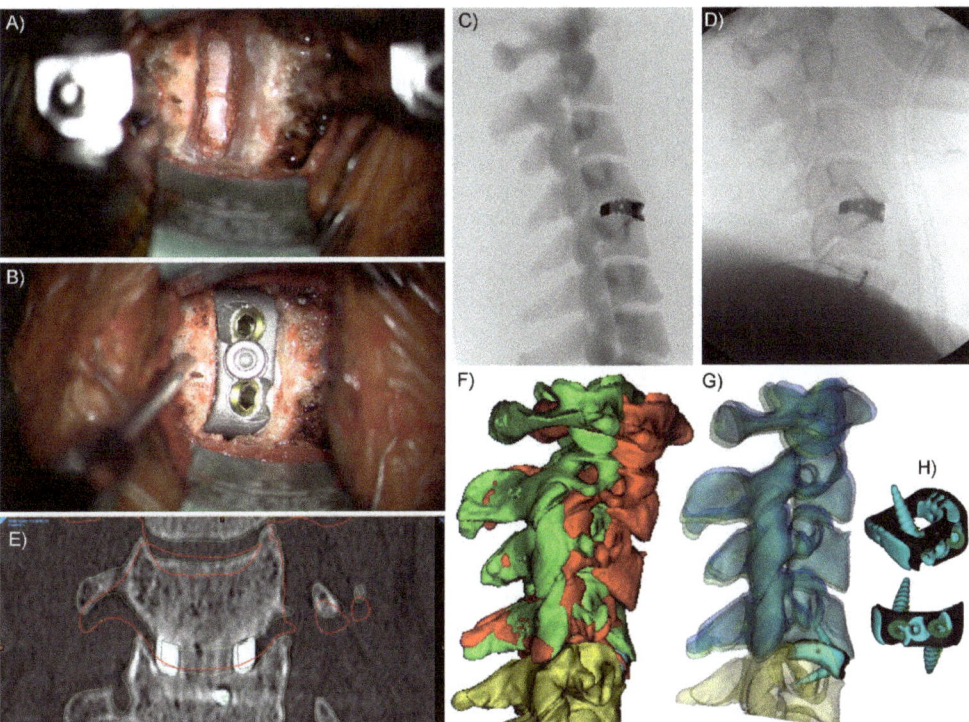

Figure 1. Stand-alone, integral screw fixation Anterior Cervical Discectomy and Fusion (ACDF) Patient-specific Implant (PSI) C4-5. (**A**) Surgical discectomy and preparation of the C4-5 interbody space (**B**) and surgical implantation of the integral screw fixation Titanium alloy PSI. (**C**) Simulated sagittal plane X-ray used intraoperatively to assess implant positioning (e.g., insertion depth), (**D**) actual intraoperative sagittal plane X-ray. (**E**) and three-month postoperative coronal plane CT slice showing fusion bone through the graft window of the Titanium PSI and no discernible subsidence. The red outlines indicate the preoperative position of the C4 vertebra. (**F**) 3D reconstructions of the cervical levels superior to the operative (C4-5) level; red is the preoperative positioning, and green is the achieved (2.5 month) postoperative positioning. (**G**) Translucent 3D reconstructions; green is the achieved (2.5 month) postoperative positioning, and blue is the virtual surgery planned (VSP) positioning. Green positioning is close to the matching blue positioning, particularly when compared to red (preoperative) positioning, which shows good surgical realisation of the plan and that anterior interbody devices can control the postoperative segment angle, as well as (height) distraction. (**H**) Blue (achieved) vs. black (planned) cage positioning within the interbody space; the cage was implanted 0.5–1 mm posterior and to the right of the plan. This was achieved through the use of VSP images (such as **C**) and as a result of the PSI conforming to the patient's anatomy, thereby auto-locating in surgery into the planned position.

3. Why Should Spinal Surgeons Use PSIs?

A range of theoretical advantages have been ascribed to PSIs, largely to do with improvements to the implant–bone interface and the overall surgical workflow. The key advantages at the implant–bone interface centre around endplate matching, which refers to the matching of the contacting surfaces of the implant and the patient anatomy. This minimises the need for endplate preparation, thereby preserving bone integrity, improving force distribution and osseointegration, as well as improving the primary stabilisation and minimising stress shielding [1,5,8,21]. The ability to manipulate the surface porosity of Titanium PSIs may additionally enhance osseointegration [21]. An improved surgical workflow is largely thought to be a result of the faster implant fit and reduced need for endplate preparation, as well as the associated preoperative planning and biomodelling (Figures 2 and 3), thereby possibly reducing operative times, blood loss, fluoroscopy use and, ultimately, costs [1,5,20,21]. Custom features may provide specific further advantages. For example, pre-planned screw trajectories and screw lengths may improve the primary stabilisation and reduce the risk of a screw exiting the bone and damaging neurovascular structures [8], as well as possibly reduce the time required to achieve screw fixation. While the current literature is undoubtedly lacking, the growing number of early reports, from multiple authors from multiple centres [5–12], detailing the successful application of spinal PSIs to a range of clinical scenarios is encouraging.

The characteristic customisability of PSIs may lend them particularly suited to spinal surgery, given the inherently complex anatomy of the spine, consisting of 33 vertebrae with up to seven joints at each vertebral level [22–24], as well as the often complex distortion produced by common pathologies, including degeneration, malignancy and deformity [11]. While, in this setting, PSIs are intuitively more likely to be superior tools in comparison to OTS generic options, the customisability of PSIs also provides spinal surgeons with new avenues of combating some of the key challenges they routinely face. Cage subsidence can significantly reverse the surgically gained improvements to disc and neuroforaminal heights, thereby potentially leading to poorer clinical outcomes [25]. Guided by an understanding of the risk factors and mechanisms associated with cage subsidence [25], including cage design and bone quality, this not uncommon postoperative complications may be minimised through careful cage design and the minimal endplate preparation afforded by PSIs [6–8]. In cervical surgery, 3DP can allow for patient-specific, truly zero profile implants that may minimise the dysphagia and dysphonia associated with conventional instrumentation [20,26].

Spinal reconstructive surgery, particularly as indicated by primary osseous malignancy, often involves significant bone loss and may involve physiologically complex anatomy, such as the high cervical spine. These challenging operating conditions may commonly result in profound instability and instrument-related complications. PSIs have been described as a potential way of combating this by allowing for strong primary stabilisation, filling of the defect and deformity correction [6,7,27]. Figure 3 provides an example of our relevant clinical experience. Wei et al. also suggested that PSIs may be less prone to instrument failure secondary to postoperative radiotherapy, in comparison to the reported issues with conventional reconstructive methods [7]. The ability to tailor implants to the exact size required is also hugely useful in the case of severe, progressed and/or recurrent presentations, where no appropriately large OTS implant may exist [10,11]. PSIs are particularly useful in managing infections, as bone infections can cause large defects, significant bone loss and irregular bone surfaces [11]. While a PSI can fill this defect, as described by Chung et al. [11], and also likely achieve good primary stabilisation, PSIs with antimicrobial properties have also been described. As the surface porosity of these implants would allow for a drug delivery system to be included, the risk of new-onset Surgical Site Infection or recurrent infection can be minimised in these cases, thereby preventing subsequent dismal outcomes [28,29].

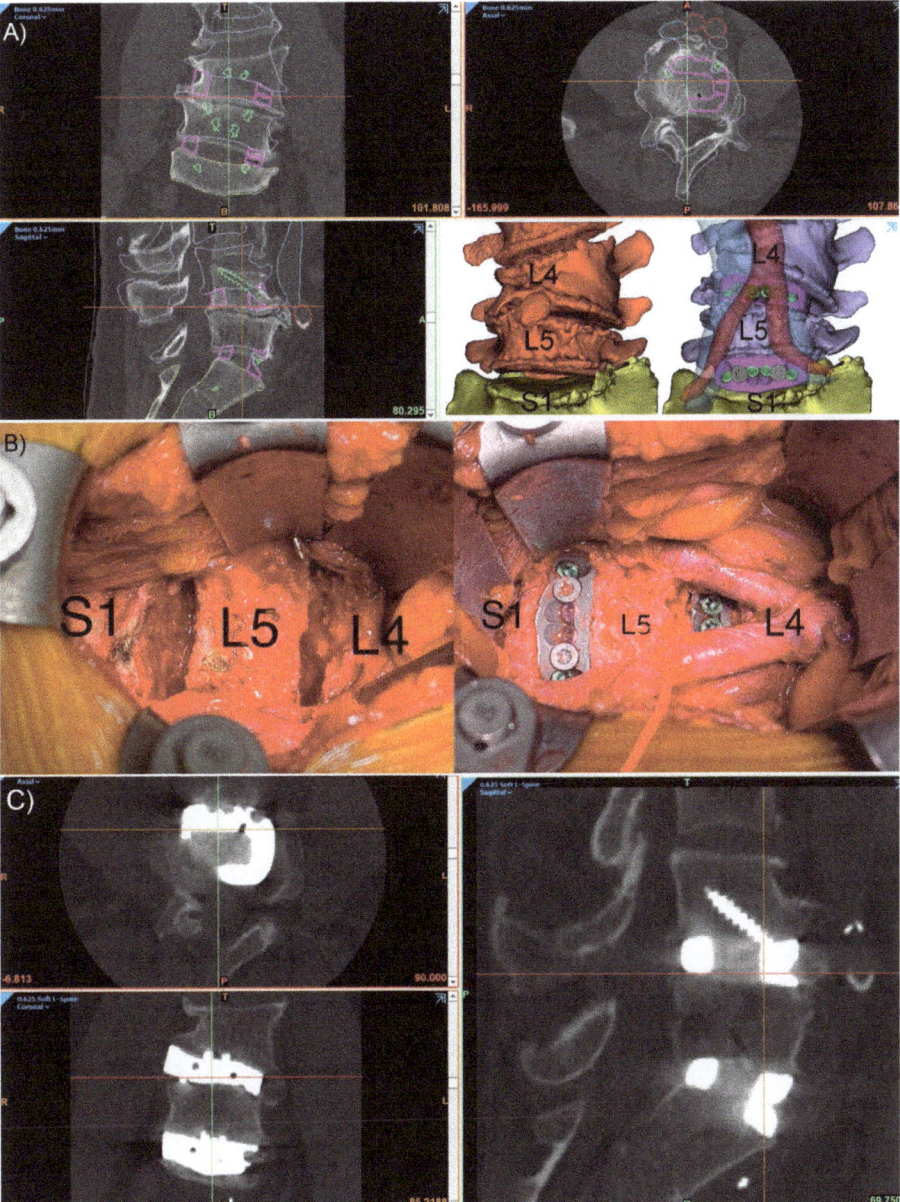

Figure 2. Integral screw fixation, stand-alone Anterior Lumbar Interbody Fusion (ALIF) patient-specific implants (PSIs) L4-5 and L5-S1, in an L4 congenital hemivertebra patient. (**A**) Preoperative CT with planned device (purple outlines), screws (green outlines), vertebral positions (blue outlines) and major vessels (inferior vena cava, blue, and aorta, red). The bottom right panel in (**A**) shows the preoperative pathological anatomy (red) and the planned postoperative state (blue) with translucent aorta (red) and inferior vena cava (blue) shown. (**B**) The intraoperative L4-L5 and L5-S1 discectomies (**left**) and final surgical reconstruction (**right**) with the aortic bifurcation at the L4 level shown. (**C**) Three-month postoperative CT of the construct showing good positioning of the devices, with no evidence of device migration or micromotion, and interbody fusion bone forming through the graft windows of both PSIs.

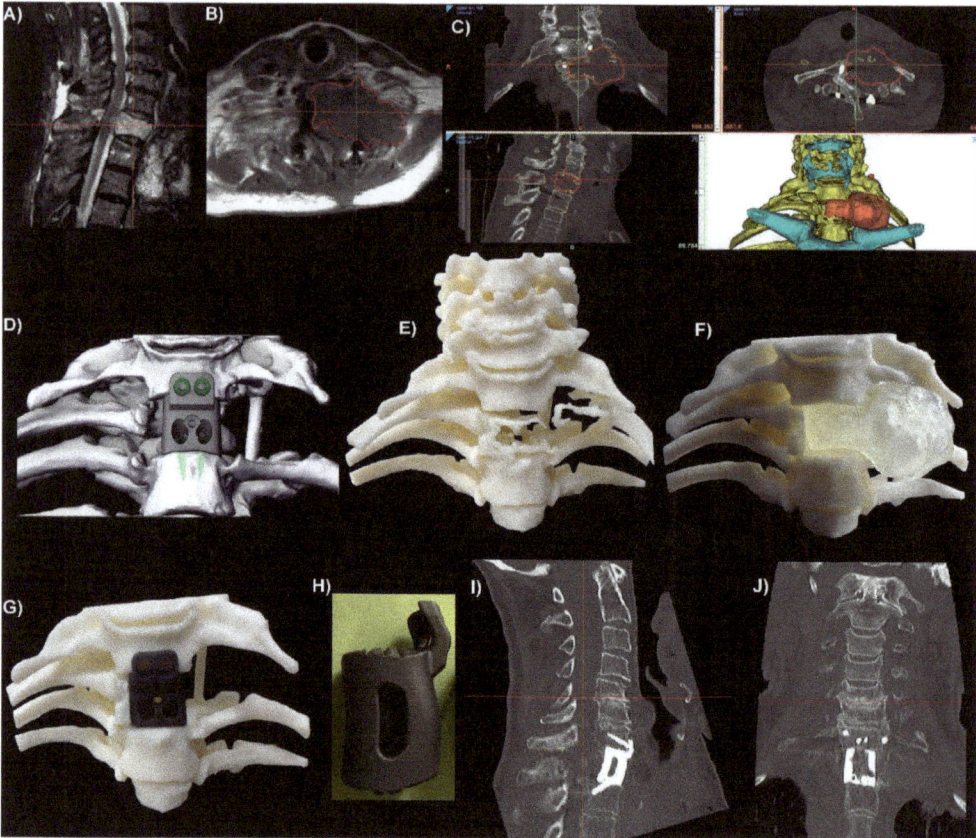

Figure 3. Integral screw fixation thoracic (T1) corpectomy/vertebrectomy patient-specific implant (PSI). (**A**) Sagittal plane MRI slice showing a tumour in the T1 vertebral body. (**B**) Axial plane MRI slice with red outlines showing the tumour. (**C**) CT slices and 3D reconstruction of the anatomy. The hyoid and sternum are shown in cyan. The position of T1 relative to the sternum meant that access to insert screws up into C7 would be difficult, so a custom anterior plate was integrated into the interbody device with anterior–posterior screw trajectories planned for C7. (**D**) Virtual Surgical Plan tumour resection and surgical reconstruction using the PSI and integral screws. (**E**) 3D-Printed 'biomodel' of the vertebral and rib bone showing the lytic effects of the tumour on the T1 vertebral and rib bone. (**F**) 3D-Printed biomodels of the vertebral bone with a removable tumour (opaque, colourless). (**G**) Same bone biomodel as (**F**) with the tumour removed and a 3D-Printed resin 'demo' PSI in position. (**H**) Sagittal plane viewpoint of the Titanium alloy (Ti_6Al_4V) PSI. One-day postoperative sagittal (**I**) and coronal (**J**) plane CT slices of the level showing good positioning and contact between the PSI and bone.

4. What Are the Issues?

The key issue facing Spinal PSIs is the lack of quality, long-term data demonstrating their utility, safety and superiority over OTS alternatives, likely in terms of patient, surgical and economic outcomes. While PSIs have a longer and more extensive history of application elsewhere in orthopaedics, such as to Total Knee Arthroplasty (TKA), concerningly the current body of evidence, though including some encouraging recent results highlighting the improved precision afforded by PSIs in TKA [30–32], does not clearly demonstrate the superiority of PSIs and, thus, fails to validate the theoretical benefits of their use [33,34]. Evidently, significant further research is required in this area, particularly of the longer-term outcomes, as well as in light of emerging evidence regarding the specific preoperative factors affecting surgical outcomes and the importance of careful patient selection [35].

While further research is clearly needed, a number of issues complicate this pursuit. The literature is currently focussed on complex cases, with inherently limited external validity. This limits the extent to which clinicians can apply these early results to clinical scenarios they encounter, as well of researchers to justify larger, comparative studies in less complex, more routine patients. The wide spectrum of patho-anatomical complexity also complicates certain essential analyses, including between PSIs in standard and complex cases, as well as between PSIs and OTS implants in cases of similar complexity. It is clear that a method of describing patho-anatomical complexity, perhaps through a qualitative grade or a quantitative index, is needed to further the literature. Researchers should also ensure that key PSI design and manufacture parameters are clearly reported and that only fundamentally similar PSIs are compared. As PSIs may sometimes make certain operations possible [9], comparisons against an OTS implant which would not have actually been used, are invalid. As other 3DP-related tools are often used alongside PSIs, including biomodels and custom instruments [20], certain analyses will likely be confounded, including assessing the impact of PSIs alone on surgical outcomes. However, given their routinely combined use, simply assessing for the overall impact of a patient-specific procedure may still be meaningful.

The other broad category of issues facing spinal PSIs revolve around the practicality of their use. PSI design and manufacture can be resource-intensive, requiring specialised skills and equipment [1,5]. However, this will likely be less important in the future considering further growth of the literature, growing familiarity and the rapid pace of development in the manufacturing fields, as well as the possible development of user-friendly holistic software solutions [3,8] and the emergence of private companies offering an integrated suite of these services [9]. The inflexibility of PSIs has also been criticised. A number of requirements must be met, including good quality imaging, careful computer processing and relatively short imaging-to-operation times, to ensure that the implants are still patient-specific [21]. Additionally, cancelled or delayed operations, as well as intraoperative positioning and both intended and inadvertent surgical remodelling, may additionally compromise the specificity and insertion of these implants [1,11]. Therefore, a number of PSIs in different sizes are often required to allow for the best fit to be determined intraoperatively [8], and OTS alternatives may also be kept on-hand.

The regulatory environment has been highlighted as a key potential obstacle for surgeons. While likely to evolve, it may be restrictive and challenging to navigate [1,5,9], though this may also be attenuated with time, mounting evidence and wider familiarity. As highlighted by Willemsen et al., the existing regulatory environment may frustrate the current use of PSIs for cases with a degree of urgency, including when dealing with malignancy or spinal instability [9]. This is particularly problematic given that these cases, often with complex and large defects, may stand to greatly benefit from this technology. While Willemsen et al. framed their devices as custom-made or personalised and so avoided the more complex and time-consuming reporting otherwise required for medical devices, these kinds of exemptions, though appropriate for select cases, would represent an abuse of the regulatory process given a sufficient patient volume and so are unsustainable in the long term. As discussed by Mobbs et al., clearly researchers, clinicians and regulators must strike a balance between lax oversight, culminating in unsafe devices being used and excessive restrictions stifling innovation, delaying state-of-the-art care options and denying patients the best management in their clinical context [21]. Table 1 summarises the key considerations for spinal surgeons regarding PSI use.

Table 1. Summary of the key advantages and disadvantages, including largely theoretical points, associated with patient-specific implant use by spinal surgeons.

Advantages	Disadvantages
Easier Implantation	Lack of Quality Data
Minimal Endplate Preparation	Research Challenges
Improved Device–Bone Load Distribution	Skilled Labour and Equipment Requirements
Improved Primary Stabilisation	Increased Preoperative Planning
Range of Customisable Features	Reduced Intraoperative Flexibility
Enhanced Osseointegration	Multiple Implants Need to be Produced Per Case
Minimised Operative Time	Off the Shelf Devices Often Also Kept on Hand
Tailor to Specific Operative Challenges and Clinical Scenarios	Challenging Regulatory Environment

5. Discussion

The growing interest in personalised medicine is clear. Driven by advances in the basic sciences and technology, clinicians are trying to optimise management, eliminate trial and error and, ultimately, improve outcomes. This is particularly evident in medical specialties, as evidenced by the emergence of pharmacogenomics and pharmacodiagnostics in lieu of traditional algorithmic and iterative approaches [36]. Wearable devices for continuous and objective patient monitoring present another excellent example of this technology-driven, highly patient-centred approach [37]. The personalised care paradigm has now increasingly begun to shape the surgical fields [3,38–40], with 3DP proving to be a versatile tool.

While some patient-specific 3D-Printed developments, namely biomodels and custom instruments, are likely to persist given the practically negligible potential for serious harm and the reasonable benefits provided in planning, training and education, as well as possibly reducing operative times [20], PSIs present a much greater challenge given their inherently invasive and essentially permanent nature. In short, the stakes are much greater. Ultimately, the turning point for PSIs will likely be the verdict of quality, long-term data investigating their outcomes in comparison to OTS generics. This evidence, alongside economic considerations, particularly with future streamlining of the design and manufacturing process, will likely guide which populations receive PSIs in the future. PSIs may prove to greatly improve outcomes in comparison to OTS alternatives and be sufficiently cost-effective enough to be used for all patients. However, if only a minor improvement to outcomes, or at least noninferiority, is demonstrated, economic considerations will likely guide their use. Routine use is more likely if PSIs do significantly reduce operative times and so result in significant cost savings [20]. Otherwise, they may continue to be used only in select patients to aid with complex cases.

Regardless, it is clear that a balance must be struck in the interim. Early on, Harrington's eponymous rods were also patient-specific and used in select cases prior to the transition to larger patient groups, widespread use and acceptance [41]. On the other hand, spinal surgeons and pioneers must not allow a sound theoretical basis, successful application in other fields and encouraging early results to drive unsubstantiated, widespread application, as some argue has occurred with certain Minimally Invasive Spinal Surgeries (MISS) [42]. Further, the possibility of unforeseen implant-related complications must not be discounted, either due to issues in the planning and implementation of a PSI [6] or inherent to the implant design or material [11,18,43].

Future areas of interest include optimising materials and custom features [5,10,44], ideally with the aims of further improving outcomes and continuing to pursue solutions to problems facing the spinal surgical community. Can patient-specific arthroplasty implants for Total Disc Replacements be produced? Can PSIs be made to suit MISS, allowing for smaller incisions and less retraction? Can devices be optimised for particular surgical techniques, including for the degrees of access they allow and the accessory instrumentation they may include [45]? Can PSIs, in combination with virtual surgery planning, reduce the risks of spine surgery sufficiently to enable better surgical outcomes by less experienced surgeons/surgical teams? Can tissues be bioprinted to combat specific operative challenges and further improve outcomes [46]? For example, can bioprinted disc substitute material or an annular defect repair patch combat post-microdiscectomy height loss or recurrent disc herniation, respectively? Research in these areas will help to distinguish the exaggerated and overly optimistic predictions of the benefits and potential uses of 3DP, PSIs and associated technologies from the realistic, practical and clinically relevant applications that researchers and clinicians should explore. In summation, the great potential of this technology is clear, but further work is required to substantiate this. The spinal surgical community must ethically apply this technology to more patients and for more indications, ultimately allowing for the larger, comparative studies and scientifically sound comparisons to be made which will shed light on the role of this technology, shape the regulatory environment and, ultimately, potentially improve outcomes.

Author Contributions: Conceptualisation, T.A. and R.J.M.; methodology, T.A., W.C.H.P. and R.J.M.; investigation, T.A., W.C.H.P. and R.J.M.; resources, T.A., W.C.H.P. and R.J.M.; writing—original draft preparation, T.A.; writing—review and editing, T.A., W.C.H.P. and R.J.M.; supervision, R.J.M. and project administration, T.A. and R.J.M. All authors have read and agreed to the published version of the manuscript.

Funding: This research received no external funding.

Institutional Review Board Statement: The study was conducted according to the guidelines of the Declaration of Helsinki and approved by the Institutional Review Board (or Ethics Committee) of the South Eastern Sydney Local Health District Human Research Ethics Committee (Ethics Approval number: LNR/16/POWH/535; Date of Approval: 19 June 2018).

Informed Consent Statement: Informed consent was obtained from all patients involved in the study.

Acknowledgments: The NeuroSpine Surgery Research Group (*NSURG*) aided with the manuscript production. The Neuro Spine Clinic provided clinic assistance for the authors.

Conflicts of Interest: T.A. and R.J.M. declare no conflict of interest. W.C.H.P. is a director at 3DMorphic Pty Ltd.

References

1. Sheha, E.D.; Gandhi, S.D.; Colman, M.W. 3D printing in spine surgery. *Ann. Transl. Med.* **2019**, *7*, S164. [CrossRef]
2. Maniar, R.N.; Singhi, T. Patient specific implants: Scope for the future. *Curr. Rev. Musculoskelet. Med.* **2014**, *7*, 125–130. [CrossRef]
3. Wong, K.C. 3D-printed patient-specific applications in orthopedics. *Orthop. Res. Rev.* **2016**, *8*, 57–66. [CrossRef] [PubMed]
4. D'Urso, P.S.; Askin, G.; Earwaker, J.S.; Merry, G.S.; Thompson, R.G.; Barker, T.M.; Effeney, D.J. Spinal biomodeling. *Spine* **1999**, *24*, 1247–1251. [CrossRef] [PubMed]
5. Wilcox, B.; Mobbs, R.J.; Wu, A.-M.; Phan, K. Systematic review of 3D printing in spinal surgery: The current state of play. *J. Spine Surg.* **2017**, *3*, 433–443. [CrossRef] [PubMed]
6. Girolami, M.; Boriani, S.; Bandiera, S.; Barbanti-Bródano, G.; Ghermandi, R.; Terzi, S.; Tedesco, G.; Evangelisti, G.; Pipola, V.; Gasbarrini, A. Biomimetic 3D-printed custom-made prosthesis for anterior column reconstruction in the thoracolumbar spine: A tailored option following en bloc resection for spinal tumors: Preliminary results on a case-series of 13 patients. *Eur. Spine J.* **2018**, *27*, 3073–3083. [CrossRef] [PubMed]
7. Wei, F.; Li, Z.; Liu, Z.; Liu, X.; Jiang, L.; Yu, M.; Xu, N.; Wu, F.; Dang, L.; Zhou, H.; et al. Upper cervical spine reconstruction using customized 3D-printed vertebral body in 9 patients with primary tumors involving C2. *Ann. Transl. Med.* **2020**, *8*, 332. [CrossRef]
8. Parr, W.C.H.; Burnard, J.L.; Singh, T.; McEvoy, A.; Walsh, W.R.; Mobbs, R.J. C3-C5 Chordoma Resection and Reconstruction with a Three-Dimensional Printed Titanium Patient-Specific Implant. *World Neurosurg.* **2020**, *136*, 226–233. [CrossRef] [PubMed]
9. Willemsen, K.; Nizak, R.; Noordmans, H.J.; Castelein, R.M.; Weinans, H.; Kruyt, M.C. Challenges in the design and regulatory approval of 3D-printed surgical implants: A two-case series. *Lancet Digit. Health* **2019**, *1*, e163–e171. [CrossRef]
10. Yang, X.; Wan, W.; Gong, H.; Xiao, J. Application of Individualized 3D-Printed Artificial Vertebral Body for Cervicothoracic Reconstruction in a Six-Level Recurrent Chordoma. *Turk. Neurosurg.* **2020**, *30*, 149–155. [CrossRef]
11. Chung, K.S.; Shin, D.A.; Kim, K.N.; Ha, Y.; Yoon, D.H.; Yi, S. Vertebral Reconstruction with Customized 3-Dimensional–Printed Spine Implant Replacing Large Vertebral Defect with 3-Year Follow-up. *World Neurosurg.* **2019**, *126*, 90–95. [CrossRef]
12. Chin, B.Z.; Ji, T.; Tang, X.; Yang, R.; Guo, W. Three-Level Lumbar En Bloc Spondylectomy with Three-Dimensional-Printed Vertebrae Reconstruction for Recurrent Giant Cell Tumor. *World Neurosurg.* **2019**, *129*, 531–537. [CrossRef] [PubMed]
13. Choy, W.J.; Parr, W.C.H.; Phan, K.; Walsh, W.R.; Mobbs, R.J. 3-dimensional printing for anterior cervical surgery: A review. *J. Spine Surg.* **2018**, *4*, 757–769. [CrossRef] [PubMed]

14. Burnard, J.L.; Parr, W.C.H.; Choy, W.J.; Walsh, W.R.; Mobbs, R.J. 3D-printed spine surgery implants: A systematic review of the efficacy and clinical safety profile of patient-specific and off-the-shelf devices. *Eur. Spine J.* **2019**. [CrossRef] [PubMed]
15. Xu, N.; Wei, F.; Liu, X.; Jiang, L.; Cai, H.; Li, Z.; Yu, M.; Wu, F.; Liu, Z. Reconstruction of the Upper Cervical Spine Using a Personalized 3D-Printed Vertebral Body in an Adolescent With Ewing Sarcoma. *Spine* **2016**, *41*, E50–E54. [CrossRef]
16. Phan, K.; Sgro, A.; Maharaj, M.M.; D'Urso, P.; Mobbs, R.J. Application of a 3D custom printed patient specific spinal implant for C1/2 arthrodesis. *J. Spine Surg.* **2016**, *2*, 314–318. [CrossRef]
17. Wei, R.; Guo, W.; Ji, T.; Zhang, Y.; Liang, H. One-step reconstruction with a 3D-printed, custom-made prosthesis after total en bloc sacrectomy: A technical note. *Eur. Spine J.* **2017**, *26*, 1902–1909. [CrossRef]
18. Siu, T.L.; Rogers, J.M.; Lin, K.; Thompson, R.; Owbridge, M. Custom-Made Titanium 3-Dimensional Printed Interbody Cages for Treatment of Osteoporotic Fracture-Related Spinal Deformity. *World Neurosurg.* **2018**, *111*, 1–5. [CrossRef]
19. Choy, W.J.; Mobbs, R.J.; Wilcox, B.; Phan, S.; Phan, K.; Sutterlin, C.E., 3rd. Reconstruction of Thoracic Spine Using a Personalized 3D-Printed Vertebral Body in Adolescent with T9 Primary Bone Tumor. *World Neurosurg.* **2017**, *1032*, e1013–e1017. [CrossRef]
20. Parr, W.C.H.; Burnard, J.L.; Wilson, P.J.; Mobbs, R.J. 3D printed anatomical (bio)models in spine surgery: Clinical benefits and value to health care providers. *J. Spine Surg.* **2019**. [CrossRef]
21. Mobbs, R.J.; Parr, W.C.H.; Choy, W.J.; McEvoy, A.; Walsh, W.R.; Phan, K. Anterior Lumbar Interbody Fusion Using a Personalized Approach: Is Custom the Future of Implants for Anterior Lumbar Interbody Fusion Surgery? *World Neurosurg.* **2019**. [CrossRef]
22. Hartman, J. Anatomy and clinical significance of the uncinate process and uncovertebral joint: A comprehensive review. *Clin. Anat.* **2014**, *27*, 431–440. [CrossRef]
23. Devereaux, M.W. Anatomy and examination of the spine. *Neurol. Clin.* **2007**, *25*, 331–351. [CrossRef] [PubMed]
24. Saker, E.; Graham, R.A.; Nicholas, R.; D'Antoni, A.V.; Loukas, M.; Oskouian, R.J.; Tubbs, R.S. Ligaments of the Costovertebral Joints including Biomechanics, Innervations, and Clinical Applications: A Comprehensive Review with Application to Approaches to the Thoracic Spine. *Cureus* **2016**, *8*, e874. [CrossRef] [PubMed]
25. Yao, Y.-C.; Chou, P.-H.; Lin, H.-H.; Wang, S.-T.; Liu, C.-L.; Chang, M.-C. Risk Factors of Cage Subsidence in Patients Received Minimally Invasive Transforaminal Lumbar Interbody Fusion. *Spine* **2020**, *45*, E1279–E1285. [CrossRef] [PubMed]
26. Amin, T.; Lin, H.; Parr, W.C.H.; Lim, P.; Mobbs, R.J. Revision of a Failed C5-7 Corpectomy Complicated by Esophageal Fistula Using a 3-Dimensional−Printed Zero-Profile Patient-Specific Implant: A Technical Case Report. *World Neurosurg.* **2021**, *151*, 29–38. [CrossRef]
27. Li, X.; Wang, Y.; Zhao, Y.; Liu, J.; Xiao, S.; Mao, K. Multilevel 3D Printing Implant for Reconstructing Cervical Spine With Metastatic Papillary Thyroid Carcinoma. *Spine* **2017**, *42*, E1326–E1330. [CrossRef] [PubMed]
28. Li, Y.; Li, L.; Ma, Y.; Zhang, K.; Li, G.; Lu, B.; Lu, C.; Chen, C.; Wang, L.; Wang, H.; et al. 3D-Printed Titanium Cage with PVA-Vancomycin Coating Prevents Surgical Site Infections (SSIs). *Macromol. Biosci.* **2020**, *20*, e1900394. [CrossRef]
29. Dong, J.; Zhang, S.; Liu, H.; Li, X.; Liu, Y.; Du, Y. Novel alternative therapy for spinal tuberculosis during surgery: Reconstructing with anti-tuberculosis bioactivity implants. *Expert Opin. Drug Deliv.* **2014**, *11*, 299–305. [CrossRef]
30. Ogura, T.; Le, K.; Merkely, G.; Bryant, T.; Minas, T. A high level of satisfaction after bicompartmental individualized knee arthroplasty with patient-specific implants and instruments. *Knee Surg. Sports Traumatol. Arthrosc.* **2019**, *27*, 1487–1496. [CrossRef] [PubMed]
31. Arbab, D.; Reimann, P.; Brucker, M.; Bouillon, B.; Lüring, C. Alignment in total knee arthroplasty—A comparison of patient-specific implants with the conventional technique. *Knee* **2018**, *25*, 882–887. [CrossRef]
32. Schroeder, L.; Martin, G. In Vivo Tibial Fit and Rotational Analysis of a Customized, Patient-Specific TKA versus Off-the-Shelf TKA. *J Knee Surg.* **2019**, *32*, 499–505. [CrossRef] [PubMed]
33. Haglin, J.M.; Eltorai, A.E.M.; Gil, J.A.; Marcaccio, S.E.; Botero-Hincapie, J.; Daniels, A.H. Patient-Specific Orthopaedic Implants. *Orthop. Surg.* **2016**, *8*, 417–424. [CrossRef]
34. Schwarzkopf, R.; Brodsky, M.; Garcia, G.A.; Gomoll, A.H. Surgical and Functional Outcomes in Patients Undergoing Total Knee Replacement With Patient-Specific Implants Compared With "Off-the-Shelf" Implants. *Orthop. J. Sports Med.* **2015**, *3*. [CrossRef]
35. Rojanasopondist, P.; Galea, V.P.; Connelly, J.W.; Matuszak, S.J.; Rolfson, O.; Bragdon, C.R.; Malchau, H. What Preoperative Factors are Associated With Not Achieving a Minimum Clinically Important Difference After THA? Findings from an International Multicenter Study. *Clin. Orthop. Relat. Res.* **2019**, *477*, 1301–1312. [CrossRef]
36. Vogenberg, F.R.; Isaacson Barash, C.; Pursel, M. Personalized medicine: Part 1: Evolution and development into theranostics. *Pharm. Ther.* **2010**, *35*, 560–576.
37. Mobbs, R.J.; Ho, D.; Choy, W.J.; Betteridge, C.; Lin, H. COVID-19 is shifting the adoption of wearable monitoring and telemedicine (WearTel) in the delivery of healthcare: Opinion piece. *Ann. Transl. Med.* **2020**, *8*, 1285. [CrossRef] [PubMed]
38. Barberan-Garcia, A.; Ubré, M.; Roca, J.; Lacy, A.M.; Burgos, F.; Risco, R.; Momblán, D.; Balust, J.; Blanco, I.; Martínez-Pallí, G. Personalised Prehabilitation in High-risk Patients Undergoing Elective Major Abdominal Surgery: A Randomized Blinded Controlled Trial. *Ann. Surg.* **2018**, *267*, 50–56. [CrossRef]
39. van der Meij, E.; Anema, J.R.; Leclercq, W.K.G.; Bongers, M.Y.; Consten, E.C.J.; Schraffordt Koops, S.E.; van de Ven, P.M.; Terwee, C.B.; van Dongen, J.M.; Schaafsma, F.G.; et al. Personalised perioperative care by e-health after intermediate-grade abdominal surgery: A multicentre, single-blind, randomised, placebo-controlled trial. *Lancet* **2018**, *392*, 51–59. [CrossRef]
40. Nicolaidis, S. Personalized medicine in neurosurgery. *Metabolism* **2013**, *62* (Suppl. 1), S45–S48. [CrossRef]

41. Tarpada, S.P.; Morris, M.T.; Burton, D.A. Spinal fusion surgery: A historical perspective. *J. Orthop.* **2016**, *14*, 134–136. [CrossRef] [PubMed]
42. McClelland, S., 3rd; Goldstein, J.A. Minimally Invasive versus Open Spine Surgery: What Does the Best Evidence Tell Us? *J. Neurosci. Rural Pract.* **2017**, *8*, 194–198. [CrossRef] [PubMed]
43. Meheux, C.J.; Park, K.J.; Clyburn, T.A. A Retrospective Study Comparing a Patient-specific Design Total Knee Arthroplasty With an Off-the-Shelf Design: Unexpected Catastrophic Failure Seen in the Early Patient-specific Design. *J. Am. Acad. Orthop. Surg. Glob. Res. Rev.* **2019**, *3*. [CrossRef]
44. Tong, Y.; Kaplan, D.J.; Spivak, J.M.; Bendo, J.A. Three-dimensional printing in spine surgery: A review of current applications. *Spine J.* **2020**, *20*, 833–846. [CrossRef] [PubMed]
45. Mobbs, R.J.; Phan, K.; Malham, G.; Seex, K.; Rao, P.J. Lumbar interbody fusion: Techniques, indications and comparison of interbody fusion options including PLIF, TLIF, MI-TLIF, OLIF/ATP, LLIF and ALIF. *J. Spine Surg.* **2015**, *1*, 2–18. [CrossRef] [PubMed]
46. Martelli, N.; Serrano, C.; van den Brink, H.; Pineau, J.; Prognon, P.; Borget, I.; El Batti, S. Advantages and disadvantages of 3-dimensional printing in surgery: A systematic review. *Surgery* **2016**, *159*, 1485–1500. [CrossRef]

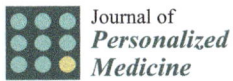
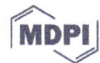

Article

Artificial Intelligence-Based Recognition of Different Types of Shoulder Implants in X-ray Scans Based on Dense Residual Ensemble-Network for Personalized Medicine

Haseeb Sultan, Muhammad Owais, Chanhum Park, Tahir Mahmood, Adnan Haider and Kang Ryoung Park *

Division of Electronics and Electrical Engineering, Dongguk University, 30 Pildong-ro 1-gil, Jung-gu, Seoul 04620, Korea; haseebsltn@gmail.com (H.S.); malikowais266@gmail.com (M.O.); pipetsupport@naver.com (C.P.); tahirmahmood.cs@gmail.com (T.M.); adnanhaider@dgu.ac.kr (A.H.)
* Correspondence: parkgr@dgu.edu; Tel.: +82-10-3111-7022; Fax: +82-2-2277-8735

Abstract: Re-operations and revisions are often performed in patients who have undergone total shoulder arthroplasty (TSA) and reverse total shoulder arthroplasty (RTSA). This necessitates an accurate recognition of the implant model and manufacturer to set the correct apparatus and procedure according to the patient's anatomy as personalized medicine. Owing to unavailability and ambiguity in the medical data of a patient, expert surgeons identify the implants through a visual comparison of X-ray images. False steps cause heedlessness, morbidity, extra monetary weight, and a waste of time. Despite significant advancements in pattern recognition and deep learning in the medical field, extremely limited research has been conducted on classifying shoulder implants. To overcome these problems, we propose a robust deep learning-based framework comprised of an ensemble of convolutional neural networks (CNNs) to classify shoulder implants in X-ray images of different patients. Through our rotational invariant augmentation, the size of the training dataset is increased 36-fold. The modified ResNet and DenseNet are then combined deeply to form a dense residual ensemble-network (DRE-Net). To evaluate DRE-Net, experiments were executed on a 10-fold cross-validation on the openly available shoulder implant X-ray dataset. The experimental results showed that DRE-Net achieved an accuracy, F1-score, precision, and recall of 85.92%, 84.69%, 85.33%, and 84.11%, respectively, which were higher than those of the state-of-the-art methods. Moreover, we confirmed the generalization capability of our network by testing it in an open-world configuration, and the effectiveness of rotational invariant augmentation.

Keywords: shoulder arthroplasty; X-ray images; implant classification; deep learning; dense residual ensemble-network; rotational invariant augmentation

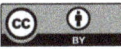

1. Introduction

The human shoulder is the most mobile joint of the body. The shoulder may be damaged owing to severe fractures or injuries to the upper arm or severe joint infection. Shoulder surgery is needed when damage to the shoulder joint progresses to such an extent that non-operative procedures cannot resolve the issue or the joint movement causes severe pain. According to the Agency for Healthcare Research and Quality, 53,000 Americans undergo shoulder replacement surgery each year [1]. Total shoulder arthroplasty (TSA) and reverse total shoulder arthroplasty (RTSA) [2] are medical procedures for treating arthritic shoulder joints. With this treatment, a prosthesis is used to repair the damaged joint of the shoulder to re-establish movement and reduce pain. TSA and RTSA are critical for shoulder pain in osteoarthritis. Proper preoperative preparation can help avoid many complications in the revision of TSA and RTSA.

One key surgical step that helps avoid more common complications is identifying prostheses to properly position them. As the morphology of the human shoulder varies from person to person, prostheses are comprised of fixtures and superstructures that can vary by their model, structure, and manufacturer. Therefore, the "one size fits all" idea is not suitable for the treatment of shoulder arthroplasty. Therefore, selecting the correct prostheses model from the right manufacturer for the right patient is very important as personalized medicine. Designing a framework for automatic selection of suitable prostheses for a patient would allow the surgeons to conduct prior and more effective decision-making.

There are many different combinations of device characteristics and surgical approaches, and surgeons often deal with a small number of implants at a time to maximize their expertise with the technology [3]. With a lack of comparable data, surgeons choose which from the few implants they currently offer are appropriate solutions for each patient, rather than choosing from the whole range of alternatives available on the market. However, in some clinical situations, surgeons may believe that only one device is the best option. Older patients, for example, are unlikely to gain additional benefits from a newer implant, but they are at higher risk of surgical problems than younger patients if revision is required [4]. In such cases, selecting a particular implant is crucial. Owing to the limited experience of surgeons with limited implants models, this makes them difficult to work in such situations. Moreover, implants are not identified by medical doctors due to incoherence in documentation and global limitations relating to access to such records, in particular by outside hospital systems [5]. With time, some models of former implants have been halted and their production cut off, whereas new models that differ somewhat from the prior models are being introduced by manufacturers. Moreover, the inclinations of doctors toward certain prostheses change over time. In an investigation carried out by arthroplasty surgeons, 88% of surgeons indicated that implant identification is a critical obstacle to the treatment of an arthroplasty patient [6]. Different prosthesis models require different systems and equipment for replacement and repair, and accurate identification of the model is mandatory. Failure to identify the correct model before surgery results in a waste of healthcare resources, time, and the health of the patient. In some situations, the manufacture and model of the implant might be obscure to surgeons and patients, for example when the original medical procedure is performed outside of the county, and the patients are unable to access their medical records. Over 40% of patients in institutions other than their original arthroplasty are less likely to access outside medical records in a timely manner [5]. As for other reasons why the prosthesis model and manufacturer are unknown, the first original surgery might be performed numerous years before the subsequent surgery, and the patient's medical information might become lost or unclear. In these cases, medical experts identify a prosthesis through a visual comparison of X-ray images and an implant atlas [7]. This task is tedious, time-consuming, dependent on the surgeon's experience, and an erroneous recognition can have certain consequences. Therefore, there is a need for an automated method for the identification of prostheses to aid surgeons with pre-operative planning and to save time and medical costs. However, high intra-class variabilities and low inter-class variabilities in shoulder implants appear in X-ray images, as shown in Figure 1, which makes this research extremely challenging.

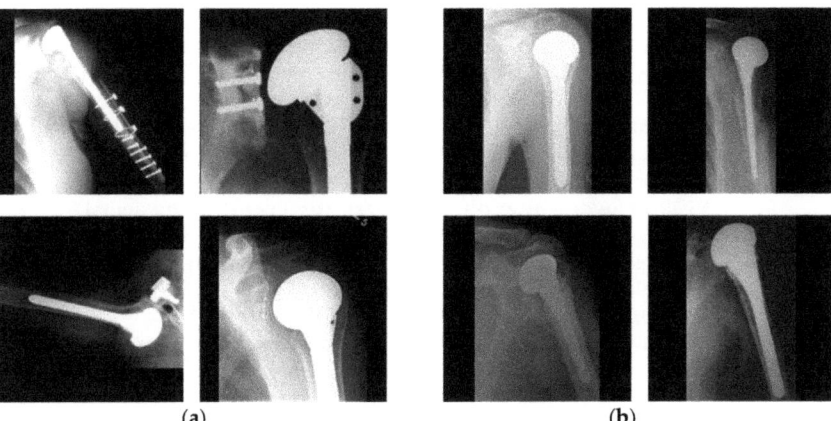

Figure 1. Examples showing high intra-class variabilities and low inter-class variabilities. Examples showing (**a**) high intra-class variability of one manufacturer (Cofield) and (**b**) low inter-class variability. In (**b**), upper-left, upper-right, lower-left, and lower-right images show the cases of four manufacturers of Cofield, Depuy, Tornier, and Zimmer, respectively.

Despite significant advancements in pattern recognition and deep learning (DL) in the medical field, there has been extremely limited research conducted on classifying shoulder implants. To address these issues, we propose a robust deep-learning-based framework comprising an ensemble of convolutional neural networks (CNNs) to classify shoulder implants in X-ray images. Compared to previous studies, our research is novel in the following five ways.

- To effectively identify shoulder implants, we propose a dense residual ensemble-network (DRE-Net) comprising two CNN models and a shallow concatenation network (SCN). Our network achieves a higher accuracy compared with state-of-the-art studies.
- We propose a rotational invariant augmentation (RIA) to tackle the overfitting problem.
- To check the generalization capability of our network, the proposed DRE-Net is analyzed in different configuration modes of open and closed worlds.
- We analyzed the impact of end-to-end and sequential training of DRE-Net on the testing accuracy of shoulder implant images.
- Our model is publicly available [8] for a fair comparison by other researchers.

The remainder of this paper proceeds as follows. In Section 2, related studies on the classification of different prostheses are described. Section 3 details our proposed classification framework for shoulder implants. In Section 4, the experimental setup and results are presented. Finally, the discussion and conclusions are presented in Sections 5 and 6, respectively.

2. Related Works

Previous studies on implant recognition have classified handcrafted feature-based and deep feature-based methods. Prior to the approach of DL strategies, previous studies have considered handcrafted feature-based methods for implant identification [9–11].

DL models have recently contributed pivotal additions in different clinical areas [12,13], including lesion classification [14,15], lesion detection [16–18], and lesion segmentation [19–22]. DL also affects every clinical specialty, including orthopedic surgery [23,24]. Plain film radiographs have been subjected to highly developed DL methods for identification of the elbow, wrist, ankle, and humerus; classification of the hip fracture types and proximal humerus; detection of the presence of arthroplasty and its type; detection of aseptic loosening; and staging the severity of knee osteoarthritis; among other applications [25–31]. In [32], a DL system was proposed to classify the knee implants of three datasets. The authors used variants of the residual network (ResNet) for different datasets and conducted a classification of two manufacturers and two models. Their network is trained to recognize only two classes, which limits its generalizability. In [33], the authors achieved 99% accuracy by using an artificial intelligence-based DL model to classify knee implants from four manufacturers. In [34], the authors used the visual geometry group (VGG)-16 and VGG-19 models by applying transfer learning to classify dental implants in panoramic X-ray images. Transfer learning with pre-trained networks is effective for learning richer features from large datasets to a small dataset to achieve a high level of accuracy. They manually segmented the panoramic images, and their network was unable to detect the uncropped panoramic image.

In [35], the authors used different CNN models, including SqueezeNet [36], GoogLeNet [37], ResNet-18 [38], MobileNet-v2 [39], and ResNet-50 [38] for the classification of dental implants in X-ray images. They used transfer learning with these pre-trained networks and achieved an accuracy of 90%–97%. In [40], they used a dense convolutional network (DenseNet)-201 [41] CNN with transfer learning to classify three total hip replacement prosthesis models in X-ray images with 100% accuracy. They implemented DenseNet-201 using two different weight initialization methods: (1) a random Gaussian distribution and (2) pre-trained weights of a CNN on the ImageNet database [42]. They demonstrated that a pretrained CNN cannot learn to identify the implant design in X-ray images well. DL also plays a vital role in the detection and classification of bone fractures [27,43]. However, this study was limited to a binary classification of broken and unbroken bones. In [44], a computer-assisted diagnosis (CAD) system based on a hierarchical CNN was designed for the classification of different types of fractures in X-ray images. However, in the case of some classes, the accuracy does not meet the expectations of physicians, and the system still needs to be improved for the classification of subclasses. A deep learning-based study was conducted on the classification of shoulder implants by four manufacturers, where the authors presented comparisons of DL models with different classifiers [45]. Nevertheless, the experiments were only conducted for a closed-world problem. They used the transfer-learning method and did not involve an open-world setting to address real-world problems. In [46], DL was used for the binary classification of shoulder implant models. They used a transfer learning approach and fine-tuned ResNet-18 for binary classification of the existence of arthroplasty implants. Similarly, they used the same approach to distinguish between TSA and RTSA. Finally, they used five fine-tuned models based on ResNet-152 to classify the five TSA models in a binary fashion. However, there is a possibility for an image to be labeled for multiple classes using this method.

To overcome these problems, we propose DRE-Net comprised of two deep CNNs and an SCN to classify shoulder implants in X-ray images. We considered a total of four different classes by manufacturers of 597 unidentified patients related to shoulder implants. We propose a deep feature-based framework for the accurate identification of shoulder implants to ease surgeons. We also address the open-world configuration and found that our model has the capability of generalizability and is therefore applicable to real-world problems.

Table 1 shows comparisons of the strengths and weaknesses of previous studies and our approach for the recognition of implants in X-ray images.

Table 1. Comparisons between our proposed and previous methods for implant recognition in X-ray images.

Category	Type	Methods	# Classes	Results	Strength	Weakness
Handcrafted feature-based	Knee	Template matching [9]	1	70% to 90% accuracies	- Uses a simple image processing technique including Sobel operator, binarization, and template matching - Computationally efficient	Requires 3D CAD models for template generation of implants
	Dental	Active contours + K-nearest neighborhood (K-NN) [10]	11	91% of the known implants are recognized	- Optimal initial location of the contour can be selected by their method - Uses simple machine learning algorithm for classification	- K-NN classifier is time-consuming for large numbers of features - Because of the large number of dental implant models, their approach returns a set of possible candidate results for identifying new implants and needs a user interaction to verify the candidate result
	Shoulder	Hough transform + histogram equalization + mean shift filter [11]	4	77% precision, and 64% F-measure	- Uses conventional image processing schemes involving bilateral filter, mean shift filter, and a median blur filter - Develops a pre-processing tool for training a classifier	Segmentation performance is dependent on the growing approach of seed region
	Knee	Pre-trained CNN [32]	2	100% sensitivity, and 100% specificity	- High classification performance - Precisely determines the presence of total knee arthroplasty (TKA) - Accurately classifies the TKA and unicompartmental knee arthroplasty (UKA)	Classification is performed in a binary fashion (the presence of implant)
		Pre-trained CNN [33]	9	99% accuracy, 95% sensitivity, and 99% specificity	High classification performance	Pre-processing is needed and computationally expensive
	Dental	Pre-trained CNN [34]	11	93.5% accuracy, 91.6% F-measures	High average classification accuracy with a small dataset of panoramas	VGG network can be replaced with the state-of-the-art networks
		Pre-trained CNN [35]	4	96% to 97% accuracies	High classification performance and computationally efficient	Their method is unable to detect several implants simultaneously
Deep feature-based	Hip	Pre-trained CNN [40]	3	100% accuracy	High classification performance	- Requires high processing power for extensive training - Uses only one post-surgery anteroposterior (AP) X-ray per patient
	Shoulder	Pre-trained CNN [46]	2	95% sensitivity, and 90% specificity to classify TSA and RTSA	- High accuracy to detect the existence of shoulder arthroplasty - High sensitivity to classify TSA and RTSA	Classification is performed in a binary fashion (the presence of implant)
		Pre-trained CNN [45]	4	80.4% accuracy, 80% precision, 75% recall, and 76% F1-score	- First deep learning based-approach to classify the manufacturers of shoulder implants - Higher classification accuracy than non-deep learning-based methods	- Accuracies are needed to be enhanced - Performance was measured only by closed-world configuration
		DRE-Net (Proposed)	4	85.92% accuracy, 84.69% F1-score, 85.33% precision, and 84.11% recall	- High classification accuracy - Applicable to real-world problems by considering both closed-world and open-world configurations	Requires more training time

3. Proposed Methods

3.1. Overview of Proposed Method

Figure 2 shows the overall procedure of our proposed method of shoulder implant classification. During the training phase, input images of 224 × 224 × 3 were augmented using the proposed RIA. This technique artificially increases the number of training datasets by the in-plane rotation of each image from 0° to 360° with an interval of 10°. In this way, in addition to the original image, we obtained 36 augmented images from one input. Training is then applied with the proposed DRE-Net, including a modified ResNet-50, a modified DenseNet-201, and an SCN for feature concatenation. During the testing phase, an image is input into the trained DRE-Net, and the final classification of the shoulder implant is conducted based on the output of DRE-Net. Detailed explanations of the proposed RIA and DRE-Net are presented in Sections 3.2 and 3.3, respectively.

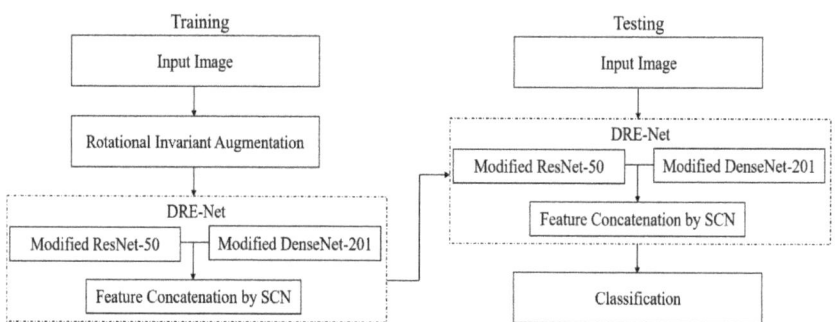

Figure 2. Overall procedure of the proposed method.

3.2. Rotational Invariant Augmentation (RIA)

The performance of a deep CNN on a dataset, including a small number of images, usually suffers from many different problems, such as an overfitting and a lack of generality. To address this issue, data augmentation has been proposed. Data augmentation includes setting up strategies that upgrade the size and worth of the training dataset with an end goal in which better DL models can be assembled utilizing such strategies [47]. Therefore, we augmented our training dataset based on the in-plane rotation. As a reason for using the in-plane rotation scheme, our dataset consists of implanted shoulder prostheses with rod-like shapes that are easily in-plane rotated in the captured X-ray images, as shown in Figure 1. Data augmentation by an in-plane rotation is applied on each image by rotating the image based on an image center of between 0° and 360°, with an interval of 10°. In this way, we obtained each image with 36 postures at different angles. Figure 3 shows the RIA samples of one image from the Cofield class.

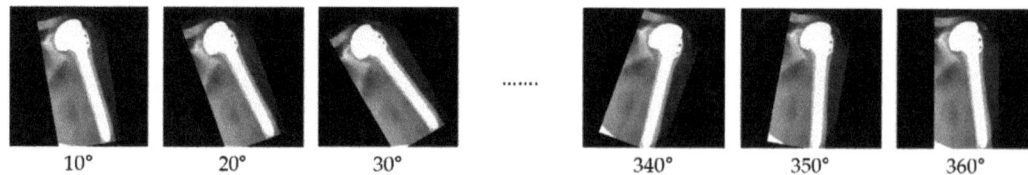

Figure 3. Examples of rotational invariant augmentation (RIA).

3.3. Classification of Shoulder Implants by DRE-Net

In machine learning, ensemble strategies merge various learning algorithms to achieve a preferable performance over any of the constituent models alone [48,49]. In the general frameworks of image classification, the main element is the optimum representation of the visual details or features. Based on this, we propose DRE-Net for the classification of shoulder implants, as shown in Figure 4. In the first stage of DRE-Net, an input image of 224 × 224 × 3 is input to two CNNs of modified ResNet-50 and DenseNet-201, which are modified by removing the fully connected layer (FCL) to extract the optimum features. Explanations of the first stage based on modified ResNet-50 and DenseNet-201 are presented in Sections 3.3.1 and 3.3.2, respectively. In the second stage of DRE-Net, the SCN obtains two feature vectors (f_1 and f_2 of Figure 4) from the first-stage networks. These features are then concatenated and passed through the FCL and SoftMax layers to classify the shoulder implant into one of the four manufacturers. Detailed explanations of our developed SCN are presented in Section 3.3.3.

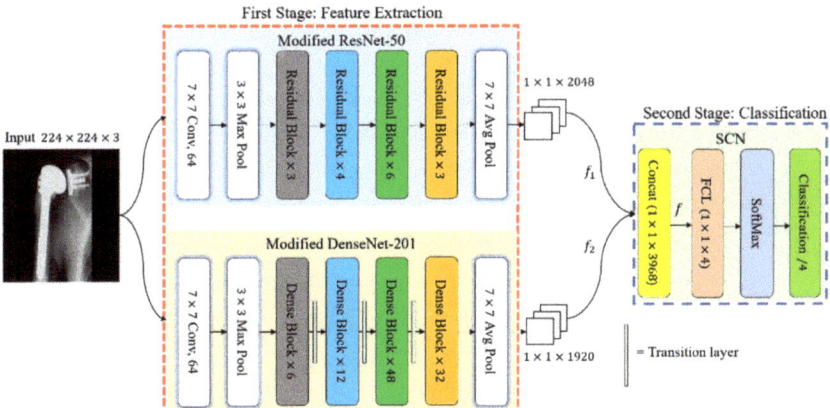

Figure 4. Diagram of our proposed DRE-Net for feature extraction and classification.

3.3.1. Feature Extraction Using Modified ResNet-50

Deep CNNs have demonstrated extreme power in representation learning because they learn the features on a pre-training task and transmit effective knowledge to the target tasks. AlexNet [50], VGG, GoogLeNet, ResNet, and DenseNet are commonly used deep CNNs for transfer learning. The experiments showed that constructing a deep network by copying layers from a learned shallow model leads to a high training error owing to vanishing gradient problems [38]. The residual network has an identity shortcut connection that skips some layers and therefore assists in shielding the network from vanishing gradient issues and improving the performance by deepening the network. Residual nets [38] were first placed in the ImageNet competition [51] for classification, localization, detection, and scoring the first position in common objects in context (COCO) competition for detection and segmentation. In our work, a state-of-the-art deep learning model of ResNet-50 pre-trained on the ImageNet dataset [42] was modified to extract the features for the classification of shoulder implant images.

As shown in Table 2, an image with a resolution of 224 × 224 × 3 was given as an input to the first layer labeled "Image Input." The second layer labeled "Conv 1" was comprised of 64 filters of 7 × 7 × 3, which exploits the input image. The convolution layer is a max-pooling layer, which reduced the dimensions of the feature map to a pixel resolution of 56 × 56 × 64. Following the max-pooling layer, the layers were grouped into four residual blocks. Each residual block was comprised of two layers of a 1×1 convolution and one layer of a 3 × 3 convolution. The first group of layers labeled "Conv 2_x" were comprised of three residual blocks, which processed the feature map and down-sampled it to a pixel resolution of 56 × 56 × 256. The output feature map of "Conv 2_x" was processed by the second group of layers labeled "Conv 3_x." This group contained four residual blocks and output a feature map with a pixel resolution of 28 × 28 × 512. Similarly, the third group of layers, labeled "Conv 4_x," contained six residual blocks. It processed the feature map of "Conv 3_x" and generated a feature map with a pixel resolution of 14 × 14 × 1024. The last group of layers labeled "Conv 5_x" contained three residual blocks. It processed the feature map of the previous layer and produced a 7 × 7 × 2048 sized feature map. Finally, the last average pooling layer named "Average Pooling" was applied with a filter size of 7 × 7 pixels and obtained a spatial feature vector f_1 of 1 × 1 × 2048. The last three layers of ResNet, labeled "FCL," "SoftMax," and "Classification Output" were removed in our modified ResNet to enhance the training convergence and extract only features not considering the classification.

Table 2. Layer configuration details of modified ResNet-50.

Layers Name	Output Feature Map Size	Kernel Size	Number of Iterations
Image Input	224 × 224 × 3	-	-
Conv 1	112 × 112 × 64	7 × 7 $conv$	1
Max Pooling	56 × 56 × 64	3 × 3 $max\ pool$	1
Conv 2_x	56 × 56 × 256	1 × 1 $conv$ 3 × 3 $conv$ 1 × 1 $conv$	3
Conv 3_x	28 × 28 × 512	1 × 1 $conv$ 3 × 3 $conv$ 1 × 1 $conv$	4
Conv 4_x	14 × 14 × 1024	1 × 1 $conv$ 3 × 3 $conv$ 1 × 1 $conv$	6
Conv 5_x	7 × 7 × 2048	1 × 1 $conv$ 3 × 3 $conv$ 1 × 1 $conv$	3
Average Pooling	1 × 1 × 2048	7 × 7 $avg\ pool$	1

3.3.2. Feature Extraction Using Modified DenseNet-201

With the rapid advancement of CNNs, they are becoming deeper, and the problem of a vanishing gradient has emerged. One solution to this problem is to introduce skip connections between layers, as in the ResNet model. These skip connections guarantee an efficient data stream among the layers in the network. To ensure the stream of maximum information among layers, all layers are associated legitimately with one another, and each layer acquires extra inputs from prior layers and gives its feature map to every single ensuing layer in the DenseNet model [41]. In our work, a state-of-the-art DenseNet-201 pre-trained on the ImageNet dataset [42] was modified to derive the features and classify the shoulder implant images.

As shown in Table 3, an image with a pixel resolution of 224 × 224 × 3 was given as an input to the first input layer called an "Image Input." The second layer, named "Conv 1," was comprised of 64 filters of 7 × 7 × 3, which exploited the input image. Following the convolution layer was a max-pooling layer, which reduced the dimensions of the feature map to 56 × 56 × 64 pixels. The layers were then grouped into four dense blocks. Each dense block included a three-sequential composite function with a convolution of 3×3, a rectified linear unit (ReLU) [52], and batch normalization (BN) [53]. The first group of layers, labeled "DenseBlock_1", which were comprised of six dense blocks, processed the feature map and down-sampled it to a pixel resolution of 28 × 28 × 128. The output feature map of "DenseBlock_1" was processed by the second group of layers, labeled "DenseBlock_2." This group contained 12 dense blocks and output a feature map with a pixel resolution of 14 × 14 × 256. Similarly, the third group of layers, labeled "DenseBlock_3," contained 48 dense blocks and processed the feature map of "DenseBlock_2." It down-sampled the features, and generated a feature map with a pixel resolution of 7 × 7 × 896. The last group of layers, labeled "DenseBlock_4", contained 32 dense blocks, processed the feature map of the previous layer, and produced a feature map with a pixel resolution of $7 \times 7 \times 1920$. Although the architecture contains dense blocks with various filters, the dimensions inside the blocks are equivalent. For compactness of the model and downsampling of the representations, the transition layer was applied between dense blocks, which comprise the convolution and pooling functions. Finally, the last average pooling layer, named "Average Pooling," was applied using a filter with a pixel resolution of 7×7, and obtained a spatial feature vector f_2 with a pixel resolution of $1 \times 1 \times 1920$. The last three layers of DenseNet, named "FCL," "SoftMax," and "Classification Output" were removed to enhance the training convergence and extract only features not considering the classification. The feature vector f_2 with 1920 dimensions was concatenated using the 2048-dimension feature vector f_1 of ResNet-50 in an SCN, and the final classification was made based on the output of the SCN, as shown in Figure 4.

Table 3. Layer configuration details of modified DenseNet-201.

Layer Name	Output Feature Map Size	Kernel Size	Number of Iterations
Image Input	$224 \times 224 \times 3$	-	-
Conv 1	$112 \times 112 \times 64$	7×7 conv	1
Max Pooling	$56 \times 56 \times 64$	3×3 max pool	1
DenseBlock_1	$56 \times 56 \times 256$	1×1 conv 3×3 conv	6
Transition Layer	$28 \times 28 \times 128$	1×1 conv 2×2 avg pool	1
DenseBlock_2	$28 \times 28 \times 512$	1×1 conv 3×3 conv	12
Transition Layer	$14 \times 14 \times 256$	1×1 conv 2×2 avg pool	1
DenseBlock_3	$14 \times 14 \times 1792$	1×1 conv 3×3 conv	48
Transition Layer	$7 \times 7 \times 896$	1×1 conv 2×2 avg pool	1
DenseBlock_4	$7 \times 7 \times 1920$	1×1 conv 3×3 conv	32
Average Pooling	$1 \times 1 \times 1920$	7×7 avg pool	1

3.3.3. Feature Concatenation and Final Classification by SCN

After extracting the feature vectors from each CNN of the first-stage networks, we further ensembled them to obtain a concatenated feature map using the proposed SCN, as shown in Figure 4. The efficiency of the ensemble learning model was substantially improved. The ensemble model allowed the true objective function to be best approximated within the space of the hypothesis, and the overall performance could be improved using various CNN features [54,55]. We propose an SCN that concatenates two sets of features into a longer feature vector. Table 4 presents the architecture of the SCN. The first layer of the SCN, called "Concat," takes the inputs from two networks of the first stage with different dimensions and concatenates them. In detail, the feature map f_1 with pixel dimensions of $1 \times 1 \times 2048$ by modified ResNet is concatenated with f_2 with pixel dimensions $1 \times 1 \times 1920$ by modified DenseNet. The Concat layer of the SCN provides a feature map f with a pixel size of $1 \times 1 \times 3968$. It then passes through the FCL. The FCL includes a limited number of neurons, taking data from one vector and returning data from another. In general, considering the jth node of the ith layer, we can obtain the following equation:

$$z_i = \sum_{l=1}^{n_{i-1}} (w_{j,l}^{[i]} a_l^{[i-1]} + b_j^{[i]}) \qquad (1)$$

where in Equation (1), $a^{[i-1]}$ is the output of the previous layer with dimensions $(n_H^{[i-1]} \times n_W^{[i-1]} \times n_C^{[i-1]})$ and is given as input to the FCL by flattening the tensor to a 1D vector with dimensions of $(n_H^{[i-1]} \times n_W^{[i-1]} \times n_C^{[i-1]}, 1)$ [56]. The learned parameters at the lth layers are weights $w_{j,l}$ with $n_{l-1} \times n_l$ parameters, and bias b_j with n_l parameters. In addition, n_H, n_W, and n_C represent the height, width, and number of channels, respectively, whereas the final output of the FCL is z_i. Subsequently, the SoftMax layer is executed. It computes the results of the FCL using the SoftMax function, which compresses the vector z of arbitrary K real numbers to a normalized vector of K real number probabilities, as a probability distribution ranging between zero and 1 with a probability equivalent to 1 [56]. The SoftMax function is as follows:

$$f(z)_i = \frac{e^{z_i}}{\sum_j^K e^{z_j}} \qquad (2)$$

where in Equation (2), K is the number of output classes, and the output $f(z)_i$ is the probability for each class. These probabilities are obtained by taking the exponential of each neuron (value) for its class, that is, e^{z_i}, and dividing by the sum of all exponentials. The denominator part acts as a normalization term to make the sum of all output values equal to 1. Finally, the classification layer computes the final probabilities to determine the class for the image.

Table 4. Layer configuration details of SCN.

Layers Name	Output Feature Map Size	Kernel Size	Number of Iterations
Concat	$1 \times 1 \times 3968$	-	1
Fully Connected	$1 \times 1 \times 4$	-	1
SoftMax	$1 \times 1 \times 4$	-	1
Classification	4	-	1

3.4. Classification Configuration

In our DRE-Net-based classification of shoulder implants, we designed two configurations of closed-world and open-world configurations. The detailed explanations are as follows: for the closed-world configuration, data from the same class are used for both training and testing. In detail, we applied a 10-fold cross-validation. Therefore, 90% of the data of each class were used for training, and the remaining 10% of the data of the same class were used for testing. This procedure was iterated 10 times, and the average accuracy of 10 trials was obtained as the final classification accuracy. Because the output classes of training and testing were the same, the final classification was made based on the output of DRE-Net, as shown in Figure 5.

For the open-world configuration, data from the same class are not used for both training and testing, which means that the classes of training and testing data are completely different, as in general content-based image retrieval systems [57]. We conducted a 2-fold cross-validation considering four output classes. Therefore, the data of classes 1 and 2 were used for training, and the remaining data of classes 3 and 4 were used for testing in the first trial. In the second trial, the training and testing data were exchanged with each other, and the same procedure was repeated. The average accuracy of the two trials was obtained as the final accuracy of classification. Because the output classes of training and testing are different, the final classification cannot be made based on the output of DRE-Net, as in the close-world configuration shown in Figure 5. Instead, the feature vector (1×3968) of one testing image is extracted from the first layer (the concatenation layer of Figure 4 and Table 4) of the SCN with trained DRE-Net, and the best matching class is determined based on the L_2-norm distance (Euclidean distance) between the extracted feature vector and mean vector of the testing classes, as shown in Figure 6. The open-world configuration can reflect the real scenario better than the closed-world configuration, because the data of the untrained class can be obtained in the medical field, as a new manufacturer appears. In this scenario, there is no need to retrain the whole network for all the previous and new classes. Only a reference mean feature vector of the new class (extracted from our network) and its corresponding label (assigned by the medical professional) need to be registered. Then, the model can also work for all the data samples of the new class. In detail, when a new implant model needs to be recognized in a testing phase, the feature vector (1×3968) of the image of the new implant model can be extracted from the first layer (the concatenation layer of Figure 4 and Table 4) of the SCN with DRE-Net without additional training. Then, the best matching class can be determined based on the L2-norm distance (Euclidean distance) between the extracted feature vector and the set of reference mean feature vectors.

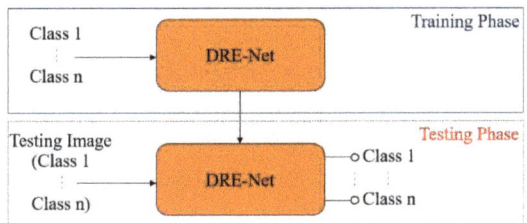

Figure 5. Diagram of closed-world configuration for classification.

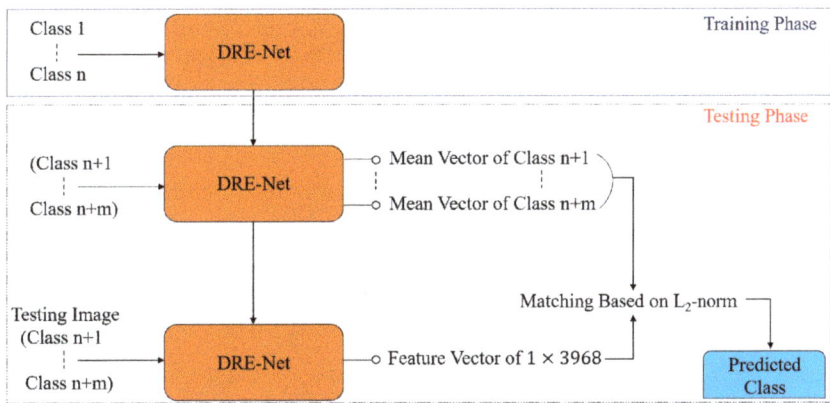

Figure 6. Diagram of open-world configuration for feature extraction and classification.

4. Experimental Setups and Results

4.1. Dataset and Experimental Setups

The dataset used in our research was collected from two different sources comprised of 597 X-ray images of shoulder implant prostheses. This is an open medical dataset that can be used for research purposes. The dataset consists of shoulder prosthesis images of 16 different models from 4 different manufacturers, which were collected from individual manufacturers, surgeons, and the University of Washington [11,45]. One image was captured from each patient in the dataset. The 597 X-ray images of implants are the sum of 83, 294, 71, and 149 of the four manufacturers, Cofield, Depuy, Tornier, and Zimmer, respectively. Figure 7 shows representatives from the dataset, including actual class labels. As shown in Figure 1, the dataset is challenging owing to (1) a high intra-class variance resulting from the various models of the same manufacturer, (2) a small inter-class variance from all X-ray scans of the implants being generally indistinguishable, and (3) a class imbalance. The intra-class variance and class imbalance problems were solved by increasing the dataset size using RIA with sufficient training.

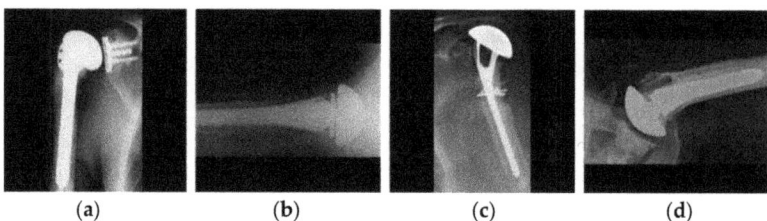

Figure 7. Examples of the dataset: shoulder implants of four different manufacturers: (**a**) Cofield, (**b**) Depuy, (**c**) Tornier, and (**d**) Zimmer.

Following the size of the input layer of our model, we resized all images of each class to spatial dimensions with a pixel resolution of 224 × 224 × 3 in a portable network graphics (PNG) file format. For the closed-world configuration, we randomly divided the dataset into 10 folds for a cross-validation, as described in Section 3.4. The number of images for the training dataset is not uniform for all classes, and this imbalance problem of the classes degrades the classification performance [58]. To eliminate this issue, we expanded the size of the training dataset by using RIA, but did not perform this augmentation with the testing dataset. Table 5 shows the detailed explanations of the 10-fold cross-validation of the training and testing datasets for the closed-world configuration. C1, C2, C3, and C4 represent the class Cofield, Depuy, Tornier, and Zimmer. We analyzed the performance of state-of-the-art methods using the same experimental protocols. In addition, state-of-the-art methods were also analyzed with online data augmentation and RIA to optimize the results.

Table 5. Summary of 10-fold cross-validation of training and testing data for closed-world configuration (unit: images).

Validation	Training		Testing				Total
	Original	Augmented	C1	C2	C3	C4	
1st fold	538	19,368	8	29	7	15	19,965
2nd fold	536	19,296	9	30	7	15	19,893
3rd fold	538	19,368	8	29	7	15	19,965
4th fold	537	19,332	8	30	7	15	19,929
5th fold	536	19,296	9	29	8	15	19,893
6th fold	539	19,404	8	29	7	14	20,001
7th fold	537	19,332	8	30	7	15	19,929
8th fold	538	19,368	8	29	7	15	19,965
9th fold	536	19,296	9	30	7	15	19,893
10th fold	538	19,368	8	29	7	15	19,965

A desktop system with the following specifications was used for all experiments in our work: 3.50 GHz Intel® (Santa Clara, CA, USA) Core™ i7–3770K central processing unit [59] with 16 GB RAM, and an NVIDIA (Santa Clara, CA, USA) GeForce GTX 1070 graphics card [60]. A deep learning toolbox with MATLAB R2019b (MathWorks, Inc., Natick, MA,

USA) [61] was used on the Windows 10 operating system to implement our RIA algorithm and DRE-Net.

4.2. Training of CNN Model

For training DRE-Net, the cross-entropy loss function was used as follows [62]:

$$CE = -\sum_{i}^{K} t_i log(f(z)_i) \qquad (3)$$

where in Equation (3), $f(z)_i$ is the probability for each class, which is defined in Equation (2). Cross entropy is simply the negative log of $f(z)_i$ for the true label class t_i. For the true label class, t_i becomes 1, whereas it becomes zero for all other classes.

Prior to training the CNNs, all of the dataset images were resized to 224 × 224 × 3 pixels. We trained different CNNs involving VGG-16, VGG-19, ResNet-18, ResNet-50, NASNet, DenseNet-201, and our deep DRE-Net for comparison. All CNNs were trained using the stochastic gradient descent (SGD) algorithm [63]. SGD is an optimization method that applies a backpropagation algorithm. The main goal of SGD is to find the optimum parameters for the model based on a mini-batch using the derivative of the loss function. SGD updates parameters, such as the weights and biases for each training instance and label. During the training of the CNN, the loss between the actual label and predicted label is calculated, and the SGD updates the parameters based on the loss function. Owing to the problems of class imbalance and the limited size of the dataset, the dataset was augmented using the proposed RIA. Owing to the small dataset, the filter weights of the first-stage networks of the modified DenseNet and ResNet were initialized using the parameters of pre-trained DenseNet-201 and ResNet-50 along with the ImageNet dataset, respectively. Transfer learning with our training data was then conducted using these CNN models. Transfer learning with pre-trained networks is effective for learning richer features from large datasets to a small dataset to achieve high accuracy. The details of the training parameters for the modified DenseNet, ResNet, and DRE-Net are listed in Table 6. The explanations of these parameters are given in [64]. In our research, we compared the accuracies from sequential training, by which modified DenseNet, ResNet, and SCN were separately trained, and the accuracies from end-to-end training, by which DRE-Net including modified DenseNet, ResNet, and SCN were trained at the same time. The training parameters of the two training cases are presented in Table 6.

Table 6. Parameters for network training.

	Methods	Number of Epochs	Mini-Batch Size	Learning Rate	Momentum Term	L2-Regularization	Learning Rate Drop Factor
Sequential training	Modified DenseNet-201	13	10	0.001	0.9	0.0001	0.1
	Modified ResNet-50	13	10	0.001	0.9	0.0001	0.1
	SCN	9	10	0.001	0.9	0.0001	0.1
End-to-end training	DRE-Net	7	10	0.001	0.9	0.0001	0.1

The graphs of the training losses and the accuracies through both sequential and end-to-end training are visualized according to the number of epochs, as shown in Figure 8. All networks were converged by increasing the accuracy to 100% while decreasing the loss to 0%, which shows that all networks were successfully trained well. However, the convergence time in terms of loss of the end-to-end training was longer than that of the modified DenseNet, ResNet, and DRE-Net when applying sequential training. In our experiments, we selected 25% of the data as a validation subset and the remaining 75% of the data as a training subset from the training data. We provide the validation losses and accuracies of the proposed SCN (Figure 8c) which shows the better testing accuracies than DRE-Net (end-to-end training) (Figure 8d). Even with the model of training accuracies at 100% (Figure 8c), we could obtain the high validation accuracy and low validation loss as shown in Figure 8e, which confirms the optimal convergence of the proposed network without causing overfitting problem with training data.

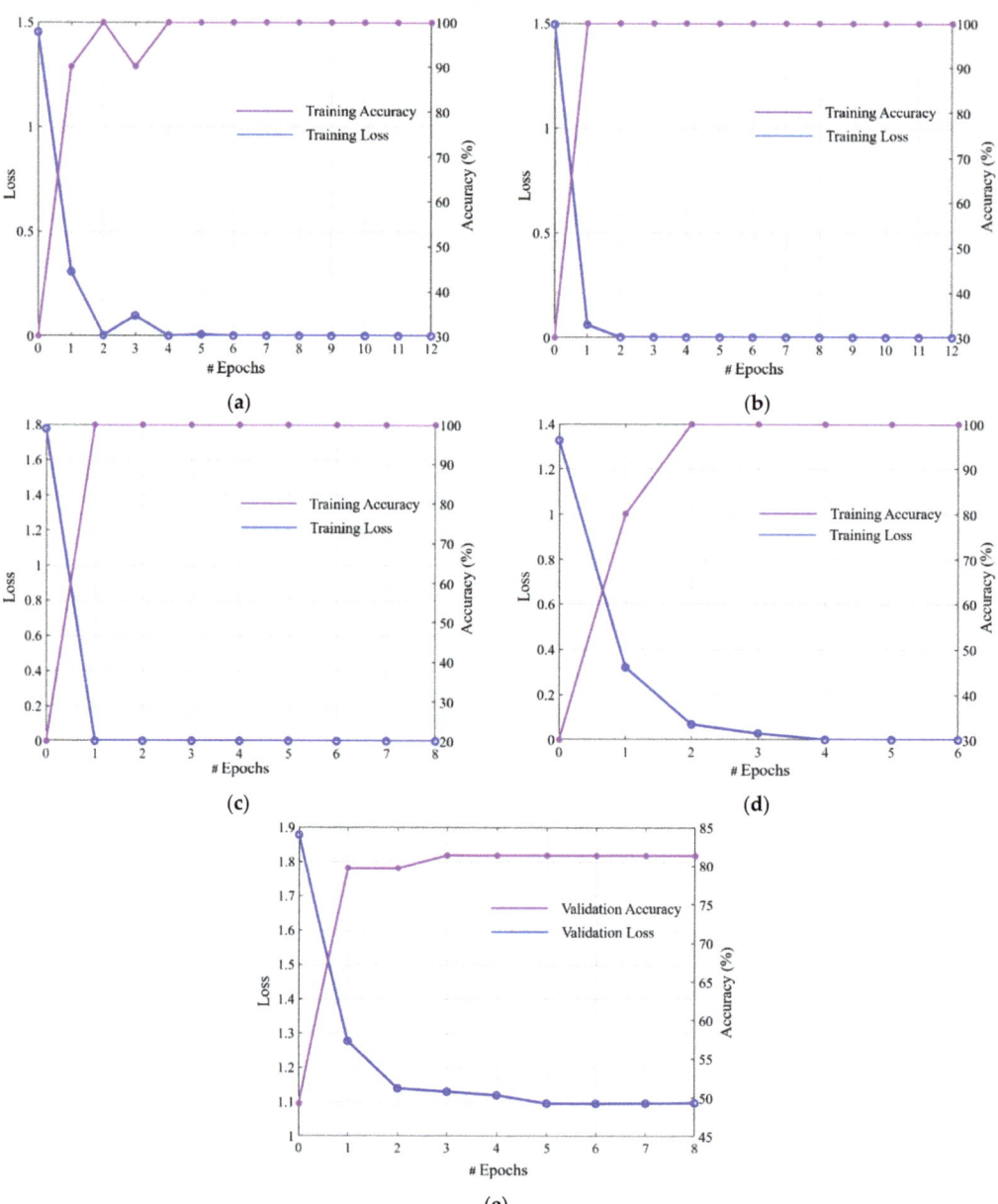

Figure 8. Plots for training losses and training accuracies: sequential training of (**a**) modified DenseNet-201, (**b**) modified ResNet-50, (**c**) SCN, (**d**) DRE-Net (end-to-end training), and (**e**) plots for validation losses and validation accuracies of SCN of (**c**).

4.3. Testing and Performance Analysis

We used four qualitative evaluation metrics to assess the performance of our classification network: the accuracy, F1-score, precision, and recall. These metrics are commonly used to evaluate classification frameworks [65] and are calculated as follows:

$$\text{Accuracy} = \frac{1}{K} \sum_{k=1}^{K} \frac{TP_k + TN_k}{TP_k + TN_k + FP_k + FN_k} \quad (4)$$

$$\text{F1-score} = 2 \times \frac{\text{Precision} \times \text{Recall}}{\text{Precision} + \text{Recall}} \quad (5)$$

$$\text{Precision} = \frac{1}{K} \sum_{k=1}^{K} \frac{TP_k}{TP_k + FP_k} \quad (6)$$

$$\text{Recall} = \frac{1}{K} \sum_{k=1}^{K} \frac{TP_k}{TP_k + TN_k} \quad (7)$$

where K represents the total number of classes, which is equivalent to 4 in our study; TP_k is the number of true positives of class k, which represents the correctly predicted image from class k; and FP_k represents the number of false positives of class k, which represents the incorrect prediction of another class into class k. In addition, TN_k represents the number of true negatives of class k, and is the result in which the other class (except for class k) is correctly predicted by the model. Finally, FN_k represents the number of false negatives of class k, which occurs when class k is incorrectly predicted into another class using the model.

4.3.1. Ablation Studies

We studied ablation studies to check the performance and contribution of each component to the overall framework. As the first ablation study, we compared the accuracies of our SCN in Figure 4 with those of the principal component analysis (PCA) + K-NN classifier. A PCA [66] followed by a K-NN [67] was utilized as a post-processing stage to generate the uncorrelated features and scale down the dimensions of the feature vector. The main purpose of applying a PCA is to analyze the discrimination of the selected features (i.e., whether features are distinctive or redundant). From the concatenation layer of a SCN, shown in Figure 4, 1×3968 features are projected into the eigenspace to obtain 3968 eigenvectors and eigenvalues of the training samples. As shown in Figure 9, different eigenvectors are selected to evaluate the PCA for computing the eigenvector (λ), which shows the best performance. As shown in Figure 9, the maximum average performance of $\lambda = 10$ was found among all eigenvectors with the training data. Then, the PCA features of the testing samples at $\lambda = 10$ were calculated and used as an input to the K-NN classifier. Detailed comparative classification results are shown in Table 7. Although the PCA can reduce the number of dimensions from 1×3968 to 1×10, the classification performance was not higher than that without the PCA-based classification framework (our SCN), as shown in Table 7. This indicates that the high-dimensional features extracted by our deep DRE-Net are already diversified.

Table 7. Performance comparisons of our proposed SCN using a PCA and a K-NN (unit: %).

Fold	Performance without a PCA (our SCN)				Performance with PCA ($\lambda = 10$) + K-NN			
	Accuracy	F1-Score	Recall	Precision	Accuracy	F1-Score	Recall	Precision
10-Fold Average	85.92	84.69	84.11	85.33	57.94	48.04	40.60	60.17

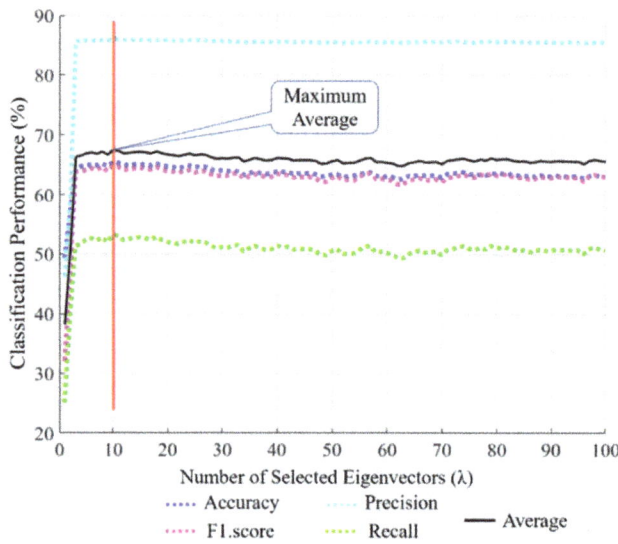

Figure 9. PCA-based performance for different numbers of eigenvectors (λ = 1, 2, 3, . . . ,100).

Table 8 shows the second ablation study of the shoulder implant classification. As shown in this table, DenseNet-201 and ResNet-50 without the proposed RIA showed lower accuracies by DenseNet-201 and ResNet-50 with RIA. However, the proposed DRE-Net, including DenseNet-201, ResNet-50, and SCN, showed the highest accuracies. The diversity of individually trained ensembles has been reported to be advantageous [68]. Therefore, we compared the results of DRE-Net using sequential and end-to-end training. The results in Table 8 suggest that ensembles of the models benefit from independent training (sequential training). End-to-end training showed a lower performance than sequential training, and the reason for this is that we used high-capacity models, and the ensemble of these models in end-to-end training shows a "model dominance" effect. Table 8 shows that there is a small difference between the results of DRE-Net (end-to-end) and ResNet-50 + RIA compared to those of DenseNet-201 + RIA. That is because DRE-Net (end-to-end) has "model dominance" effect of ResNet-50 + RIA.

Table 8. Performance comparisons of each sub-network and proposed DRE-Net by end-to-end or sequential training (unit: %).

Methods	Accuracy	F1-Score	Precision	Recall
ResNet-50 [38]	66.70	62.02	64.67	59.83
DenseNet-201 [41]	55.76	47.55	49.73	45.73
ResNet-50 + RIA	80.57	78.02	79.21	76.95
DenseNet-201 + RIA	84.75	83.76	85.21	82.42
DRE-Net (end-to-end)	81.55	79.12	80.77	77.66
DRE-Net (sequential)	85.92	84.69	85.33	84.11

Figure 10a–c present the classification performances of the second-best (DenseNet-201 + RIA) and third-best approaches (ResNet-50 + RIA) and our model (DRE-Net (sequential training)) from Table 8 in terms of a confusion matrix. The diagonal values of each table in Figure 10 show the average recall of each class. As shown in Figure 10, our model outperforms both DenseNet-201 + RIA and ResNet-50 + RIA. The reason why class 4 shows

lower accuracies by our model than with the other classes is that the data of class 4 have a higher interclass similarity with those of class 2, as explained in Section 5.

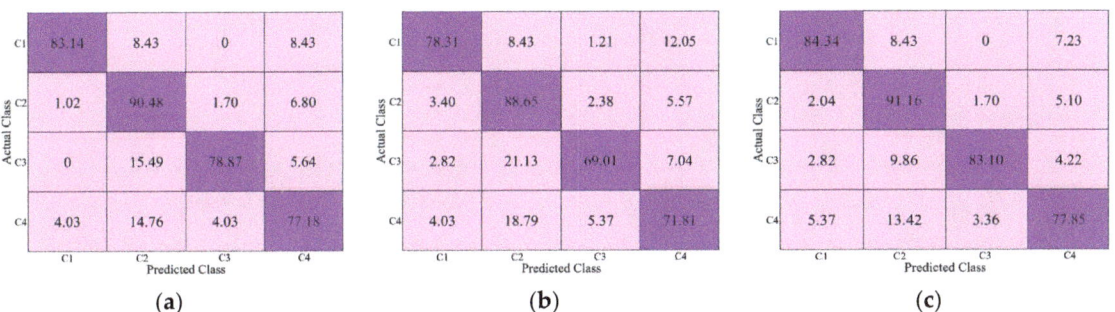

Figure 10. Confusion matrix of (**a**) DenseNet-201 + RIA, (**b**) ResNet-50 + RIA, and (**c**) DRE-Net (sequential training). C1–C4 indicate the classes of four manufacturers of Cofield, Depuy, Tornier, and Zimmer, respectively (unit: %).

4.3.2. Comparison of Proposed DRE-Net with the Subjective Evaluation

To highlight the significance of the proposed deep learning method, we additionally performed a subjective evaluation experiment considering the same experimental setup (same testing data samples and 10-fold cross validation). The graphical user interface (GUI) of the experimental protocol was designed in MATLAB R2019b (MathWorks, Inc., Natick, MA, USA) [61], as shown in Figure 11. In detail, a total of 10 individuals (without medical training) participated in this subjective evaluation and visually predicted the class label of all testing data samples one by one for each fold. The demographic details of these participants and subjective performance are given in Table 9. Participants (80% male and 20% female) from three different countries, including 50% from South Korea, 40% from Pakistan, and 10% from Iran took part in this subjective evaluation. All information for experiments was given to participants in advance. Each participant could observe both a set of random training samples of each manufacturer of Figure 11a, and one-fold testing images which is the 10% of the data of Figure 11b at the same time. In this way, each testing-fold samples were provided to each person to perform 10-fold cross validation. The group evaluated all of the testing images of each fold, and assigned the appropriate label to each sample of Figure 11b by visually comparing the training set as shown in Figure 11a. The average time calculated for the evaluation of one participant was about twenty minutes. Once all individuals had completed the evaluation, the average performance of each fold was calculated as shown in Table 9. Finally, we obtained the average performance (as confusion matrix, average accuracy, F1-score, precision, and recall) of this subjective evaluation and compared them with the proposed DRE-Net as presented in Figure 12 and Table 10. It can be observed that our proposed DRE-Net shows the superior performance over subjective evaluation with average performance gains of 33.67%, 35.15%, 36.47%, and 33.83% in terms of accuracy, F1-score, precision, and recall, respectively.

In addition, as shown in Figure 12a, the correct classification accuracy by human subject with Cofield data (C1) was 63.86% which was much lower than that by our proposed method of 84.34%. These results confirm that it is visually difficult to discriminate the data of C1 from Figure 1a, and we can tell that there exist the differences among those intra models.

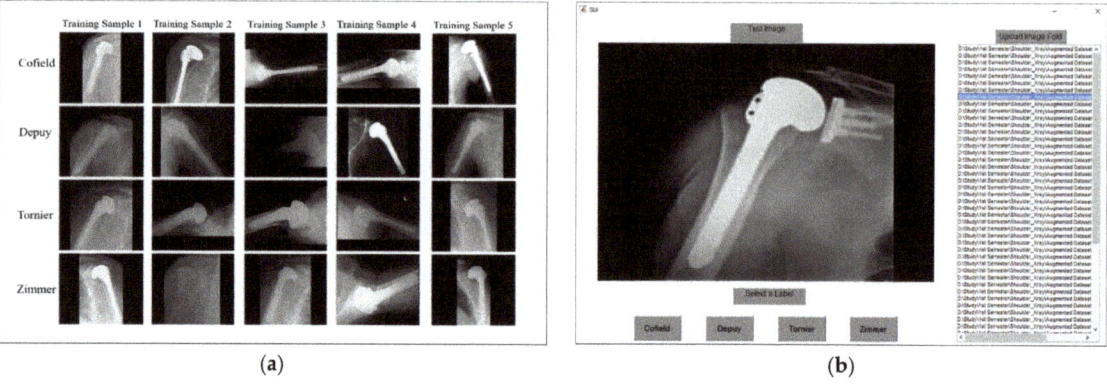

Figure 11. Graphical user interface used for subjective evaluation (**a**) random training samples of each class, which are shown to user during subjective evaluation, (**b**) interface showing all the testing data samples to user one by one for subjective class prediction.

Table 9. Demographic details of different subjects and their subjective evaluation results.

	Demographic Details			Subjective Performance (%)			
Participant Index	Age	Nationality	Sex	Accuracy	F1-Score	Precision	Recall
1	28	Pakistan	Male	57.63	53.40	53.51	53.29
2	28	Pakistan	Male	55.74	48.86	49.23	48.49
3	23	South Korea	Male	50.85	55.35	55.51	55.19
4	32	Pakistan	Male	48.33	48.43	46.90	50.06
5	27	South Korea	Male	50.82	45.58	45.51	45.66
6	29	South Korea	Male	55.17	45.67	45.13	46.23
7	42	Iran	Female	58.33	54.87	52.92	56.96
8	27	South Korea	Female	45.76	42.83	41.84	43.88
9	32	Pakistan	Male	52.46	46.77	46.63	46.90
10	28	South Korea	Male	47.46	53.68	51.47	56.09

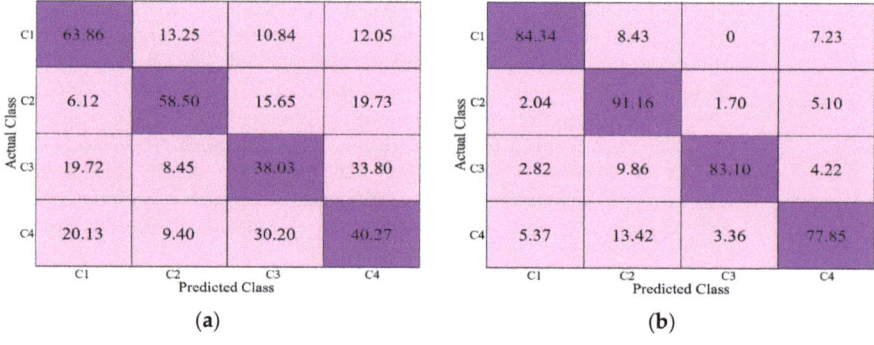

Figure 12. Performance comparison in terms of confusion matrices of (**a**) subjective method and (**b**) the proposed DRE-Net (sequential training). C1–C4 indicate the classes of four manufacturers of Cofield, Depuy, Tornier, and Zimmer, respectively (unit: %).

Table 10. Average performance comparison (10-folds) between subjective evaluation and the proposed DRE-Net (unit: %).

Methods	Accuracy	F1-Score	Precision	Recall
Subjective Method	52.25	49.54	48.86	50.28
DRE-Net (sequential)	**85.92**	**84.69**	**85.33**	**84.11**

4.3.3. Comparisons of Proposed DRE-Net with the State-of-The-Art Methods

The performances of various state-of-the-art methods [38,41,45,46,69,70] were compared with those of our approach. Table 11 shows the performance comparisons by the state-of-the-art methods and the proposed method without data augmentation, and ResNet-50 [38] outperformed the other methods. In this case, all methods were compared without a data augmentation for a fair comparison. Table 12 shows the performance comparisons by the state-of-the-art methods and the proposed method with data augmentation (through a random in-plane rotation and translation), which shows higher accuracies than those listed in Table 11. The results in most cases show that ResNet-50 [38] and DenseNet-201 [41] outperformed the other methods. In this case, all methods were compared with the data augmentation (random in-plane rotation and translation) for fair comparisons. However, our proposed model does not produce state-of-the-art results with this augmentation technique, as shown in Table 12. This demonstrates that different augmentation techniques have different impacts on the neural networks.

Table 11. Performance comparisons of state-of-the-art methods and the proposed approach without data augmentation. Averages from a 10-fold cross-validation are shown (unit: %).

Methods	Accuracy	F1-Score	Precision	Recall
VGG-16 [45,69]	58.70	45	54	45
VGG-19 [45,69]	63.60	54	61	53
ResNet-18 [38,46]	66.13	60.86	64.25	58.13
ResNet-50 [38]	**66.70**	**62.02**	**64.67**	**59.83**
NASNet [45,70]	64.50	54	62	52
DenseNet-201 [41]	55.76	47.55	49.73	45.73
Proposed	58.10	50.82	51.78	49.96

Table 12. Performance comparisons of the state-of-the-art methods and proposed approach with data augmentation by random in-plane rotation and translation. Averages from a 10-fold cross-validation are shown (unit: %).

Methods	Accuracy	F1-Score	Precision	Recall
VGG-16 [45,69]	74	69	72	68
VGG-19 [45,69]	76.20	70	75	69
ResNet-18 [38,46]	70.82	65.93	68.02	64.38
ResNet-50 [38]	80.56	**77.66**	79.49	76.02
NASNet [45,70]	80.40	76	**80**	75
DenseNet-201 [41]	**80.57**	77.60	79.05	**76.32**
Proposed	77.05	74.80	76.93	73.07

As can be seen in Table 13, when the performances are compared between the state-of-the-art methods and the proposed method with RIA, a 4.18% performance gain was shown in the average accuracy of DenseNet-201 with ResNet-50. In addition, NASNet exhibited a 1.34% performance decrease in terms of the average accuracy with ResNet-50. Among all methods applied, our approach (DRE-Net (sequential training)) outperforms all other state-of-the-art methods. In this case, all methods were compared with RIA for a fair comparison. In addition, we can confirm that the accuracies of Table 13 are higher than those of Tables 11 and 12 in most cases. For fair comparison, the weights of the CNN models were pre-trained on the ImageNet dataset, and transfer learning was performed again with our training data in all experiments presented in Tables 11–13.

Table 13. Performance comparisons of the state-of-the-art methods and proposed approach with RIA. Averages from a 10-fold cross-validation are shown (unit: %).

Methods	Accuracy	F1-Score	Precision	Recall
VGG-16 [45,69]	68.85	66.90	66.82	67.22
VGG-19 [45,69]	66.54	63.54	63.81	63.35
ResNet-18 [38,46]	77.41	74.67	76.60	73.05
ResNet-50 [38]	80.57	78.02	79.21	76.95
NASNet [45,70]	79.23	76.28	77.25	75.44
DenseNet-201 [41]	84.75	83.76	85.21	82.42
Proposed	**85.92**	**84.69**	**85.33**	**84.11**

We evaluated the deep models using a 10-fold cross-validation and calculated the mean scores. To verify that the difference between mean scores was statistically significant, a t-test [71] was conducted. This test is based on a null hypothesis (H), which states that the performances of our model and the other approaches are not expected to be different (i.e., H = 0). The T-test is carried out to verify the substantial disparity between our model and the second-best [41] and third-best [38] baseline models in Table 13. Our sample size was small and increased the complexity of the statistical analysis. In detail, as the sample size decreases, the chance that every measured mean value is the same as the real total mean value decreases and the degree of uncertainty about the true value of the mean increases. Therefore, we conducted a t-test by combining 10-fold cross-validation values of the accuracy, F1-score, precision, and recall. The null hypothesis is rejected when there is less than a 5% chance of validity. The results in Table 14 show that the p-values calculated by the second- and third-best methods with our model are 0.03 (<0.05) and 7.84×10^{-9} (<0.001%), respectively, which demonstrates the effective distinction between our model and the other approaches. The p-value (0.03) for the second-best model shows that the null hypothesis is rejected at a 97% confidence level and shows a significant difference between our approach and the second-best model. In the case of the third-best model, the p-value (7.84×10^{-9}) indicates a significant difference between our approach and the third-best model, and the null hypothesis is rejected at a 99% confidence level.

Table 14. The t-test analysis results between our model and the second-best and third-best models.

Comparisons		p-Value	Confidence Level
Proposed	Second-best	0.03	97%
Proposed	Third-best	7.84×10^{-9}	99%

5. Discussions

In this study, we implemented two spatial feature extraction networks using a densely connected convolution network and a residual neural network. In the first stage, our proposed model envisages the spatially extracted features of both networks, which eventually leads to better results compared to other state-of-the-art classification networks. In the second stage, the proposed SCN further processes the spatial features, and therefore, ideal spatial features are extracted to achieve the best result. The architecture of the modified DenseNet model is shown in Table 3, and shows various dense blocks and transition layers used to exploit the optimal spatial features of the input image and achieve superior outcomes over other CNN models.

In this section, we generate class activation maps to illustrate the performance of the achievements of the modified DenseNet. Figure 13 shows the discriminative image regions used by the modified DenseNet to identify the class. The activation maps calculated for each dense block are represented using a pseudo color scheme [72]. The left column in Figure 13 shows the input images of four classes (C1–C4) given to DenseNet to learn its features, and it can be seen that the activation maps (F_1, F_2, ..., F_5) become salient after processing through each dense block. Finally, we can obtain class-specific regions (activation map F_5) that provide the specific visual pattern for each class, which ensures that DenseNet learns the features well. Similarly, we generated class activation maps to illustrate the performance of the modified ResNet. The architecture of the modified ResNet model is listed in Table 2, and shows various residual blocks used to exploit the optimal spatial features of the input image. Figure 14 shows the discriminative image regions used by the modified ResNet to identify the class. The left column in Figure 14 shows the input images of four classes (C1–C4) given to ResNet to learn its features and activation maps calculated by each residual block, which are represented by a pseudo color scheme [72]. The activation maps (F_1, F_2, ..., F_5) become prominent after processing through the residual blocks. Ultimately, we can obtain class-specific regions (activation map F_5) that provide a specific visual pattern for each class. However, as shown in Figure 14, the activation map for class 4 (Zimmer) does not clearly match visually distinct patterns. For a fair comparison between first-stage networks, we used the same input images of different classes to generate activation maps in Figures 13 and 14. The activation maps for class 4 generated by DenseNet and ResNet are quite different. The activation map generated by DenseNet for class 4 is the representation of its visually discriminated region, as shown in the last row of Figure 13, whereas that generated by ResNet for the same class shows a deviation from the discriminated region, as shown in the last row of Figure 14. This indicates that ResNet made predictions not on the head of the implants, which is a discriminated part, but on the background. Therefore, ResNet does not make a decision well for class 4 to learn the features. Moreover, as shown in Figure 10, the confusion matrix of the first-stage networks shows that ResNet has 5.37% less average recall than DenseNet for class 4. In addition, the activation map generated by ResNet-50 for class 3, as shown in the third row of Figure 14, is not focused on the head and is larger than that generated by DenseNet-201, shown in the third row of Figure 13. Therefore, the recall of ResNet-50 is much lower than that of DenseNet-201, as indicated in Figure 10. A similar analysis can be made for class 1. The activation map generated by ResNet-50 for class 1, as shown in the first row of Figure 14, does not accurately exist in the head area compared to that by DenseNet-201, as shown in the first row of Figure 13. Therefore, the recall of ResNet-50 is lower than that of DenseNet-201, as shown in Figure 10.

Finally, the final class activation maps (F_5) of the first-stage networks are processed by the proposed SCN for final classification after passing through their respective average pooling layers. A class activation map for the second-stage network cannot be generated. The reason for this is that, in the second stage network, the feature vector is $1 \times 1 \times 4$, and it lacks the visual information. Moreover, the ability of visual object detection by convolution layer was lost when FCL was used for classification in the second stage network. The fundamental difference between the SCN and first-stage networks is the processing of the feature maps. DenseNet and ResNet extract and process the feature maps of an image independently, whereas SCN combines the connectivity of both networks and processes their feature maps. In this way, an optimal representation of the spatial features is generated, which ultimately leads to a better performance in the classification of various types of shoulder prostheses.

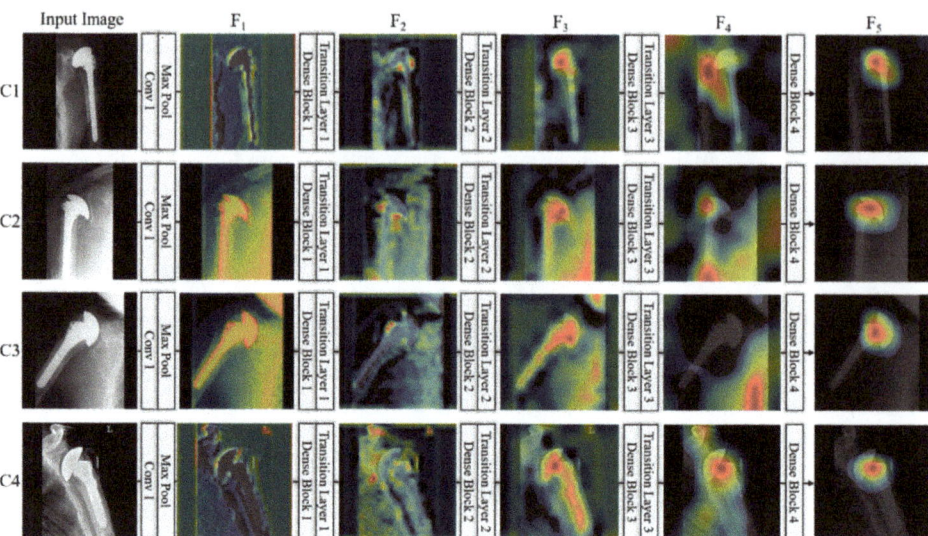

Figure 13. Class activation maps for given inputs of four classes (C1–C4), which are extracted from modified DenseNet-201 of Table 3. C1–C4 indicate the classes of four manufacturers, Cofield, Depuy, Tornier, and Zimmer, respectively.

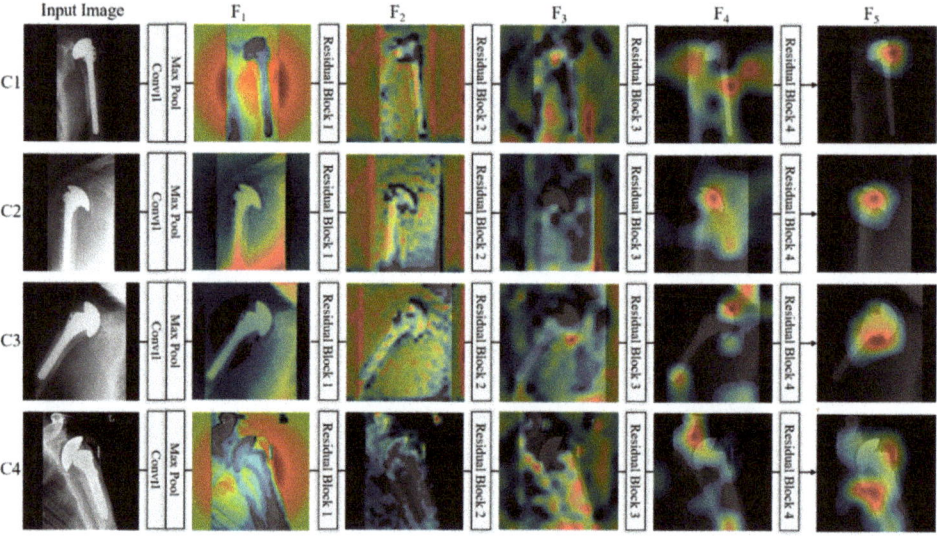

Figure 14. Class activation maps for given inputs of four classes (C1–C4), which are extracted from modified ResNet-50 of Table 2. C1–C4 indicate the classes of the four manufacturers, Cofield, Depuy, Tornier, and Zimmer, respectively.

We also computed the performance of our proposed network for an open-world configuration. For the open-world configuration, we conducted two-fold experiments by splitting the datasets into two halves, as explained in Section 3.4. The first half was used for training, while the other half was used for testing. Similar to the closed-world configuration, the training dataset in the open-world configuration is augmented using RIA. The main step in the open-world setup is to judge the real class label of the query image by calculating its similarity score with the class mean features. Thus, the Euclidean distance can be used to predict a class label for the query image. Owing to the limited number of classes (i.e., 4), we used two-fold cross-validation. Table 15 displays the details of the two-fold cross-validation of the training and testing datasets for the open-world configuration. Table 16 shows the experimental results of our proposed model, and the second- and third-best models are shown in Table 13 for the open-world configuration. There is a 0.72% performance gain in the average accuracy of our model over the second-best model and 2.4% over the third-best model.

Table 15. Summary of two-fold cross-validation of training and testing data for open-world configuration (unit: images).

Validation	Training			Testing		
	Classes	Original	Augmented	Classes	Original	Total
1st fold-A	Cofield, Depuy	377	13,572	Tornier, Zimmer	220	14,169
1st fold-B	Tornier, Zimmer	220	7920	Cofield, Depuy	377	8517
2nd fold-A	Tornier, Cofield	154	5544	Zimmer, Depuy	443	3585
2nd fold-B	Zimmer, Depuy	443	15,948	Tornier, Cofield	154	16,545

Table 16. Comparison of our proposed model with the second- and third-best models of Table 13 for open-world configuration (unit: %).

CNN Model	Accuracy	F1-Score	Precision	Recall
ResNet-50 [38]	74.96	67.14	67.78	66.51
DenseNet-201 [41]	76.64	71.31	70.64	72.05
Proposed	77.36	70.85	71.22	70.49

In this section, we also measured the performance of the proposed network in terms of confusion matrices considering open-world setting, as shown in Figure 15. In the 1st fold-A and -B, Tornier (C3), Zimmer (C4) (Figure 15b) and Cofield (C1), Depuy (C2) (Figure 15a) are used in testing, respectively. Similarly, in the 2nd fold-A and -B, Depuy (C2), Zimmer (C4) (Figure 15c) and Cofield (C1), Tornier (C3) (Figure 15d) are used in testing, respectively. As shown in these figures, the average value of correct classification ((84.01 + 51.68)/2(%)) with the testing of C2 and C4 (Figure 15c) is lower than those with the testing of C1 and C2 (Figure 15a) and C1 and C3 (Figure 15d). However, it is higher than that with the testing of C3 and C4 (Figure 15b). These results mean that the similarity between C2 and C4 does not give much effect on testing by open-world configuration compared to that by closed-world configuration. That is because the number of classes in the testing of open-world configuration (two classes) is half of that of closed-world configuration (four classes), which increases the inter-distance between two classes and consequently reduces the effect of similarity of C2 and C4 on testing accuracy of open-world configuration. In the open-world configuration mode, which is more complicated and challenging than the closed-world configuration mode, our model performs the best and is likely applicable to real-world problems as well.

We analyzed the false-positive and false-negative cases of our classifier and found that the reasons for the erroneous classification are structural similarities of the prostheses and the limited size of the dataset. For example, in Figure 10, the confusion matrix of our proposed model shows a lower average recall of class 4 (Zimmer) than that of the other classes. This is because the size (the number of images) of class 4 is two times less than that of class 2 (Depuy) with a high inter-class similarity between them, as can be seen in Figure 16. However, we maintain the sizes of the classes using RIA, although the class imbalance problem remains. It should be considered that the class imbalance problem is still an open issue [73], and thus various solutions are not guaranteed to be optimal. In addition, we analyzed the two-fold experiments for the open-world configuration owing to the limited number of classes. We plan to increase the number of folds in the future by increasing the number of classes. We trained two separate CNNs to extract the features and ensemble them using an SCN. This approach increases the training time owing to the large number of parameters required but makes the model more robust.

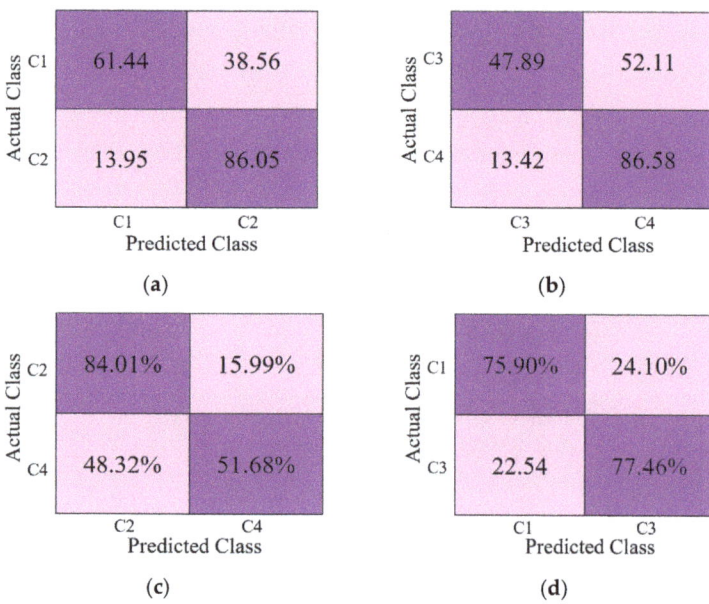

Figure 15. Performance of the proposed network considering open-world setting as confusion matrices (a) 1st fold-A (using C1 and C2 in testing), (b) 1st fold-B (using C3 and C4 in testing), (c) 2nd fold-A (using C2 and C4 in testing), and (d) 2nd fold-B (using C1 and C3 in testing).

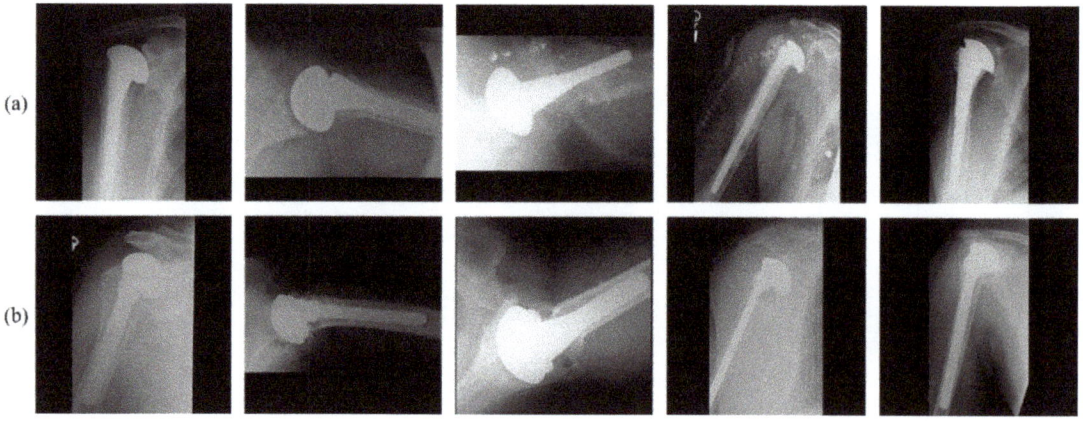

Figure 16. The high inter-class similarity between the two classes: (a) class 2 (Depuy) and (b) class 4 (Zimmer).

6. Conclusions

In this study, we proposed the use of DRE-Net by combining features for shoulder implant classification in X-ray images based on two independent models: modified

ResNet-50 and DenseNet-201. This framework automatically detects the prostheses by the manufacturer and aids the surgeons to fit it in the patient's body by their anatomy as personalized medicine. We analyzed the application of different deep learning models for the classification of shoulder implants by the manufacturer, and compared them with the ensemble of two deep learning models. The ensemble of models using the proposed SCN minimizes the weaknesses of each individually and takes advantage of the strengths of both. To further improve the efficiency of the classification, we proposed the application of RIA and increased the results by 8.87%. We discovered that independent (sequential) training of ensemble models shows better performance than end-to-end training. Although the dataset is relatively small, we obtained the optimum results for shoulder implant classification by integrating transfer learning, ensemble learning, feature concatenation, and RIA. We also examined our model for an open-world configuration and achieved the best results compared to the other deep models, which demonstrates the generalizability of our approach. As reported in previous research [11,45,46], the usage of computer-based algorithms can do better to identify shoulder arthroplasty implants compared to medical experts, which can reduce the risk of delayed operations, perioperative morbidity, and overuse of resources due to lack of correct identification of shoulder arthroplasty implants. Based on these motivations, previous research [11,45,46] has also studied the computer-based algorithms for the identification of shoulder implants. This study is helpful for personalized shoulder arthroscopy and researchers working on X-ray image-based implant recognition.

In the future, we plan to upgrade the results and reduce the training time of the proposed technique by establishing a custom-built model. We also plan to extend this work by adding additional manufacturers and classifying shoulder implants using the models. In addition, the class imbalance problem and increased number of classes for open-world configurations will also researched in the future.

Author Contributions: H.S., M.O. and K.R.P. designed the overall framework. In addition, H.S. and K.R.P. wrote and revised the paper. C.P., T.M. and A.H. helped the comparative analysis and experiments. All authors have read and agreed to the published version of the manuscript.

Funding: This work was supported in part by the National Research Foundation of Korea (NRF) funded by the Ministry of Science and ICT (MSIT) through the Basic Science Research Program (NRF-2020R1A2C1006179), in part by the MSIT, Korea, under the ITRC (Information Technology Research Center) support program (IITP-2021-2020-0-01789) supervised by the IITP (Institute for Information & Communications Technology Planning & Evaluation), and in part by the NRF funded by the MSIT through the Basic Science Research Program (NRF-2019R1A2C1083813).

Institutional Review Board Statement: Not applicable.

Informed Consent Statement: Not applicable.

Data Availability Statement: Not applicable.

Acknowledgments: Not applicable.

Conflicts of Interest: The authors declare no conflict of interest.

References

1. OrthoInfo, AAOS. Shoulder Joint Replacement. Available online: https://www.orthoinfo.org/en/treatment/shoulder-joint-replacement/ (accessed on 5 February 2021).
2. Wicha, M.; Tomczyk-Warunek, A.; Jarecki, J.; Dubiel, A. Total Shoulder Arthroplasty, an Overview, Indications and Prosthetic Options. *Wiad. Lek.* **2020**, *73*, 1870–1873. [CrossRef]
3. Burns, L.R.; Housman, M.G.; Booth, R.E.J.; Koenig, A. Implant Vendors and Hospitals: Competing Influences over Product Choice by Orthopedic Surgeons. *Health Care Manag. Rev.* **2009**, *34*, 2–18. [CrossRef]
4. Mahomed, N.N.; Barrett, J.A.; Katz, J.N.; Phillips, C.B.; Losina, E.; Lew, R.A.; Guadagnoli, E.; Harris, W.H.; Poss, R.; Baron, J.A. Rates and Outcomes of Primary and Revision Total Hip Replacement in the United States Medicare Population. *JBJS* **2003**, *85*, 27–32. [CrossRef]

5. Dy, C.J.; Bozic, K.J.; Padgett, D.E.; Pan, T.J.; Marx, R.G.; Lyman, S. Is Changing Hospitals for Revision Total Joint Arthroplasty Associated with More Complications? *Clin. Orthop. Relat. Res.* **2014**, *472*, 2006–2015. [CrossRef]
6. Wilson, N.A.; Jehn, M.; York, S.; Davis, C.M. Revision Total Hip and Knee Arthroplasty Implant Identification: Implications for Use of Unique Device Identification 2012 AAHKS Member Survey Results. *J. Arthroplast.* **2014**, *29*, 251–255. [CrossRef]
7. Branovacki, G. *Ortho Atlas: Hip Arthroplasty U.S. Femoral Implants 1938–2008*; Ortho Atlas Publishing: Chicago, IL, USA, 2008.
8. CNN Models for Shoulder Implants Recognition with Algorithms. Available online: http://dm.dgu.edu/link.html (accessed on 6 February 2021).
9. Bredow, J.; Wenk, B.; Westphal, R.; Wahl, F.; Budde, S.; Eysel, P.; Oppermann, J. Software-Based Matching of X-ray Images and 3D Models of Knee Prostheses. *Technol. Health Care* **2014**, *22*, 895–900. [CrossRef]
10. Morais, P.; Queirós, S.; Moreira, A.H.J.; Ferreira, A.; Ferreira, E.; Duque, D.; Rodrigues, N.F.; Vilaça, J.L. Computer-Aided Recognition of Dental Implants in X-ray Images. In Proceedings of the SPIE 9414, Medical Imaging: Computer-Aided Diagnosis, Orlando, FL, USA, 20 March 2015; Volume 9414, p. 94142E.
11. Stark, M.B.C.G. Automatic Detection and Segmentation of Shoulder Implants in X-ray Images. Master Thesis, San Francisco State University, San Francisco, CA, USA, 2018.
12. Litjens, G.; Kooi, T.; Bejnordi, B.E.; Setio, A.A.A.; Ciompi, F.; Ghafoorian, M.; van der Laak, J.A.W.M.; van Ginneken, B.; Sánchez, C.I. A Survey on Deep Learning in Medical Image Analysis. *Med. Image Anal.* **2017**, *42*, 60–88. [CrossRef] [PubMed]
13. Koteluk, O.; Wartecki, A.; Mazurek, S.; Kołodziejczak, I.; Mackiewicz, A. How Do Machines Learn? Artificial Intelligence as a New Era in Medicine. *J. Pers. Med.* **2021**, *11*, 32. [CrossRef]
14. Owais, M.; Arsalan, M.; Choi, J.; Mahmood, T.; Park, K.R. Artificial Intelligence-Based Classification of Multiple Gastrointestinal Diseases Using Endoscopy Videos for Clinical Diagnosis. *J. Clin. Med.* **2019**, *8*, 986. [CrossRef]
15. Owais, M.; Arsalan, M.; Choi, J.; Park, K.R. Effective Diagnosis and Treatment through Content-Based Medical Image Retrieval (CBMIR) by Using Artificial Intelligence. *J. Clin. Med.* **2019**, *8*, 462. [CrossRef]
16. Mahmood, T.; Arsalan, M.; Owais, M.; Lee, M.B.; Park, K.R. Artificial Intelligence-Based Mitosis Detection in Breast Cancer Histopathology Images Using Faster R-CNN and Deep CNNs. *J. Clin. Med.* **2020**, *9*, 749. [CrossRef] [PubMed]
17. Suh, Y.J.; Jung, J.; Cho, B.-J. Automated Breast Cancer Detection in Digital Mammograms of Various Densities via Deep Learning. *J. Clin. Med.* **2020**, *10*, 211. [CrossRef]
18. Arsalan, M.; Baek, N.R.; Owais, M.; Mahmood, T.; Park, K.R. Deep Learning-Based Detection of Pigment Signs for Analysis and Diagnosis of Retinitis Pigmentosa. *Sensors* **2020**, *20*, 3454. [CrossRef]
19. Arsalan, M.; Owais, M.; Mahmood, T.; Cho, S.W.; Park, K.R. Aiding the Diagnosis of Diabetic and Hypertensive Retinopathy Using Artificial Intelligence-Based Semantic Segmentation. *J. Clin. Med.* **2019**, *8*, 1446. [CrossRef]
20. Arsalan, M.; Kim, D.S.; Owais, M.; Park, K.R. OR-Skip-Net: Outer Residual Skip Network for Skin Segmentation in Non-Ideal Situations. *Expert Syst. Appl.* **2020**, *141*, 112922. [CrossRef]
21. Arsalan, M.; Owais, M.; Mahmood, T.; Choi, J.; Park, K.R. Artificial Intelligence-Based Diagnosis of Cardiac and Related Diseases. *J. Clin. Med.* **2020**, *9*, 871. [CrossRef]
22. Arsalan, M.; Kim, D.S.; Lee, M.B.; Owais, M.; Park, K.R. FRED-Net: Fully Residual Encoder–Decoder Network for Accurate Iris Segmentation. *Expert Syst. Appl.* **2019**, *122*, 217–241. [CrossRef]
23. Olczak, J.; Fahlberg, N.; Maki, A.; Razavian, A.S.; Jilert, A.; Stark, A.; Sköldenberg, O.; Gordon, M. Artificial Intelligence for Analyzing Orthopedic Trauma Radiographs: Deep Learning Algorithms-Are They on Par with Humans for Diagnosing Fractures? *Acta Orthop.* **2017**, *88*, 581–586. [CrossRef]
24. Bini, S.A. Artificial Intelligence, Machine Learning, Deep Learning, and Cognitive Computing: What Do These Terms Mean and How Will They Impact Health Care? *J. Arthroplast.* **2018**, *33*, 2358–2361. [CrossRef]
25. Tiulpin, A.; Thevenot, J.; Rahtu, E.; Lehenkari, P.; Saarakkala, S. Automatic Knee Osteoarthritis Diagnosis from Plain Radiographs: A Deep Learning-Based Approach. *Sci. Rep.* **2018**, *8*, 1727. [CrossRef]
26. Chung, S.W.; Han, S.S.; Lee, J.W.; Oh, K.-S.; Kim, N.R.; Yoon, J.P.; Kim, J.Y.; Moon, S.H.; Kwon, J.; Lee, H.-J.; et al. Automated Detection and Classification of the Proximal Humerus Fracture by Using Deep Learning Algorithm. *Acta Orthop.* **2018**, *89*, 468–473. [CrossRef]
27. Lindsey, R.; Daluiski, A.; Chopra, S.; Lachapelle, A.; Mozer, M.; Sicular, S.; Hanel, D.; Gardner, M.; Gupta, A.; Hotchkiss, R.; et al. Deep Neural Network Improves Fracture Detection by Clinicians. *Proc. Natl. Acad. Sci. USA* **2018**, *115*, 11591–11596. [CrossRef] [PubMed]
28. Kitamura, G.; Chung, C.Y.; Moore, B.E. Ankle Fracture Detection Utilizing a Convolutional Neural Network Ensemble Implemented with a Small Sample, De Novo Training, and Multiview Incorporation. *J. Digit. Imaging* **2019**, *32*, 672–677. [CrossRef]
29. Rayan, J.C.; Reddy, N.; Kan, J.H.; Zhang, W.; Annapragada, A. Binomial Classification of Pediatric Elbow Fractures Using a Deep Learning Multiview Approach Emulating Radiologist Decision Making. *Radiol. Artif. Intell.* **2019**, *1*, e180015. [CrossRef]
30. Borjali, A.; Chen, A.F.; Muratoglu, O.K.; Morid, M.A.; Varadarajan, K.M. Detecting Mechanical Loosening of Total Hip Replacement Implant from Plain Radiograph Using Deep Convolutional Neural Network. *arXiv* **2019**, arXiv:1912.00943v1. Available online: https://arxiv.org/abs/1912.00943 (accessed on 7 February 2021).
31. Krogue, J.D.; Cheng, K.V.; Hwang, K.M.; Toogood, P.; Meinberg, E.G.; Geiger, E.J.; Zaid, M.; McGill, K.C.; Patel, R.; Sohn, J.H.; et al. Automatic Hip Fracture Identification and Functional Subclassification with Deep Learning. *Radiol. Artif. Intell.* **2020**, *2*, e190023. [CrossRef]

32. Yi, P.H.; Wei, J.; Kim, T.K.; Sair, H.I.; Hui, F.K.; Hager, G.D.; Fritz, J.; Oni, J.K. Automated Detection & Classification of Knee Arthroplasty Using Deep Learning. *Knee* **2020**, *27*, 535–542. [CrossRef]
33. Karnuta, J.M.; Luu, B.C.; Roth, A.L.; Haeberle, H.S.; Chen, A.F.; Iorio, R.; Schaffer, J.L.; Mont, M.A.; Patterson, B.M.; Krebs, V.E.; et al. Artificial Intelligence to Identify Arthroplasty Implants from Radiographs of the Knee. *J. Arthroplast.* **2021**, *36*, 935–940. [CrossRef]
34. Sukegawa, S.; Yoshii, K.; Hara, T.; Yamashita, K.; Nakano, K.; Yamamoto, N.; Nagatsuka, H.; Furuki, Y. Deep Neural Networks for Dental Implant System Classification. *Biomolecules* **2020**, *10*, 984. [CrossRef]
35. Kim, J.-E.; Nam, N.-E.; Shim, J.-S.; Jung, Y.-H.; Cho, B.-H.; Hwang, J.J. Transfer Learning via Deep Neural Networks for Implant Fixture System Classification Using Periapical Radiographs. *J. Clin. Med.* **2020**, *9*, 1117. [CrossRef]
36. Iandola, F.N.; Han, S.; Moskewicz, M.W.; Ashraf, K.; Dally, W.J.; Keutzer, K. SqueezeNet: AlexNet-Level Accuracy with 50× Fewer Parameters and <0.5 MB Model Size. *arXiv* **2016**, arXiv:1602.07360v4. Available online: https://arxiv.org/abs/1602.07360 v4?source=post_page (accessed on 9 February 2021).
37. Szegedy, C.; Liu, W.; Jia, Y.; Sermanet, P.; Reed, S.; Anguelov, D.; Erhan, D.; Vanhoucke, V.; Rabinovich, A. Going Deeper with Convolutions. In Proceedings of the IEEE Conference on Computer Vision and Pattern Recognition, Boston, MA, USA, 7–12 June 2015; pp. 1–9. [CrossRef]
38. He, K.; Zhang, X.; Ren, S.; Sun, J. Deep Residual Learning for Image Recognition. In Proceedings of the IEEE Conference on Computer Vision and Pattern Recognition, Las Vegas, NV, USA, 27–30 June 2016; pp. 770–778. [CrossRef]
39. Sandler, M.; Howard, A.; Zhu, M.; Zhmoginov, A.; Chen, L.-C. MobileNetV2: Inverted Residuals and Linear Bottlenecks. In Proceedings of the IEEE Conference on Computer Vision and Pattern Recognition, Salt Lake City, UT, USA, 18–23 June 2018; pp. 4510–4520. [CrossRef]
40. Borjali, A.; Chen, A.F.; Muratoglu, O.K.; Morid, M.A.; Varadarajan, K.M. Detecting Total Hip Replacement Prosthesis Design on Plain Radiographs Using Deep Convolutional Neural Network. *J. Orthop. Res.* **2020**, *38*, 1465–1471. [CrossRef]
41. Huang, G.; Liu, Z.; van der Maaten, L.; Weinberger, K.Q. Densely Connected Convolutional Networks. In Proceedings of the IEEE Conference on Computer Vision and Pattern Recognition, Honolulu, HI, USA, 21–26 July 2017; pp. 4700–4708. [CrossRef]
42. Deng, J.; Dong, W.; Socher, R.; Li, L.-J.; Li, K.; Fei-Fei, L. ImageNet: A Large-scale Hierarchical Image Database. In Proceedings of the IEEE Conference on Computer Vision and Pattern Recognition, Miami, FL, USA, 20–25 June 2009; pp. 248–255.
43. Pranata, Y.D.; Wang, K.-C.; Wang, J.-C.; Idram, I.; Lai, J.-Y.; Liu, J.-W.; Hsieh, I.-H. Deep Learning and SURF for Automated Classification and Detection of Calcaneus Fractures in CT Images. *Comput. Meth. Programs Biomed.* **2019**, *171*, 27–37. [CrossRef]
44. Tanzi, L.; Vezzetti, E.; Moreno, R.; Aprato, A.; Audisio, A.; Massè, A. Hierarchical Fracture Classification of Proximal Femur X-ray Images Using a Multistage Deep Learning Approach. *Eur. J. Radiol.* **2020**, *133*, 109373. [CrossRef]
45. Urban, G.; Porhemmat, S.; Stark, M.; Feeley, B.; Okada, K.; Baldi, P. Classifying Shoulder Implants in X-ray Images Using Deep Learning. *Comp. Struct. Biotechnol. J.* **2020**, *18*, 967–972. [CrossRef] [PubMed]
46. Yi, P.H.; Kim, T.K.; Wei, J.; Li, X.; Hager, G.D.; Sair, H.I.; Fritz, J. Automated Detection and Classification of Shoulder Arthroplasty Models Using Deep Learning. *Skelet. Radiol.* **2020**, *49*, 1623–1632. [CrossRef] [PubMed]
47. Shorten, C.; Khoshgoftaar, T.M. A Survey on Image Data Augmentation for Deep Learning. *J. Big Data* **2019**, *6*, 60. [CrossRef]
48. Polikar, R. Ensemble Based Systems in Decision Making. *IEEE Circuits Syst. Mag.* **2006**, *6*, 21–45. [CrossRef]
49. Rokach, L. Ensemble-Based Classifiers. *Artif. Intell. Rev.* **2010**, *33*, 1–39. [CrossRef]
50. Krizhevsky, A.; Sutskever, I.; Hinton, G.E. ImageNet Classification with Deep Convolutional Neural Networks. In Proceedings of the 25th International Conference on Neural Information Processing Systems, Lake Tahoe, NV, USA, 3–8 December 2012; pp. 1097–1105. [CrossRef]
51. ImageNet. Available online: http://www.image-net.org/ (accessed on 7 February 2021).
52. Glorot, X.; Bordes, A.; Bengio, Y. Deep Sparse Rectifier Neural Networks. In Proceedings of the 14th International Conference on Artificial Intelligence and Statistics, Fort Lauderdale, FL, USA, 11–13 April 2011; pp. 315–323.
53. Ioffe, S.; Szegedy, C. Batch Normalization: Accelerating Deep Network Training by Reducing Internal Covariate Shift. In Proceedings of the International Conference on Machine Learning, Lille, France, 7–9 July 2015; pp. 448–456.
54. Zheng, L.; Zhao, Y.; Wang, S.; Wang, J.; Tian, Q. Good Practice in CNN Feature Transfer. *arXiv* **2016**, arXiv:1604.00133v1. Available online: https://arxiv.org/abs/1604.00133 (accessed on 9 February 2021).
55. Kawahara, J.; Hamarneh, G. Multi-Resolution-Tract CNN with Hybrid Pretrained and Skin-Lesion Trained Layers. In Proceedings of the International Workshop on Machine Learning in Medical Imaging, Athens, Greece, 17 October 2016; pp. 164–171.
56. Goodfellow, I.; Bengio, Y.; Courville, A. *Deep Learning*; MIT Press: Cambridge, MA, USA, 2016; Volume 1.
57. Heesch, D. A Survey of Browsing Models for Content Based Image Retrieval. *Multimed. Tools Appl.* **2008**, *40*, 261–284. [CrossRef]
58. Buda, M.; Maki, A.; Mazurowski, M.A. A Systematic Study of the Class Imbalance Problem in Convolutional Neural Networks. *Neural Netw.* **2018**, *106*, 249–259. [CrossRef]
59. Intel®Core™ i7-3770K Processor. Available online: https://ark.intel.com/content/www/us/en/ark/products/65523/intel-core-i7-3770k-processor-8m-cache-up-to-3-90-ghz.html (accessed on 1 December 2020).
60. GeForce GTX 1070. Available online: https://www.geforce.com/hardware/desktop-gpus/geforce-gtx-1070/specifications (accessed on 1 December 2020).
61. Deep Learning Toolbox. Available online: https://www.mathworks.com/products/deep-learning.html (accessed on 1 December 2020).

62. Heaton, J. *Artificial Intelligence for Humans, Volume 3—Deep Learning and Neural Networks*; Heaton Research, Inc.: St. Louis, MO, USA, 2013; ISBN 978-1-5057-1434-0.
63. Ruder, S. An Overview of Gradient Descent Optimization Algorithms. *arXiv* **2017**, arXiv:1609.04747v2. Available online: https://arxiv.org/abs/1609.04747 (accessed on 9 February 2021).
64. Options for Training Deep Learning Neural Network. Available online: https://www.mathworks.com/help/deeplearning/ref/trainingoptions.html (accessed on 13 February 2021).
65. Hossin, M. A Review on Evaluation Metrics for Data Classification Evaluations. *Int. J. Data Min. Knowl. Manag. Process* **2015**, *5*, 1–11. [CrossRef]
66. Abdi, H.; Williams, L.J. Principal Component Analysis. *WIREs Comput. Stat.* **2010**, *2*, 433–459. [CrossRef]
67. Cover, T.; Hart, P. Nearest Neighbor Pattern Classification. *IEEE Trans. Inf. Theory* **1967**, *13*, 21–27. [CrossRef]
68. Kuncheva, L.I.; Whitaker, C.J. Measures of Diversity in Classifier Ensembles and Their Relationship with the Ensemble Accuracy. *Mach. Learn.* **2003**, *51*, 181–207. [CrossRef]
69. Simonyan, K.; Zisserman, A. Very Deep Convolutional Networks for Large-Scale Image Recognition. *arXiv* **2015**, arXiv:1409.1556v6. Available online: https://arxiv.org/abs/1409.1556 (accessed on 11 February 2021).
70. Zoph, B.; Vasudevan, V.; Shlens, J.; Le, Q.V. Learning Transferable Architectures for Scalable Image Recognition. In Proceedings of the IEEE Conference on Computer Vision and Pattern Recognition, Salt Lake City, UT, USA, 18–23 June 2018; pp. 8697–8710. [CrossRef]
71. Livingston, E.H. Who Was Student and Why Do We Care so Much about His T-Test? *J. Surg. Res.* **2004**, *118*, 58–65. [CrossRef]
72. Zhou, B.; Khosla, A.; Lapedriza, A.; Oliva, A.; Torralba, A. Learning Deep Features for Discriminative Localization. In Proceedings of the IEEE Conference on Computer Vision and Pattern Recognition, Las Vegas, NV, USA, 27–30 June 2016; pp. 2921–2929.
73. Krawczyk, B. Learning from Imbalanced Data: Open Challenges and Future Directions. *Prog. Artif. Intell.* **2016**, *5*, 221–232. [CrossRef]

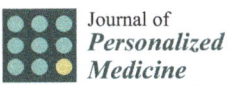

Article

The Orthopedic-Vascular Multidisciplinary Approach Improves Patient Safety in Surgery for Musculoskeletal Tumors: A Large-Volume Center Experience

Andrea Angelini [1,2], Michele Piazza [3], Elisa Pagliarini [1,2], Giulia Trovarelli [1,2], Andrea Spertino [3] and Pietro Ruggieri [1,2,*]

1. Department of Orthopedics and Orthopedic Oncology, University of Padua, Via Giustiniani 2, 35128 Padova, Italy; andrea.angelini@unipd.it (A.A.); dr.elisa.pagliarini@gmail.com (E.P.); giuliatrovarelli87@gmail.com (G.T.)
2. Department of Surgery, Oncology and Gastroenterology, University of Padova, 35128 Padova, Italy
3. Department of Vascular and Endovascular Surgery, University of Padua, 35128 Padova, Italy; michele.piazza@unipd.it (M.P.); andrea.spertino@gmail.com (A.S.)
* Correspondence: pietro.ruggieri@unipd.it; Tel.: +39-049-821-3311 or +39-333-326-6234

Abstract: Objective: Wide-margin resection is mandatory for malignant bone and soft tissue tumors. However, this increases the complexity of resections, especially when vessels are involved. Patients in this high-risk clinical setting could be surgically treated using the multidisciplinary orthopedic-vascular approach. This study was carried out in this healthcare organization to evaluate patient safety in term of oncologic outcomes and reduction of the complication rate. **Materials and Methods:** We retrospectively reviewed 74 patients (37 males, 37 females; mean age 46 years, range 9–88) who underwent surgical excision for bone/soft tissue malignant tumors closely attached to vascular structures from October 2015 to February 2019. Vascular surgery consisted of isolation of at least one vessel (64 patients), bypass reconstruction (9 patients), and end-to-end anastomosis (1 patient). Mean follow-up was 27 months. Patients' demographics, tumor characteristics, adjuvant treatments, type of orthopedic and vascular procedures, and oncologic and functional outcomes and complications were recorded. **Results:** Overall survival was 85% at 3 years follow-up. In total, 22 patients experienced at least one major complication requiring further surgery and 13 patients experienced at least one minor complication, whereas 17 reported deviations from the normal postoperative course without the need for pharmacological or interventional treatment. Major complications were higher in pelvic resections compared to limb-salvage procedures ($p = 0.0564$) and when surgical time was more than 4 h ($p = 0.0364$) at univariate analysis, whereas the most important multivariate independent predictors for major complications were pelvic resection ($p = 0.0196$) and preoperative radiotherapy ($p = 0.0426$). **Conclusions:** A multidisciplinary ortho-vascular approach for resection of malignant bone and soft tissue tumors tightly attached to important vascular structures should be considered a good clinical practice for patient safety.

Keywords: limb salvage; patient safety management; vascular bypass; soft tissue sarcoma; vascular reconstruction

1. Introduction

Patient care is changing over time because of the improvement of technology, pharmacology, and surgical techniques. The most important predictor of local recurrence after surgical excision of bone and soft tissue malignant tumors is negative resection margins. Before the advent of chemotherapy, the primary surgical treatment for bone tumors of the extremities was amputation, whereas today, secondary to the advances in adjuvant treatments and surgical techniques, limb-salvage surgery has been shown to be feasible with adequate margins in >90% of cases [1–3]. However, involvement of neurovascular

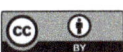

bundles challenges negative resection margins. The pioneers in the field of musculoskeletal oncology anticipated the essential role of the multidisciplinary orthopedic and vascular surgery approach to treat patients with bone and soft tissue malignant tumors [4]. It is clear that the proper management of major vessels is part of the routine work of an orthopedic oncology surgeon, but this poses challenges to patient safety with a need for change in the way we approach patient care in surgery. A surgical team in which orthopedic and vascular surgeons cooperate has been associated with decreased morbidity and complications, and improved outcomes for the patients [5–9].

We performed a retrospective analysis of patients who underwent surgical excision for bone/soft tissue malignant tumors closely attached to vascular structures, using a multidisciplinary orthopedic and vascular surgery approach and aiming to evaluate patient safety in terms of oncologic outcomes and reduction of the complication rate.

2. Materials and Methods

We retrospectively studied all patients with malignant bone and soft tissue tumors that were treated using a multidisciplinary approach combining the expertise of orthopedic oncology and vascular surgeons from October 2015 to February 2019. We intentionally excluded from the analysis all patients treated after February 2019 to have a potential minimum follow-up of 2 years. From a total of 493 operations for musculoskeletal tumors, in 393 operations a vascular surgeon was not required, in 24 operations a vascular surgeon was on call but never scrubbed-in, and in 2 operations a vascular surgeon was called in emergency for intraoperative vascular complications (Figure 1).

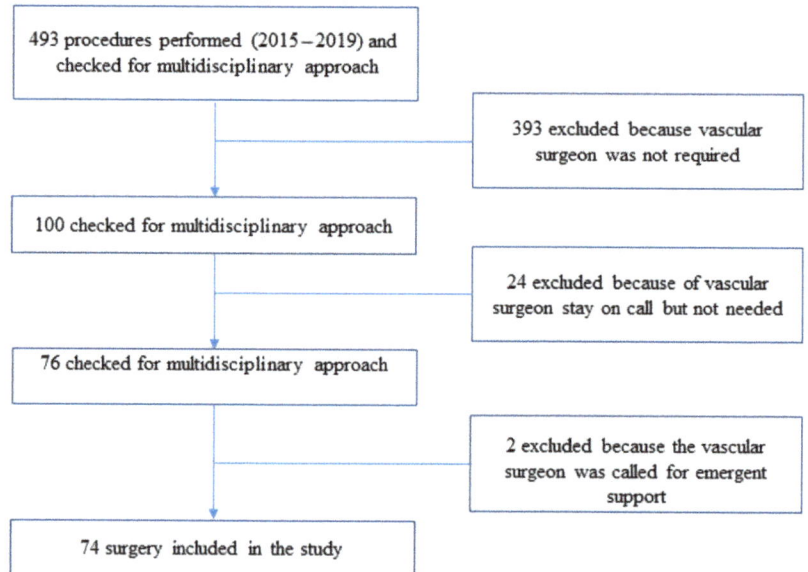

Figure 1. Patients' cohort selection process.

The above exclusions left us with 74 patients (37 male and 37 female patients; mean age, 46 years; age range, 9–88 years) who underwent combined ortho-vascular surgery that required orthopedic oncology en bloc tumor resection and vascular surgery for the protection/isolation and/or reconstruction of major vessels. The mean follow-up was 27 months (range, 24–44 months). All patients or their relatives gave written informed consent for their data to be included in scientific studies. An Institutional Review Board/Ethics Committee approval was not required for our retrospective study with fully anonymized clinical routine data.

Details of patients' age, gender, comorbidities, tumor histology, grade, staging and site, medical history, imaging studies, and oncological management, including resection and reconstruction, vascular reconstruction, additional procedures, and the need for adjuvant treatments (radiation therapy and chemotherapy), were recorded and analyzed: 33 patients had at least one cardiovascular risk factor including smoking, obesity, type 2 diabetes mellitus, arterial hypertension, and hyper-cholesterol; 1 patient had coronary artery disease; 4 patients had peripheral arterial disease; and 3 patients had a history of deep venous thrombosis; furthermore, 14 patients were classified as American Society of Anesthesiologists (ASA) physical status classification system 1, 45 patients as ASA 2, and 15 patients as ASA 3 (Table 1).

Table 1. Demographic details of the patients ($n = 74$) included in this series.

Data	Patients (n)	%
Age (mean years)	46 (range, 9–88)	-
Gender (male/female)	37/37	-
Obesity	16	21.6
Hypertension	15	20.3
Smoking	13	17.6
Dyslipidemia	6	8.1
Type II diabetes	4	5.4
Peripheral arterial disease	4	5.4
Coronary artery disease	1	1.4
Previous deep vein thrombosis	3	4.1
>1 cardiovascular risk factors	45	60.8
American Society of Anesthesiologists (ASA) Score 1	14	18.9
American Society of Anesthesiologists (ASA) Score 2	45	60.8
American Society of Anesthesiologists (ASA) Score 3	15	20.3
Bone tumors	54	73
Symptoms:		
Pain	38	70.4
Swelling	8	14.8
Functional limitation	9	16.7
Pathological fracture	7	13
Asymptomatic	9	16.7
Histological diagnosis:		
Osteosarcoma	19	35.1
Chondrosarcoma	16	29.6
Ewing's sarcoma	3	5.6
Chordoma	1	1.9
Metastatic bone disease	11	20.4
Hematological malignancies	4	7.4
Site:		
Proximal tibia	15	27.8
Proximal femur	12	22.2
Pelvis/sacrum	9	16.7
Distal femur	9	16.7
Proximal humerus	6	11.1
Scapula	1	1.9
Humeral shaft	1	1.9
Proximal tibia/distal tibia	1	1.9
Soft tissue tumors	20	27
Symptoms:		
Mass/Swelling	13	65
Pain	8	40

Table 1. Cont.

Data	Patients (n)	%
Functional limitation	2	10
Asymptomatic	3	15
Histological diagnosis:		
Synovial sarcoma	7	35
Leiomyosarcoma	2	10
Liposarcoma	2	10
Pleomorphic sarcoma	2	10
Other	7	35
Site:		
Thigh	9	45
Popliteal fossa	3	15
Hip	2	10
Buttocks	2	10
Forearm	2	10
Knee	1	5
Pelvis	1	5
Metastases at time of surgery (bone and soft tissue tumors)	10	13.5
Lung metastases:	9	12.2
Skip metastases	1	1.4

All patients underwent preoperative radiographic (for bone tumors), computed tomography (CT), and magnetic resonance (MR) imaging staging. The average tumor volume was 297 cc (median, 102 cc; range, 3–4082 cc), which was an average of 162 cc (median, 102 cc; range, 12–942 cc) for bone tumors and an average of 599 cc (median, 133 cc; range, 3–4082 cc) for soft tissue tumors. The average maximum diameter of the tumor was 8.9 cm (median, 8 cm; range, 3–30 cm), which was an average of 8.0 cm (median, 7 cm; range, 3.2–15 cm) for bone tumors and an average of 11.2 cm (median, 12 cm; range, 3–30 cm) for soft tissue tumors. The difference in volume and diameter between bone and soft tissue tumors was not statistically significant ($p = 0.123$ and $p = 0.063$, respectively). In 67 patients a needle or trocar biopsy was done preoperatively; in 7 patients, biopsy was not done because the tumor had pathognomonic characteristics on imaging (2 patients) or was an obvious local recurrence (5 patients). CT angiography was routinely performed to assess the vascular anatomy and its relation to the tumor in order to plan an adequate dissection or possible reconstruction. In patients with inconclusive CT angiography, digital subtraction angiography was performed.

Perioperative adjuvant treatments included chemotherapy in 28 patients, radiotherapy in 16 patients, combined chemotherapy and radiotherapy in 12 patients, and selective arterial embolization in 6 patients. Surgical treatments included removal of primary tumors in 57 patients and local recurrences in 17 patients. Additionally, seven patients were treated with forequarter amputation (two cases) or hindquarter amputation (five cases) as primary treatment. Reconstruction of bone defects after tumor resection was done in 51 patients with a megaprosthesis (41 patients), a custom-made 3D-printed pelvic prosthesis (7 patients), an expandable proximal tibia megaprosthesis (1 patient), a conventional revision hip prosthesis (1 patient), and a massive distal femur bone allograft (1 patient). Surgical margins were histologically defined on the basis of the worst margin on the specimen according to Enneking [10]: wide if a continuous shell of healthy tissue could be demonstrated around the tumor (53 patients; 72%), marginal if the plane of resection was along the pseudocapsule (15 patients; 20%), and intralesional when pathological tissue was present in a margin (6 patients; 8%). Moreover, the surgical margins were also identified according to the R categories defined by the Union for International Cancer Control (UICC), with R0 representing no macroscopic or microscopic residual tumor postoperatively (68 patients;

92%), R1 microscopic (4 patients; 5%), and R2 macroscopic residual tumor (2 patients; 3%), respectively [11].

Vascular surgery during en bloc tumor resection included isolation of at least one vessel strictly related to the tumor with the possibility of preserving it in 64 patients, bypass vascular reconstruction in 9 patients, and end-to-end vascular anastomosis in 1 patient. In four patients the major artery only was reconstructed (Type II reconstruction) [12], and in five patients the major artery and vein were reconstructed (Type I reconstruction) [12]. The contralateral great saphenous vein was used for the bypass venous reconstruction in all patients, and for the arterial bypass reconstruction in eight patients (Figure 2); a polytetrafluoroethylene (PTFE) vascular graft was used for a femoro-popliteal arterial bypass in one patient because the contralateral great saphenous vein was not adequate.

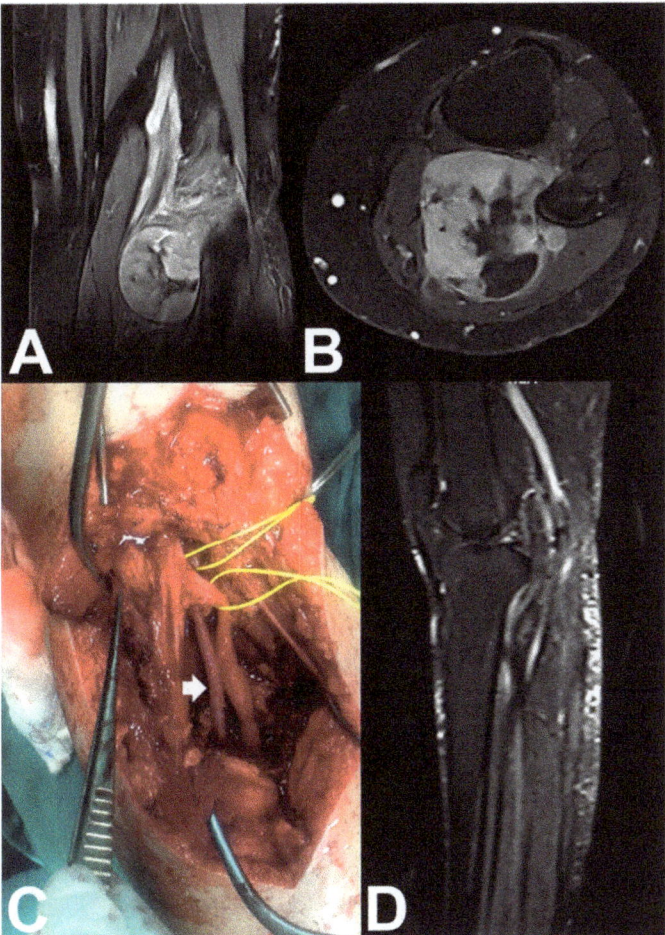

Figure 2. (**A**) Coronal and (**B**) axial T2-weighted MR images of the left knee of a 55-year-old woman with a popliteal fossa synovial sarcoma. (**C**) En bloc (marginal) tumor resection was done after identification and preservation of the peroneal and tibial nerves (lower vessel-loop), ligation without reconstruction of the popliteal vein, identification of the popliteal artery (upper vessel-loop), and arterial bypass reconstruction with the tibial artery using a contralateral great saphenous vein graft (white arrow) without venous bypass reconstruction. (**D**) Sagittal T2-weighted MR image shows tumor resection and limb preservation with patent anastomosis.

After the ortho-vascular surgery, plastic surgery wound coverage was necessary in 21 patients using the medial gastrocnemius flap (13 patients) or local myocutaneous flaps (8 patients). The mean duration of the ortho-vascular surgery was 270 min (range, 65–770 min), and the mean blood loss was 770 mL (range, 50–4600 mL). As expected, the surgical time and blood loss was higher for major resections and reconstructions such as pelvic tumors resections.

Routine follow-up examinations were performed every 3 months for the first 2 years, every 6 months for the next 3 years, and then annually. Follow-up examinations included physical examination and functional evaluation, imaging studies, and disease-specific imaging. Oncologic results were evaluated with respect to local recurrence, metastasis, or death, and the patients were classified as having no evidence of disease (NED), being disease free after treatment of local recurrence (NED-LR) or metastasis (NED-M), being alive with disease because of local recurrence or metastasis (AWD), and being dead of disease (DWD). Survival was defined as the time from surgery to last follow-up or death. Complications were recorded and graded according to the Clavien–Dindo classification of surgical complications [8,9]. In summary, complications were divided in five grades: Grade (I)—any deviation from the normal postoperative course without the need for pharmacological or interventional treatment; Grade (II)—requiring pharmacological treatment with drugs; Grade (III)—requiring surgical, endoscopic, or radiological intervention; Grade (IV)—life-threatening complication requiring intermediate care (IC)/intensive care unit (ICU); Grade (V)—death [8].

Categorical variables were expressed as percentages of the total patients in a category. The mean, standard deviation, and range of all continuous variables were calculated. The effect level of clinical characteristics on outcomes was evaluated using the univariate Kaplan–Meier analysis as a time-event analysis. Comparison of the curves was done in a bivariate analysis with the log-rank test. Logistic binary regression was used for analyzing if there one or more independent variables that influence the rate of major complications (measured as a dichotomous variable). Differences were considered statistically significant when the p value was less than 0.05. The data were recorded in a Microsoft Excel1 2003 spreadsheet and analyzed using Med-Calc software version 11.1 (MedCalc Software, Mariakerke, Belgium).

3. Results

3.1. Oncological Outcome

Mean follow-up was 27 months. At 3 years of follow-up, the overall survival of the patients was 85% (Figure 3).

At the last follow-up, 39 patients were NED, 7 patients were NED-LR, 3 patients were NED-M, 1 patient was NED-LR/M, 17 patients were AWD, and 7 patients were DWD. The overall survival to local recurrence was 64% (Figure 4) and the overall survival to metastasis was 58% (Figure 5). We observed that patients with no evidence of disease at the last follow-up were 16% (1/6 patients) in those treated with intralesional margins, 67% (10/15 patients) in marginal margins, and 55% (29/53 patients) in wide margins.

3.2. Complication Rate

In total, 22 patients experienced at least one major complication (Grade III), 13 patients experienced at least one minor complication (Grade II), whereas 17 reported deviation from the normal postoperative course without the need for pharmacological or interventional treatment (Grade I) (Table 2).

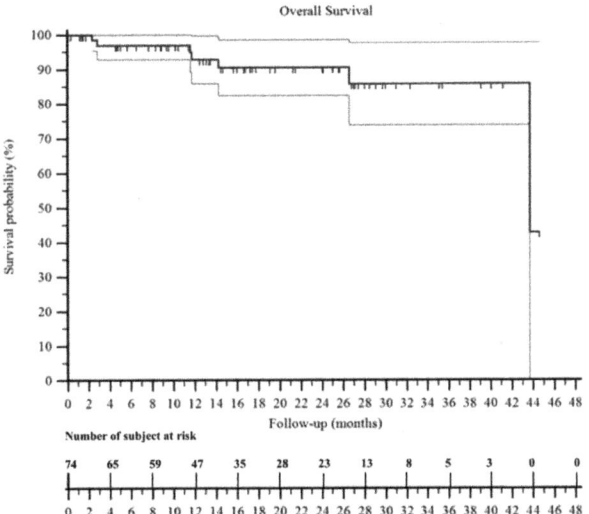

Figure 3. A Kaplan–Meier curve shows the overall survival of the patients included in this series. It was 92% at 2 years and 85% at 3 years. The two surrounding thin black lines represent the 95% confidence intervals.

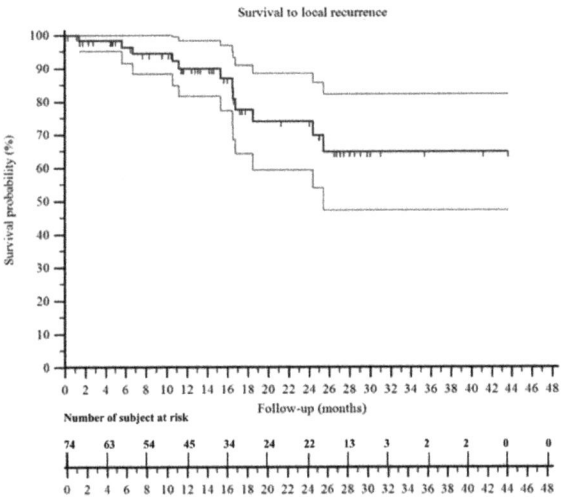

Figure 4. A Kaplan–Meier curve shows the survival to local recurrence of the patients included in this series. It was 74% at 2 years and 64% at 3 years. The two surrounding thin black lines represent the 95% confidence intervals.

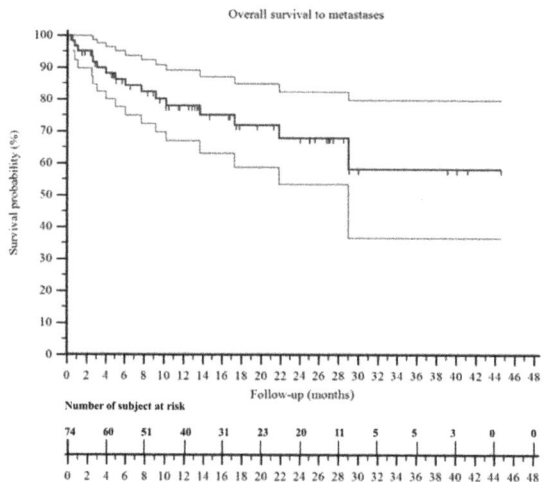

Figure 5. A Kaplan–Meier curve shows the survival to metastasis of the patients included in this series. It was 68% at 2 years and 58% at 3 years. The two surrounding thin black lines represent the 95% confidence intervals.

No patient experienced limb ischemia during the follow up, even if in two patients, a subtotal occlusion of the venous bypass was observed at the Doppler ultrasonography that, however, did not require any further management for the patients. Deep hematoma and wound-related problems with/without infection were the most common major complications (Table 2). A deep hematoma or sieroma was observed in five patients, but revision operation in these patients showed active bleeding from the dissected tissues without any bypass leakage. Wound dehiscence was treated with surgical debridement and pedicle flaps, especially in the four cases with large wound necrosis. One patient with major complication (deep infection) underwent final amputation after several inefficient surgical debridements.

Wound dehiscence was the most common minor complication (five patients), followed by superficial infection and sieroma (two patients each) that were treated effectively conservatively with wound dressing and pharmacological treatment. Four patients experienced deep vein thrombosis (DVT) treated with drugs, but none of these patients had a vascular reconstruction. Edema of the limb was observed in six patients with vascular reconstructions at the early postoperative period and was treated successfully with compression stockings. Temporary sensory nerve deficits (paresthesia, hypoesthesia) were reported in 19 patients, and temporary motor deficits (muscles weakness and atrophy) in 12 patients. Seven amputees reported phantom limb pain for which they took analgesic therapy. The most important univariate predictors for major ortho-vascular complications were a pelvic resection compared to a limb-salvage resection ($p = 0.0564$), as well as a surgical time of more than 4 h ($p = 0.0364$) (Table 3). The most important multivariate independent predictors for major ortho-vascular complications were pelvic resection ($p = 0.0196$) and preoperative radiotherapy ($p = 0.0426$) (Table 4).

Table 2. Complications of ortho-vascular surgery in the patients included in this series, classified according to the Clavien–Dindo system.

Data	* Postop	Early	Late	N. Events/n. pts	Relative %**	Absolute %°°
Grade I						
Edema of the limb (13)	7	6	-	15/17	42.50%	22.90%
Delayed wound healing (4)	4	-	-			
Grade II						
Subtotal bypass occlusion (2)	-	2	-			
Superficial infection (2)	1	1	-			
Wound dehiscence and partial necrosis (5)	4	1	-	16/13	32.50%	17.60%
Sieroma or haematoma (2)	-	2	-			
Deep vein thrombosis (4)	2	2	-			
Periprosthetic fracture with cast (1)	-	-	1			
Grade III						
Deep hematoma or sieroma (5)	4	1	-			
Complete wound dehiscence (11)	7	3	1			
Wound necrosis and infection (4)	2	2	-	28/22	55%	29.70%
Active bleeding (1)	1	-	-			
Deep infection (6)	2	-	4			
Prosthetic dislocation (1)	-	-	1			
Grade IV						
Myocardial infarction (1)	1	-	-	2	5%	2.70%
Systemic sepsis (1)	-	1	-			
Grade V	-	-	-	-	-%	-%

* Postoperative (<1 month from surgery), early onset (between 1 and 6 months), late (after 6 months). ** Relative percentage of subtype complication on 40 patients (that reported almost one complication). °° Absolute percentage of subtype complication on 74 patients (entire series).

Table 3. Risk factors for major complications (Grade III Clavien–Dindo) of ortho-vascular surgery in the patients included in this series.

Variables	Cut Off n. Events/pts Hazard Ratio (95%CI)	Cut Off n. Events/pts Hazard Ratio (95% CI)	p-Value
Age	<65 years 17/57 (29.8%) HR 1.0231	>65 years 5/17 (29.4%) HR 0.9775	0.9641
Gender	Female 14/37 (37.8%) HR 2.0658	Male 8/37 (21.6%) HR 0.4841	0.0914
Cardiovascular risk factors	Yes 13/45 (28.9%) HR 0.9124	No 9/29 (31.0%) HR 1.0960	0.8347
Type 2 diabetes mellitus	Yes 1/4 (25.0%) HR 1.3288	No 21/70 (30.0%) HR 0.7526	0.7487
Obesity	Yes 5/16 (31.2%) HR 2.0448	No 17/58 (29.3%) HR 0.8547	0.1726
Preoperative radiotherapy	Yes 8/16 (50.0%) HR 2.3397	No 14/58 (24.1%) HR 0.4274	0.1
Neoplasia volume	<100 mL 12/38 (31.6%) HR 1.1961	>100 mL 10/36 (27.8%) HR 0.8360	0.6754
Intervention time	Less 4 h 6/35 (17.1%) HR 0.4083	>4 h 16/39 (41.0%) HR 2.4491	0.0364 *
Vascular bypass	Yes 4/9 (44.4%) HR 2.1040	No 18/65 (27.7%) HR 0.4753	0.2772
Flap (yes vs. no)	Yes 8/21 (38.1%) HR 1.6540	No 14/53 (26.4%) HR 0.6046	0.2984
Tumor site (pelvis vs. other sites)	Pelvis 6/10 (60.0%) HR 3.0753	Other sites 16/64 (25.0%) HR 0.3252	0.0564 *

Table 4. Logistic regression analysis to evaluate independent variables as predictors for major complications (Grade III Clavien–Dindo) in the entire series.

Variables	Odds ratio	C.I. 95%	p-Value
Age (<65 years)	1.4684	0.2550–8.4556	$p = 0.6671$
Gender (F)	2.3379	0.6725–8.1272	$p = 0.1816$
Cardiovascular risk factors	1.4685	0.3449–6.2517	$p = 0.6032$
Type 2 diabetes mellitus	1.4414	0.0613–33.8653	$p = 0.8204$
Obesity	2.3910	0.1913–29.8893	$p = 0.4988$
Preoperative radiotherapy	4.7287	1.0535–21.2256	$p = 0.0426$ *
Tumor volume > 100 mL	1.2882	0.3609–4.5978	$p = 0.6965$
Surgical time > 4 h	2.0073	0.4204–9.5837	$p = 0.3823$
Vascular bypass	1.8550	0.2875–11.9707	$p = 0.5160$
Flap reconstruction	3.2670	0.7090–15.0548	$p = 0.1288$
Site (pelvis)	10.6054	1.4601–77.0316	$p = 0.0196$ *

* statistically significant.

4. Discussion

Musculoskeletal tumors are a rare heterogeneous group of neoplasms. Appropriate management of the patients from the diagnosis and treatment to the follow-up should be done in specialized centers, which can ensure extensive experience and a multidisciplinary approach based on a team composed by orthopedic oncology surgeons, vascular surgeons, and plastic surgeons, if necessary, to aim for the best successful surgical results and adequate margins achieving acceptable outcomes [13]. This has been shown in the present study; a combined ortho-vascular approach for malignant bone and soft tissue tumor patients provided the best surgical outcome with a low rate of major local complications. The retrospective design of the study and heterogeneous group of patients are limitations with possible selection biases; however, retrospective studies are useful for the evaluation of treatment approaches. Moreover, the number of samples and the heterogeneity in diagnoses are related to the rarity of individual tumors, despite the fact that our institute is a national reference center. Because of the relatively small number of patients in some of our histologic subtypes, we could not analyze all confounding variables with a multivariate regression model; in fact, we had the choice to reduce the number of variables to increase the value of our analysis and focused the results on complications. Moreover, we did not want to run a large number of post hoc analyses to assess the influence of some variables on oncologic outcome (such as chemotherapy induced necrosis, surgical margins, etc.) that have been clearly studied before. Finally, the lack of a control group did not allow for a rigorous interpretation of the clinical significance of oncological and vascular outcomes.

Vascular surgery contribution in orthopedic oncology surgery relates to intraoperative support in tumor resection and vascular reconstructions. Preoperative ortho-vascular planning aims to study the patency of the contralateral great saphenous vein and preparation of sterile field for harvesting, if necessary, to insert temporary shunts after resection of the tumor en bloc with the vessels, which makes reconstruction of bone defects with megaprostheses easier and allows for the perfusion of the limb before vascular reconstruction, as well as to preserve the popliteal artery branch to the medial gastrocnemius muscle head in proximal tibia reconstructions when a rotating flap of the medial gastrocnemius muscle is required [13]. Awad et al. evaluated their experience including a vascular surgeon in a multidisciplinary team for treatment of 63 patients with soft tissue sarcomas [7]. A vascular surgeon was requested for bypass reconstruction (12.5%), vessel reconstruction (25%), and vessel ligation (62.5%) [7]. In studies on soft tissue tumors of the lower extremities the incidence of vascular reconstructions was 4%–9% [14–17]. Most clinical studies regarding cooperation with vascular surgeons in orthopedic oncology included only patients that required vascular reconstruction with bypass after the en bloc excision of a tumor involving vascular bundles. Fortner et al., in 1977, were the first to demonstrate the feasibility of vascular reconstruction after en bloc tumor resection [18]. Vessel en bloc excision with the tumor specimen allows for wide margins without violating the tumor capsule, while at the same time, vessel reconstruction provides for restoration of the limb's vascularization. In that study, in a small sample size, the authors reported no case of leg ischemia or gangrene; edema was the most common complication [19]. Other studies confirmed that tumor involvement of the vascular bundle is not an absolute indication for amputation, provided that vascular bypass can be performed [14,19,20]; in these studies, the local recurrence and metastases rate of the patients treated with en bloc resection involving major vessels was similar to those of patient treated differently.

On the other hand, the role of venous reconstruction in vascular surgery for tumors is not clear. Fortner et al. recommended routine venous reconstruction to avoid edema to the limb [18]. Another study in 23 patients with bone and soft tissue sarcomas treated with en bloc resection with arterial and venous reconstruction reported a higher incidence and a longer duration of edema in the group of patients treated with arterial reconstruction only [21]. Similarly, Hohenberger et al. in 20 cases of soft tissue sarcomas treated with en bloc resection, including neuro-vascular bundle and reconstruction with bypass (arterial bypass in 9 patients and venous bypass in 11 patients), reported edema in only 2 cases; they observed that in the case of resection of the external iliac vein or the superficial femoral vein, the ability of the great saphenous vein and lymphatic vessels is adequate if not resected with the tumor specimen [19]. Other authors reported no significant difference in complications and function in a comparison study between 12 patients treated with arterial reconstruction and 13 patients with both venous and arterial reconstruction [17]. Faenza et al. observed that venous reconstruction has some advantages postoperatively, but in the long term, they observed edema developing in all their patients [22]. Therefore, when resection is extensive and involves superficial and deep veins, venous reconstruction is recommended [19,23–26]; the superficial femoral vein and the popliteal vein should not be reconstructed, especially if the great saphenous vein is preserved [27], and if the vein is occluded, there is an absolute contraindication to its reconstruction [24]. In the present study and our practice, venous bypass reconstruction was performed when a significant compromise of the venous flow was expected after resection; in two patients, subtotal occlusion of the bypass was diagnosed at follow-up, without any complications, and in one patient, the venous reconstruction was not performed because the vein was compromised.

Currently, the most used grafts for vascular bypasses are the autologous vein and the synthetic grafts (ePTFE or Dacron). Some authors suggested the use of autologous large saphenous vein bypass [28], whereas other authors did not find any differences in terms of long-term patency between synthetic prostheses and autologous vein grafts [12]. The main concern for synthetic vascular grafts is the risk of infection. Adelani et al. in 14 patients with soft tissue sarcomas treated by resection and vascular bypass reconstructions reported no superiority of the autologous vein prosthesis over the synthetic prosthesis relative to the risk of infection, even if the latter appeared to increase the risk of wound dehiscence [29]. Other studies reported that autologous vein prosthesis has a higher long-term patency rate and lower risk of infection [12,19,25,26,30–34]. In our practice, the contralateral great saphenous vein was used as the first choice; a synthetic graft was used only in one patient because the contralateral great saphenous vein was too short after harvesting. Synthetic vascular grafts are a valid alternative in cases where an autologous vein is not available or there is a significant discrepancy in the diameters of the vessels to be reconstructed. A further aspect to consider for the choice of synthetic vascular grafts is the anatomical site; above the knee both autologous vein and synthetic vascular grafts can be used, while below the knee autologous veins are preferable [19,27].

Vascular reconstructions in orthopedic oncology surgery do not have a negative effect on the survival of the patients. Some authors reported a significantly lower survival of patients treated with vascular reconstructions, even if a selection bias of a locally more aggressive neoplasm should be considered [15]. Poultsides et al. compared the outcomes of two groups of soft tissue sarcoma patients [14]. The first group included 50 patients undergoing resection and vascular reconstruction and the second group included 100 patients without vascular reconstructions; they reported no statistically significant differences in the 5-year overall survival between the two study groups (group I, 59%; group II, 53%; $p = 0.067$) [14]. In the present study, the overall survival was good; however, we did not include a control group for comparison analysis. Moreover, the well-known role of surgical margins for local control and overall survival on malignant tumors should be considered in oncologic outcome. In our series we included several histotypes, with sometimes challenging surgeries, which justifies the relative low incidence of consecutively NED patients (55%) with adequate margins. Different scores have been used for the evaluation of the function of the patients with musculoskeletal tumors [3,35,36]. Ghert et al. compared the function of the patients after lower limb soft tissue sarcoma surgery, with and without vascular reconstruction. They found no statistically significant difference of function between the group with vascular reconstructions (mean score, 78.5%) and the group without vascular reconstructions (mean score, 82.2%) [37]. Other authors reported similar results with respect function in sarcoma patients with resection and vascular reconstructions (mean score, 70%–80% [12,31,38,39]. In the present study, we did not evaluate the function of the patients because data on parameters of function were not available for the majority of the patients. We observed a significant number of patients with temporary sensory and motor nerve deficits that seemed not to be related to the vascular reconstructions themselves considering the self-limiting duration of the symptoms.

Complications do occur in tumor surgery as well as in vascular repair/reconstructions. However, amputation as definitive surgery is rarely required for vascular complications after tumor resection with vascular reconstructions [12,16,27,40]. Awad et al. reported a 17.7% rate of complications, mainly superficial infections (54.5%), deep infections (27.3%), seromas (9%), and local flap necrosis (9%); in their series, complications were more common in patients undergoing hip disarticulation and hemipelvectomy [7]. We concur with this report; in the present study, the rate of complications was higher in the group of patients with pelvic surgery, maybe due to the high complexity of this type of surgery. However, we did not find a significant association between vascular reconstructions and major complications, as previously reported by other authors [14,15,30,31,40]. Davis et al. observed that the wound-healing time in patients with resection and vascular reconstruction was almost twice than that of the group of patients without vascular reconstructions (88 vs. 39 days; $p < 0.002$) with a significantly higher number of revision operations for wound complications [15]. Radiotherapy is an important predictor for major complications in tumor surgery with and without vascular reconstructions [3,15,41]. We strongly recommend a combined plastic surgery approach with soft tissue reconstruction in cases where the risk of complications is high due to a wider resection area, poor coverage of megaprostheses and allografts, and previous radiotherapy [13,26].

5. Conclusions

Although the lack of a control group and limitations of this study prevent us from a statistical demonstration on improved overall survival, the multidisciplinary orthovascular approach for the surgical treatment of patients with musculoskeletal tumors tightly attached to important vascular structures should be considered a good clinical practice for patient safety. Both consultation and cooperation with vascular surgeons are paramount, not only if vascular reconstruction is planned, but in all cases of complex tumor resections close to vascular bundles that may require intraoperative vascular surgery support for possible vascular reconstruction. In this scenario, the outcome of the patients is hypothetically expected to improve without increasing the rate of vascular reconstruction-related complications, even if further, more focused studies should be performed before including this combined approach in the routine management of these patients.

Author Contributions: Conceptualization, A.A. and P.R.; methodology, A.A. and M.P.; validation, A.A., M.P. and P.R.; formal analysis, A.A and M.P.; investigation, E.P.; data curation, E.P., G.T. and A.S.; writing—original draft preparation, A.A. and E.P.; writing—review and editing, A.A. and M.P.; supervision, A.A. and M.P.; project administration, P.R.; funding acquisition, P.R. All authors have read and agreed to the published version of the manuscript.

Funding: This study was financed by research projects of the University of Padova: in part by the project "Nuovi approcci ricostruttivi con impianti protesici dopo resezione per tumori ossei. Analisi prospettica dei risultati oncologici e funzionali"; PI Ruggieri Pietro (prot n. DOR1970520/19), and in part by the project "New approaches and concepts in bone metastases: from bone remodeling markers to clinical implications in oligometastases"; PI Ruggieri Pietro (prot. n. BIRD205407).

Institutional Review Board Statement: Ethical review and approval were waived for this study because of an Institutional Review Board/Ethics Committee approval was not required for retrospective study with fully anonymized clinical routine data.

Informed Consent Statement: Informed consent was obtained from all subjects involved in the study. All patients or their relatives gave written informed consent for their data to be included in scientific studies.

Data Availability Statement: Data and material are available on request.

Conflicts of Interest: On behalf of all authors, the corresponding author states that there is no conflict of interest.

References

1. Mavrogenis, A.F.; Angelini, A.; Errani, C.; Rimondi, E. How should musculoskeletal biopsies be performed? *Orthopedics* **2014**, *37*, 585–588. [CrossRef] [PubMed]
2. Blakely, M.L.; Spurbeck, W.W.; Pappo, A.S.; Pratt, C.B.; Rodriguez-Galindo, C.; Santana, V.M.; Merchant, T.E.; Prichard, M.; Rao, B.N. The impact of margin of resection on outcome in pediatric nonrhabdomyosarcoma soft tissue sarcoma. *J. Pediatr. Surg.* **1999**, *34*, 672–675. [CrossRef]
3. Davis, A.M.; Kandel, R.A.; Wunder, J.S.; Unger, R.; Meer, J.; O'Sullivan, B.; Catton, C.N.; Bell, R.S. The impact of residual disease on local recurrence in patients treated by initial unplanned resection for soft tissue sarcoma of the extremity. *J. Surg. Oncol.* **1997**, *66*, 81–87. [CrossRef]
4. Campanacci, M. *Bone and Soft Tissue Tumors: Clinical Features, Imaging, Pathology and Treatment*; Springer: New York, NY, USA, 1999; pp. 1–70.
5. Mogannam, A.C.; Chavez de Paz, C.; Sheng, N.; Patel, S.; Bianchi, C.; Chiriano, J.; Teruya, T.; Abou-Zamzam, A.M., Jr. Early vascular consultation in the setting of oncologic resections: Benefit for patients and a continuing source of open vascular surgical training. *Ann. Vasc. Surg.* **2015**, *29*, 810–815. [CrossRef]
6. Manzur, M.F.; Ham, S.W.; Elsayed, R.; Abdoli, S.; Simcox, T.; Han, S.; Rowe, V.; Weaver, F.A. Vascular surgery: An essential hospital resource in modern health care. *J. Vasc. Surg.* **2017**, *65*, 1786–1792. [CrossRef]
7. Awad, N.; Lackman, R.; McMackin, K.; Kim, T.W.; Lombardi, J.; Caputo, F. Multidisciplinary Approach to Treatment of Soft Tissue Sarcomas Requiring Complex Oncologic Resections. *Ann. Vasc. Surg.* **2018**, *53*, 212–216. [CrossRef]
8. Clavien, P.A.; Sanabria, J.R.; Strasberg, S.M. Proposed classification of complications of surgery with examples of utility in cholecystectomy. *Surgery* **1992**, *111*, 518–526.
9. Dindo, D.; Demartines, N.; Clavien, P.A. Classification of surgical complications: A new proposal with evaluation in a cohort of 6336 patients and results of a survey. *Ann. Surg.* **2004**, *240*, 205–213. [CrossRef]
10. Enneking, W.F. A system of staging musculoskeletal neoplasms. *Clin. Orthop. Relat. Res.* **1986**, *204*, 9–24. [CrossRef]
11. Wittekind, C.; Compton, C.; Quirke, P.; Nagtegaal, I.; Merkel, S.; Hermanek, P.; Sobin, L.H. A uniform residual tumor (R) classification: Integration of the R classification and the circumferential margin status. *Cancer* **2009**, *115*, 3483–3488. [CrossRef]
12. Schwarzbach, M.H.; Hormann, Y.; Hinz, U.; Bernd, L.; Willeke, F.; Mechtersheimer, G.; Böckler, D.; Schumacher, H.; Herfarth, C.; Büchler, M.W.; et al. Results of limb-sparing surgery with vascular replacement for soft tissue sarcoma in the lower extremity. *J. Vasc. Surg.* **2005**, *42*, 88–97. [CrossRef] [PubMed]
13. Angelini, A.; Tiengo, C.; Sonda, R.; Berizzi, A.; Bassetto, F.; Ruggieri, P. One-Stage Soft Tissue Reconstruction Following Sarcoma Excision: A Personalized Multidisciplinary Approach Called "Orthoplasty". *J. Pers. Med.* **2020**, *10*, 278. [CrossRef] [PubMed]
14. Poultsides, G.A.; Tran, T.B.; Zambrano, E.; Janson, L.; Mohler, D.G.; Mell, M.W.; Avedian, R.S.; Visser, B.C.; Lee, J.T.; Ganjoo, K.; et al. Sarcoma Resection With and Without Vascular Reconstruction: A Matched Case-control Study. *Ann. Surg.* **2015**, *262*, 632–640. [CrossRef]
15. Davis, L.A.; Dandachli, F.; Turcotte, R.; Steinmetz, O.K. Limb-sparing surgery with vascular reconstruction for malignant lower extremity soft tissue sarcoma. *J. Vasc. Surg.* **2017**, *65*, 151–156. [CrossRef]
16. Radaelli, S.; Fiore, M.; Colombo, C.; Ford, S.; Palassini, E.; Sanfilippo, R.; Stacchiotti, S.; Sangalli, C.; Morosi, C.; Casali, P.G.; et al. Vascular resection en-bloc with tumor removal and graft reconstruction is safe and effective in soft tissue sarcoma (STS) of the extremities and retroperitoneum. *Surg. Oncol.* **2016**, *25*, 125–131. [CrossRef] [PubMed]
17. Tsukushi, S.; Nishida, Y.; Sugiura, H.; Nakashima, H.; Ishiguro, N. Results of limb-salvage surgery with vascular reconstruction for soft tissue sarcoma in the lower extremity: Comparison between only arterial and arterovenous reconstruction. *J. Surg. Oncol.* **2008**, *97*, 216–220. [CrossRef]
18. Fortner, J.G.; Kim, D.K.; Shiu, M.H. Limb-preserving vascular surgery for malignant tumors of the lower extremity. *Arch. Surg.* **1977**, *112*, 391–394. [CrossRef] [PubMed]
19. Hohenberger, P.; Allenberg, J.R.; Schlag, P.M.; Reichardt, P. Results of surgery and multimodal therapy for patients with soft tissue sarcoma invading to vascular structures. *Cancer* **1999**, *85*, 396–408. [CrossRef]
20. Bianchi, C.; Ballard, J.L.; Bergan, J.H.; Killeen, J.D. Vascular reconstruction and major resection for malignancy. *Arch. Surg.* **1999**, *134*, 851–855. [CrossRef] [PubMed]
21. Umezawa, H.; Sakuraba, M.; Miyamoto, S.; Nagamatsu, S.; Kayano, S.; Taji, M. Analysis of immediate vascular reconstruction for lower-limb salvage in patients with lower-limb bone and soft-tissue sarcoma. *J. Plast. Reconstr. Aesthet. Surg.* **2013**, *66*, 608–616. [CrossRef] [PubMed]
22. Faenza, A.; Ferraro, A.; Gigli, M.; De Paolis, M.; Errani, C.; Mercuri, M. Vascular homografts for vessel substitution in skeletal and soft tissue sarcomas of the limbs. *Transplant. Proc.* **2005**, *37*, 2692–2693. [CrossRef]
23. Bonardelli, S.; Nodari, F.; Maffeis, R.; Ippolito, V.; Saccalani, M.; Lussardi, L.; Giulini, S. Limb salvage in lower-extremity sarcomas and technical details about vascular reconstruction. *J. Orthop. Sci.* **2000**, *5*, 555–560. [CrossRef]
24. Wortmann, M.; Alldinger, I.; Böckler, D.; Ulrich, A.; Hyhlik-Dürr, A. Vascular reconstruction after retroperitoneal and lower extremity sarcoma resection. *Eur. J. Surg. Oncol.* **2017**, *43*, 407–415. [CrossRef] [PubMed]

25. McKay, A.; Motamedi, M.; Temple, W.; Mack, L.; Moore, R. Vascular reconstruction with the superficial femoral vein following major oncologic resection. *J. Surg. Oncol.* **2007**, *96*, 151–159. [CrossRef] [PubMed]
26. Muramatsu, K.; Ihara, K.; Miyoshi, T.; Yoshida, K.; Taguchi, T. Clinical outcome of limb-salvage surgery after wide resection of sarcoma and femoral vessel reconstruction. *Ann. Vasc. Surg.* **2011**, *25*, 1070–1077. [CrossRef]
27. Kawai, A.; Hashizume, H.; Inoue, H.; Uchida, H.; Sano, S. Vascular reconstruction in limb salvage operations for soft tissue tumors of the extremities. *Clin. Orthop. Relat. Res.* **1996**, *332*, 215–222. [CrossRef]
28. Baxter, B.T.; Mahoney, C.; Johnson, P.J.; Selmer, K.M.; Pipinos, I.I.; Rose, J.; Neff, J.R. Concomitant arterial and venous reconstruction with resection of lower extremity sarcomas. *Ann. Vasc. Surg.* **2007**, *21*, 272–279. [CrossRef]
29. Adelani, M.A.; Holt, G.E.; Dittus, R.S.; Passman, M.A.; Schwartz, H.S. Revascularization after segmental resection of lower extremity soft tissue sarcomas. *J. Surg. Oncol.* **2007**, *95*, 455–460. [CrossRef]
30. Karakousis, C.P.; Karmpaliotis, C.; Driscoll, D.L. Major vessel resection during limb-preserving surgery for soft tissue sarcomas. *World J. Surg.* **1996**, *20*, 345–349. [CrossRef]
31. Koperna, T.; Teleky, B.; Vogl, S.; Windhager, R.; Kainberger, F.; Schatz, K.D.; Kotz, R.; Polterauer, P. Vascular reconstruction for limb salvage in sarcoma of the lower extremity. *Arch. Surg.* **1996**, *131*, 1103–1107. [CrossRef]
32. Nishinari, K.; Krutman, M.; Aguiar Junior, S.; Pignataro, B.S.; Yazbek, G.; Zottele, B.G.A.; Teivelis, M.P.; Wolosker, N. Surgical outcomes of vascular reconstruction in soft tissue sarcomas of the lower extremities. *J. Vasc. Surg.* **2015**, *62*, 143–149. [CrossRef]
33. Leggon, R.E.; Huber, T.S.; Scarborough, M.T. Limb salvage surgery with vascular reconstruction. *Clin. Orthop. Relat. Res.* **2001**, *387*, 207–216. [CrossRef] [PubMed]
34. Park, D.; Cho, S.; Han, A.; Choi, C.; Ahn, S.; Min, S.I.; Ha, J.; Min, S.K. Outcomes after Arterial or Venous Reconstructions in Limb Salvage Surgery for Extremity Soft Tissue Sarcoma. *J. Korean Med. Sci.* **2018**, *33*, e265. [CrossRef]
35. Enneking, W.F.; Dunham, W.; Gebhardt, M.C.; Malawar, M.; Pritchard, D.J. A system for the functional evaluation of reconstructive procedures after surgical treatment of tumors of the musculoskeletal system. *Clin. Orthop. Relat. Res.* **1993**, *286*, 241–246. [CrossRef]
36. Ruggieri, P.; Mavrogenis, A.F.; Mercuri, M. Quality of life following limb-salvage surgery for bone sarcomas. *Expert Rev. Pharmacoecon. Outcomes Res.* **2011**, *11*, 59–73. [CrossRef]
37. Ghert, M.A.; Davis, A.M.; Griffin, A.M.; Alyami, A.H.; White, L.; Kandel, R.A.; Ferguson, P.; O'Sullivan, B.; Catton, C.N.; Lindsay, T.; et al. The surgical and functional outcome of limb-salvage surgery with vascular reconstruction for soft tissue sarcoma of the extremity. *Ann. Surg. Oncol.* **2005**, *12*, 1102–1110. [CrossRef] [PubMed]
38. Akgül, T.; Sormaz, İ.C.; Aksoy, M.; Uçar, A.; Özger, H.; Eralp, L. Results and functional outcomes of en-bloc resection and vascular reconstruction in extremity musculoskeletal tumors. *Acta Orthop. Traumatol. Turc.* **2018**, *52*, 409–414. [CrossRef] [PubMed]
39. Emori, M.; Hamada, K.; Omori, S.; Joyama, S.; Tomita, Y.; Hashimoto, N.; Takami, H.; Naka, N.; Yoshikawa, H.; Araki, N. Surgery with vascular reconstruction for soft-tissue sarcomas in the inguinal region: Oncologic and functional outcomes. *Ann. Vasc. Surg.* **2012**, *26*, 693–699. [CrossRef] [PubMed]
40. Cetinkaya, O.A.; Celik, S.U.; Kalem, M.; Basarir, K.; Koksoy, C.; Yildiz, H.Y. Clinical Characteristics and Surgical Outcomes of Limb-Sparing Surgery with Vascular Reconstruction for Soft Tissue Sarcomas. *Ann. Vasc. Surg.* **2019**, *56*, 73–80. [CrossRef]
41. Haubner, F.; Ohmann, E.; Pohl, F.; Strutz, J.; Gassner, H.G. Wound healing after radiation therapy: Review of the literature. *Radiat. Oncol.* **2012**, *7*, 162. [CrossRef]

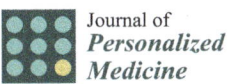 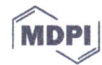

Article

Highly Cancellous Titanium Alloy (TiAl$_6$V$_4$) Surfaces on Three-Dimensionally Printed, Custom-Made Intercalary Tibia Prostheses: Promising Short- to Intermediate-Term Results

Wiebke K. Guder *[ ], Jendrik Hardes, Markus Nottrott, Lars E. Podleska and Arne Streitbürger

Department of Orthopedic Oncology, University Hospital Essen, Hufelandstrasse 55, 45147 Essen, Germany; jendrik.hardes@uk-essen.de (J.H.); markus.nottrott@uk-essen.de (M.N.); lars-eric.podleska@uk-essen.de (L.E.P.); arne.streitbuerger@uk-essen.de (A.S.)
* Correspondence: wiebke.guder@uk-essen.de

Abstract: Custom-made, three-dimensionally-printed (3D) bone prostheses gain increasing importance in the reconstruction of bone defects after musculoskeletal tumor resections. They may allow preservation of little remaining bone stock and ensure joint or limb salvage. However, we believe that by constructing anatomy-imitating implants with highly cancellous titanium alloy (TiAl$_6$V$_4$) surfaces using 3D printing technology, further benefits such as functional enhancement and reduction of complications may be achieved. We present a case series of four patients reconstructed using custom-made, 3D-printed intercalary monobloc tibia prostheses treated between 2016 and 2020. The mean patient age at operation was 30 years. Tumor resections were performed for Ewing sarcoma ($n = 2$), high-grade undifferentiated pleomorphic bone sarcoma ($n = 1$) and adamantinoma ($n = 1$). Mean resection length was 17.5 cm and mean operation time 147 min. All patients achieved full weight-bearing and limb salvage at a mean follow-up of 21.25 months. One patient developed a non-union at the proximal bone-implant interface. Alteration of implant design prevented non-union in later patients. Mean MSTS and TESS scores were 23.5 and 88. 3D-printed, custom-made intercalary tibia prostheses achieved joint and limb salvage in this case series despite high, published complication rates for biological and endoprosthetic reconstructions of the diaphyseal and distal tibia. Ingrowth of soft tissues into the highly cancellous implant surface structure reduces dead space, enhances function, and appears promising in reducing complication rates.

Keywords: highly cancellous; implant surface; tibia; titanium alloy; 3D printing; megaendoprosthesis; orthopedic oncology

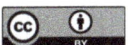

1. Introduction

Personalized, custom-made implants have gained importance in the reconstruction of bone defects after musculoskeletal tumor resections. Megaendoprostheses are a well-established and accepted reconstruction technique of osteoarticular defects of the hip, knee, and glenohumeral joint [1]. However, depending on the amount of remaining bone stock and soft tissue coverage, standard megaendoprosthetic implants are either unavailable or associated with higher complication rates in more distally located sites such as the distal tibia and ankle [2–7]. Since three-dimensional (3D) computer-assisted design (3D-CAD) and 3D-printing technology were introduced in the production process of orthopedic implants, the availability of patient-individualized stems and anatomy-imitating implants in complex anatomic and biomechanical sites has improved the rates of joint and limb salvage of both osteoarticular and intercalary reconstructions [8–10].

3D printing technology also has its implications in improving osseointegration by creating implant designs with highly cancellous surfaces [11,12].

To our knowledge, the ingrowth of soft tissues into highly cancellous implant surfaces as a means of reducing dead space around megaendoprostheses, improving periprosthetic infection rates and enhancing functional outcome remains largely unexplored. Soft tissue attachment to titanium implants has only been investigated in the context of intraosseous transcutaneous amputation prostheses to serve as a barrier for exogenous agents such as bacteria [13].

For this reason, we present the short- to intermediate-term results of a case series of four patients treated by intercalary tumor resection for tumors of the distal tibia and reconstruction using a novel, custom-made 3D-printed monobloc implant design and a highly porous surface. The presented implant design avoids distal tibia resection—in favor of intercalary resection—in all cases despite little remaining bone stock above the ankle joint.

2. Materials and Methods

Four patients, who underwent tibial intercalary resection for malignant primary bone tumors, were reconstructed using 3D-printed intercalary monobloc tibia megaendoprostheses with highly cancellous titanium alloy surfaces ($TiAl_6V_4$) between 2016 and 2020.

Patient data were prospectively collected and retrospectively analyzed.

2.1. Patient Characteristics

The mean patient age at the time of operation was 30 years (range 19–54 years). In all cases, the diagnosis of a malignant primary bone tumor was confirmed by incisional biopsy. Histological diagnoses in decreasing order were Ewing sarcoma ($n = 2$), high-grade undifferentiated pleomorphic bone sarcoma (UPS), and adamantinoma in one case each. Three patients received neoadjuvant and adjuvant chemotherapy. None of the patients received (neo-)adjuvant radiation treatments of the primary tumor site. Comorbidities were absent in all treated patients.

Three patients underwent tumor resection and reconstruction using an intercalary tibia monobloc implant within the same operation, one patient was temporarily reconstructed using a polymethyl methacrylate (PMMA) spacer and underwent definite reconstruction after completion of chemotherapy. The mean tumor resection and reconstruction length was 17.5 cm with a mean of 28.75 mm remaining distal tibia. Bone growth stimulants or postoperative drugs to enhance tissue growth were not administered. The mean operation time was 147 min. All monobloc prostheses were implanted in a non-cemented fashion. Local muscle flaps were performed for adequate soft tissue coverage of the implants. All patients ambulated with partial weight-bearing of 20 kg using crutches for 6 weeks after the operation. Weight-bearing was then increased at increments of 10 kg on a weekly basis.

All four patients were alive at the time of retrospective analysis without evidence of disease at a mean follow-up of 21.25 months (range 5–52 months).

Patient and operation-specific data are detailed in Table 1.

Table 1. Patient and operation-specific characteristics.

#	1	2	3	4
Age (years)	25	19	22	54
Diagnosis	Adamantinoma	Ewing	Ewing	UPS
Grading	low-grade	high-grade	high-grade	high-grade
Resection length (mm)	175	200	160	165
Remaining distal tibia (mm)	5	30	45	35
Operation time (minutes)	NA	210	125	106
Margin (R)	0	0	0	0
Chemotherapy	-	+	+	+
Radiation	-	-	-	-
Complication	Non-union (proximal)	-	-	-
MSTS	20	29	25	20

Table 1. Cont.

#	1	2	3	4
TESS	86	100	96	70
Follow-up (months)	52	18	10	5

number.

2.2. Indication

To be eligible for reconstruction using a custom-made 3D printed intercalary titanium alloy implant with a highly cancellous surface, patients had to meet the following criteria:

- Primary malignant bone tumor of the diaphysis and metaphysis of the distal tibia;
- Remaining bone stock in the distal tibia excluded use of off-the-shelf intercalary tibial megaendoprosthetic implants and stems;
- Absence of comorbidities affecting bone and wound healing, such as diabetes mellitus, peripheral artery occlusive disease, or positive smoking history;
- Patient consent to undergo this reconstruction rather than below-knee amputation or other biological reconstruction.

2.3. Pre-Operative Planning and Production

Custom-made 3D-printed intercalary tibia monobloc titanium aluminum vanadium alloy (TiAl$_6$V$_4$) implants with highly cancellous implant surfaces were planned on preoperative computed tomography (CT) scans (DICOM format, reconstruction matrix 512 × 512, slice thickness ≤ 1 mm). Osteotomy levels were defined using corresponding pre-treatment magnetic resonance imaging (MRI) studies and measured by distance to the adjacent joint line. 3D-CAD of the implants was performed by Implantcast Inc. (Buxtehude, Germany) as specified and approved by the operating surgeon before production using electron beam melting technology (EBM®) commenced (Figure 1). Implants were gamma-sterilized using the same parameters established for off-the-shelf implants.

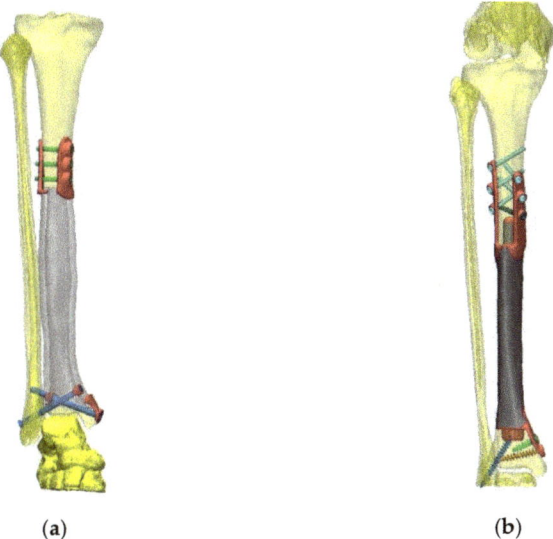

Figure 1. 3D-CADs based on computed tomography datasets (**a**) Patient #1: hollow implant with a highly cancellous implant surface and extracortical plates with supplementary interlocking screw options at proximal and distal implant-bone interface; (**b**) Patient #4: solid implant with a highly cancellous implant surface, small solid proximal and hollow distal stem and plates with interlocking screw options at the proximal and distal implant-bone interface.

2.4. Implant Properties and Highly Cancellous Implant Surface (EPORE®, Implantcast, Buxtehude, Germany)

All custom-made 3D-printed intercalary tibia monobloc titanium alloy (TiAl$_6$V$_4$) implants were designed imitating the individual patient's bone geometry and dimensions (Table 2).

Table 2. Mechanical Implant Properties.

#	1	2	3	4
Reconstruction Length (mm)	175	200	160	165
Implant body	hollow	solid	solid	solid
Proximal stem (mm)	none	Solid 14 × 20	solid 14 × 28	solid 11 × 25
Proximal extracortical plates (mm)				
medial	41	55	60	67
lateral	38	65	55	76
Distal stem (mm)	none	none	none	hollow 20 × 10
Distal extracortical plates (mm)				
medial	12	25	38	28
ventral	-	18	28	-

\# number.

Implants were manufactured with a highly cancellous implant surface (EPORE®) characterized by trabeculae with a diameter of 330–390 μm to imitate trabecular bone and promote tissue ingrowth (Figure 2).

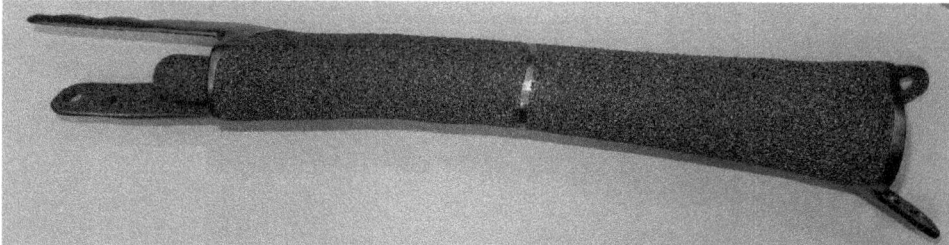

Figure 2. Photograph of a finished monobloc solid body implant (Patient #2) with highly cancellous implant surface on stem, bone-facing extracortical plates, and implant body.

The implant was designed with a hollow prosthetic body for patient #1, while a solid body was used for following implants.

Stems or extracortical plates with supplementary interlocking screw options were used to anchor the implants to adjacent bone at implant-bone interfaces. At the proximal interface, solid stem designs were used; distally hollow stems were planned whenever feasible depending on remaining bone stock.

2.5. Surgical Technique

The stem length of tibial monobloc implants with a proximal and distal stem is a limiting factor for successful implantation. If the stem dimensions are chosen too long, they will pose an obstacle to repositioning the tibia. For this reason, the implant design of the monobloc implant of patient #4 included a distal stem with a length of only 10 mm. After resection of the distal diaphyseal tibia, axial, angular, and rotational maneuverability of the lower leg are increased even when an intact fibula remains. Therefore, in the case of patient #4, the proximal stem was implanted first while the remaining distal tibia and foot were lowered and rotated to the side as much as possible to prevent interference with the proximal implantation. When resetting the distal tibia with the distal implant interface and stem, the existing soft tissue expansibility was used to gain the leeway necessary for implanting the 10 mm distal stem. If implantation of the distal stem had proven impossible for a lack of leeway, an additional fibular osteotomy would have been performed to gain more clearance. As the maximum amount of contrivable clearance is limited, implantation of longer implant stems would need to be planned with a modular implant design.

2.6. Bone Ingrowth

Bone ingrowth at the implant-bone interfaces was assessed clinically and radiographically. An absence of pain or instability (after full weight-bearing was achieved) served as a clinical indicator for bone ingrowth. Radiographic criteria on postoperative plain radiographs included correct implant positioning without dislocation or signs for aseptic loosening. In the event of clinical or radiographic symptoms, additional CT imaging of the reconstruction was performed.

2.7. Complication Assessment

Complications were categorized according to the Henderson classification [14].

2.8. Functional Assessment

The Musculoskeletal Tumor Society (MSTS) score and Toronto Extremity Salvage Score (TESS) were used to assess functional outcomes [15,16]. The respective questionnaires were handed out in paper form and completed by patients as part of their outpatient follow-up examinations.

3. Results

In the four patients—reconstructed using custom-made 3D-printed intercalary megaendoprostheses with a highly cancellous implant surface—distal tibia resection and below-knee amputation were avoided in all cases (Figure 3).

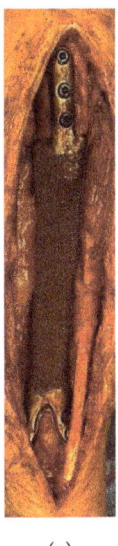
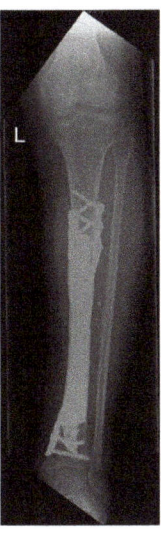

(a) (b)

Figure 3. Patient #3: Reconstruction after implantation of a monobloc intercalary distal tibia implant: (**a**) intraoperative image; (**b**) postoperative radiograph of the tibia anterior-posterior (a.p.) view. L means left.

3.1. Bone Ingrowth

Primary ingrowth of the implant occurred in all patients at both implant-bone interfaces except for the proximal osteotomy line of patient #1. A partial non-union observed in this patient is more comprehensively analyzed in Section 3.3. At the current follow-up, we did not observe differences in osseointegration among treated patients (regardless of age at operation).

3.2. Soft Tissue Ingrowth

A complete ingrowth of muscular tissue into the highly cancellous implant surface was confirmed in one patient who underwent a revision for partial non-union (Figure 4).

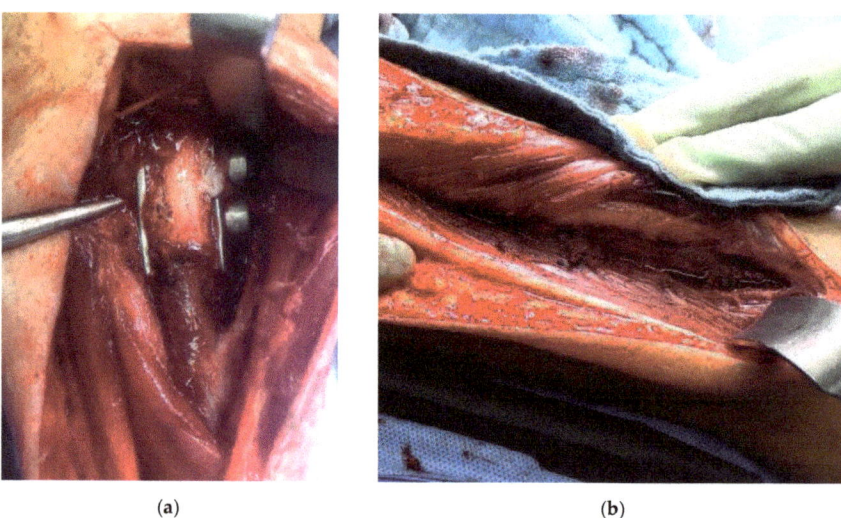

(a)   (b)

Figure 4. Patient #1: Intraoperative images during revision operation nine months after primary reconstruction: (**a**) view of proximal implant-tibia interface with visibility of partial non-union and soft tissue ingrowth into the highly cancellous implant surface; (**b**) complete ingrowth of muscles and soft tissues into the highly cancellous implant body surface.

3.3. Complications

The first patient reconstructed using a highly cancellous 3D-printed monobloc intercalary tibia implant developed an incomplete non-union at the proximal bone-implant interface (Henderson Type 3—structural failure). Two extracortical plates with supplementary interlocking screws bridging the bone-implant interface were used to anchor the implant to the proximal tibial diaphysis without a central stem. This anchorage design was chosen to allow filling the hollow implant body with autologous iliac crest graft (Figure 5). Operative revision and additional plating of the bone implant interface while retaining the original implant were performed 9 months after primary reconstruction (Figure 6). In addition, the ipsilateral fibula was osteotomized and fixed to the tibial column using screw osteosyntheses after roughening the facing bone cortices to encourage bone union. A hypertrophic pseudarthrosis recurred at the tibial bone-implant interface while the fibular transfer consolidated and continues to stabilize the reconstruction by taking part of the load. The patient currently has full weight bearing using a light brace and declines further operative revision as her activities of daily life are not impaired and she has no athletic ambitions. Implant design has been adapted to include a central stem and solid implant body at the proximal bone-implant interface. After this alteration, non-union and hypertrophic pseudarthrosis were avoided in later patients.

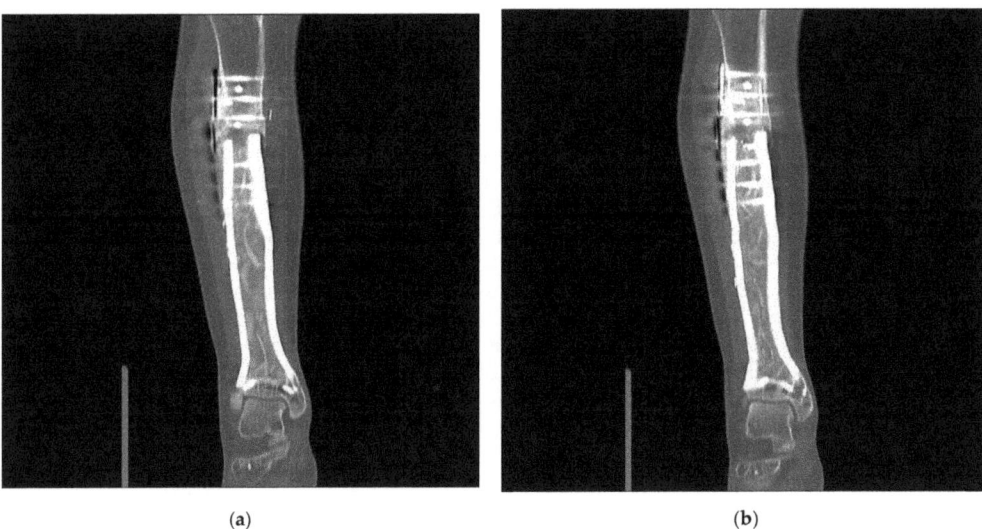

Figure 5. Patient #1: Computed tomography scan 43 months after primary reconstruction: (**a,b**) coronar view of the implant with the depiction of the bone graft-loaded hollow implant cavity and persistent non-union of the proximal implant-bone interface.

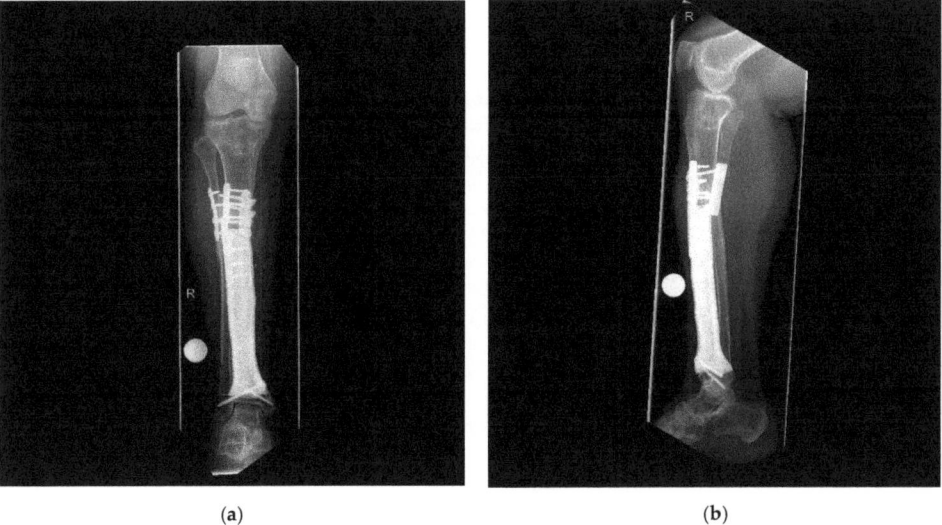

Figure 6. Patient #1: Postoperative radiographs after osteosynthetic plating of the proximal implant-bone interface (**a**) a.p. view; (**b**) lateral view. R means right.

Soft tissue failure (Henderson type 1), aseptic loosening (Henderson type 2), periprosthetic infections (Henderson type 4), or local recurrence (Henderson type 5) were not observed in this collective.

3.4. Functional Outcome

All patients have achieved full weight-bearing and returned to their activities of daily life. The mean MSTS and TESS scores were 23.5 and 88, respectively. Patient #4 completed the functional questionnaire three months after the operation when presenting at the outpatient clinic for her first postoperative follow-up. She has not completed a functional rehabilitation program due to ongoing adjuvant chemotherapy yet.

4. Discussion

In this study, we present the short- to intermediate-term outcomes of four patients reconstructed using 3D-printed patient-individualized intercalary tibia monobloc prostheses with highly cancellous implant surfaces. From our point of view, complete ingrowth of soft tissues into the highly cancellous implant surface and continued joint salvage of the ankle joint despite little remaining bone stock are the most significant findings of this study.

The rationale for using titanium aluminum vanadium alloy ($TiAl_6V_4$) implants for the presented implant design were based on two main considerations: biocompability and choice of available production technique. Titanium alloys are a certified and reliable material with good biocompability for non-cemented reconstructions. They also have sufficient stability and processed using EBM allows for highly porous implant surfaces.

Periprosthetic infection is a serious problem affecting primary and revision total joint arthroplasties [17,18], but infection rates of megaendoprosthetic reconstructions are even higher despite implant features such as silver coating [19]. Possible reasons are larger reconstruction lengths with larger implant surfaces, longer operation times, and frequently immunocompromised patients. McConoughey et al., report that bacteria are often introduced into the wound in their planktonic form, growing in joint fluids before colonizing an implant. Later, they form biofilms to avoid exposure to high doses of antibiotics, develop resistance, and persist in a dormant state [20].

Complete ingrowth of soft tissues into the implant surface, as observed in this study, addresses many known causes and promotive factors in the development of periprosthetic infection: reduction of (a) dead space, (b) scar tissue formation surrounding the implants at a distance, and (c) excessive joint fluid formation around the implant.

In a study by Cordero et al., rough titanium alloy surfaces have shown a higher tendency of bacterial colonization when compared with smooth surfaces [20,21]. However, soft tissue ingrowth and accessibility of implant surfaces for immune cells may balance this observed disadvantage. While we concede that a lack of periprosthetic infection in the presented case series is not sufficient to make any firm conclusions about the impact of soft tissue ingrowth on implant surfaces, highly cancellous implant surfaces seem a feasible implant modification warranting further research.

Bone and soft tissue ingrowth also have implications for functional outcomes. MSTS and TESS scores of 23.5 and 88 in this study were satisfactory and most likely caused by the preservation of the ankle joint as well as soft tissue ingrowth. They compete with or exceed functional outcomes observed after biological and endoprosthetic intercalary or osteoarticular distal tibia reconstructions. Tanaka et al. reported MSTS scores of nineteen patients ranging between 93–100% after reconstruction with vascularized fibula grafts in intercalary femur and tibia defects. They also observed a union rate of 79% after a mean time of 7.8 months, which necessitated long periods of partial to no weight-bearing [22]. Khira et al., published a mean MSTS score of 84 (80–92) in their collective of patients reconstructed using vascularized fibula grafts with an Ilizarov external fixator for large tibial bone defects [23]. Intercalary or osteoarticular distal tibia allografts (optionally augmented with vascularized fibula grafts or composite prostheses) are another biological reconstruction option reported by Donati et al. However, they were rarely indicated for the ankle joint compared with other locations ($n = 3$). Complications included non-union (49%) and fracture (27%) observed in all reconstructed sites ($n = 112$) [24].

Abudu et al. reported their results for endoprosthetic replacement of the distal tibia and ankle joint ($n = 5$). While function was excellent to begin with, it deteriorated over time. Yet, patients maintained a mean Enneking score of 50% in this study [5]. In 2017, Yang et al. documented a median MSTS score of 66% in eight patients treated by custom-made distal tibia megaprosthesis [2]. Lee et al. assessed a mean MSTS score of 24.2 in six patients treated with the custom-made, hinged distal tibia and ankle prostheses. Among complications, talar collapse and wound infection were noted [6]. Shekkeris et al. reported that two of six patients treated by endoprosthetic distal tibia replacement went on to have below-knee amputation for persistent infection after a mean of 16 months in their study. The mean MSTS and TESS score of patients retaining the implants was 70% and 71% [3]. The most common complication after endoprosthetic intercalary reconstruction observed by Streitbürger et al. was aseptic loosening. Alteration of stem design to fit biomechanical demands of epi- or metaphyseal stem anchorage showed a tendency to improve implant longevity, though. [10].

The complication rates presented in the above-mentioned studies prove that reconstruction of bone defects of the distal tibia after tumor resections remains challenging regardless of the reconstruction technique chosen. Furthermore, the authors agree that below-knee amputation remains a valid treatment choice. The implant design presented in this case series achieved joint and limb salvage at a low complication rate and satisfactory functional outcomes with an early return to full weight-bearing. For this reason, increased consideration of biomechanical demands on implants and further technological advancements of 3D-printing seem a promising research avenue to increase the role of megaendoprosthetic reconstructions in this challenging location.

5. Conclusions

Reconstruction of the diaphyseal and distal tibia using custom-made 3D-printed intercalary implants proves to be a feasible treatment strategy in this case series. Considering that functional outcome after below-knee amputation leads to acceptable results and lower complication rates compared with other limb salvaging biological and standard megaendoprosthetic approaches, a low complication rate and good functional outcome in this case series emphasize that limb salvage using 3D-printed custom-made implants should be considered when counseling patients despite a lack of long-term experiences. However, observation of these patients with regard to long-term functional results and complication rates is necessary. Highly cancellous implant body designs should be considered in other megaendoprosthetic implant sites as well and future studies investigating this design's advantages and complications seem warranted.

Author Contributions: Conceptualization, W.K.G., J.H. and A.S.; methodology, not applicable; software, not applicable; validation, W.K.G., J.H. and A.S.; formal analysis, W.K.G.; investigation, W.K.G.; resources, W.K.G.; data curation, W.K.G.; writing—original draft preparation, W.K.G.; writing—review and editing, W.K.G., J.H., M.N., L.E.P. and A.S.; visualization, W.K.G.; supervision, not applicable; project administration, W.K.G.; funding acquisition, not applicable. All authors have read and agreed to the published version of the manuscript.

Funding: This research received no external funding.

Institutional Review Board Statement: The study was conducted according to the guidelines of the Declaration of Helsinki, and approved by the Ethics Committee of the University of Duisburg-Essen (protocol code 21-9859-BO, approved 16 February 2021).

Informed Consent Statement: Informed consent was obtained from all subjects involved in the study.

Data Availability Statement: The data presented in this study are available on reasonable request from the corresponding author.

Conflicts of Interest: The authors W.G., M.N. and L.P. declare no conflict of interest. The authors J.H. and A.S. received research grants from "implantcast" company and financial support for attending symposia. The company "implantcast" had no role in the design of the study; in the collection, analyses, or interpretation of data; in the writing of the manuscript, or in the decision to publish the results.

References

1. Hardes, J.; Guder, W.; Dudda, M.; Nottrott, M.; Podleska, L.-E.; Streitbürger, A. Aktuelle Ergebnisse der Tumorendoprothetik bei Jugendlichen und Erwachsenen. *Orthopäde* **2019**, *48*, 744–751. [CrossRef] [PubMed]
2. Yang, P.; Evans, S.; Khan, Z.; Abudu, A.; Jeys, L.; Grimer, R. Reconstruction of the Distal Tibia Following Resection of Aggressive Bone Tumours Using a Custom-made Megaprosthesis. *J. Orthop.* **2017**, *14*, 406–409. [CrossRef] [PubMed]
3. Shekkeris, A.S.; Hanna, S.A.; Sewell, M.D.; Spiegelberg, B.G.I.; Aston, W.J.S.; Blunn, G.W.; Cannon, S.R.; Briggs, T.W.R. Endoprosthetic Reconstruction of the Distal Tibia and Ankle Joint after Resection of Primary Bone Tumours. *J. Bone Jt. Surgery. Br. Vol.* **2009**, *91*, 1378–1382. [CrossRef] [PubMed]
4. Zhao, Z.; Yan, T.; Guo, W.; Yang, R.; Tang, X.; Wang, W. Surgical Options and Reconstruction Strategies for Primary Bone Tumors of Distal Tibia: A Systematic Review of Complications and Functional Outcome. *J. Bone Oncol.* **2019**, *14*, 100209. [CrossRef]
5. Abudu, A.; Grimer, R.J.; Tillman, R.M.; Carter, S.R. Endoprosthetic Replacement of the Distal Tibia and Ankle Joint for Aggressive Bone Tumours. *Int. Orthop.* **1999**, *23*, 291–294. [CrossRef]
6. Lee, S.H.; Kim, H.-S.; Park, Y.-B.; Rhie, T.-Y.; Lee, H.K. Prosthetic Reconstruction for Tumours of the Distal Tibia and Fibula. *J. Bone Jt. Surgery. Br. Vol.* **1999**, *81*, 803–807. [CrossRef]
7. Natarajan, M.V.; Annamalai, K.; Williams, S.; Selvaraj, R.; Rajagopal, T.S. Limb Salvage in Distal Tibial Osteosarcoma Using a Custom Mega Prosthesis. *Int. Orthop.* **2000**, *24*, 282–284. [CrossRef]
8. Feng, D.; He, J.; Zhang, C.; Wang, L.; Gu, X.; Guo, Y. 3D-Printed Prosthesis Replacement for Limb Salvage after Radical Resection of an Ameloblastoma in the Tibia with 1 Year of Follow Up: A Case Report. *Yonsei Med J.* **2019**, *60*, 882–886. [CrossRef]
9. Angelini, A.; Kotrych, D.; Trovarelli, G.; Szafrański, A.; Bohatyrewicz, A.; Ruggieri, P. Analysis of Principles Inspiring Design of Three-dimensional-printed Custom-made Prostheses in Two Referral Centres. *Int. Orthop.* **2020**, *44*, 829–837. [CrossRef]
10. Streitbürger, A.; Hardes, J.; Nottrott, M.; Guder, W.K. Reconstruction Survival of Segmental Megaendoprostheses: A Retrospective Analysis of 28 Patients Treated for Intercalary Bone Defects after Musculoskeletal Tumor Resections. *Arch. Orthop. Trauma Surg.* **2020**, 1–16. [CrossRef]
11. Fang, C.; Cai, H.; Kuong, E.; Chui, E.; Siu, Y.C.; Ji, T.; Drstvenšek, I. Surgical Applications of Three-dimensional Printing in the Pelvis and Acetabulum: From Models and Tools to Implants. *Unfallchirurg* **2019**, *122*, 278–285. [CrossRef]
12. Crovace, A.M.; Lacitignola, L.; Forleo, D.M.; Staffieri, F.; Francioso, E.; Di Meo, A.; Becerra, J.; Crovace, A.; Santos-Ruiz, L. 3D Biomimetic Porous Titanium (Ti_6Al_4V ELI) Scaffolds for Large Bone Critical Defect Reconstruction: An Experimental Study in Sheep. *Animals* **2020**, *10*, 1389. [CrossRef] [PubMed]
13. Chen, G.J.; Wang, Z.; Bai, H.; Li, J.M.; Cai, H. A Preliminary Study on Investigating the Attachment of Soft Tissue onto Micro-arc Oxidized Titanium Alloy Implants. *Biomed. Mater.* **2009**, *4*, 015017. [CrossRef] [PubMed]
14. Pala, E.; Trovarelli, G.; Calabrò, T.; Angelini, A.; Abati, C.N.; Ruggieri, P. Survival of Modern Knee Tumor Megaprostheses: Failures, Functional Results, and a Comparative Statistical Analysis. *Clin. Orthop. Relat. Res.* **2015**, *473*, 891–899. [CrossRef] [PubMed]
15. Enneking, W.F.; Dunham, W.; Gebhardt, M.C.; Malawar, M.; Pritchard, D.J. A System for the Functional Evaluation of Reconstructive Procedures After Surgical Treatment of Tumors of the Musculoskeletal System. *Clin. Orthop. Relat. Res.* **1993**. [CrossRef]
16. Davis, A.M.; Wright, J.G.; Williams, J.I.; Bombardier, C.; Griffin, A.; Bell, R.S. Development of a Measure of Physical Function for Patients with Bone and Soft Tissue Sarcoma. *Qual. Life Res.* **1996**, *5*, 508–516. [CrossRef] [PubMed]
17. Jämsen, E.; Huhtala, H.; Puolakka, T.; Moilanen, T. Risk Factors for Infection after Knee Arthroplasty. *JBJS* **2009**, *91*, 38–47. [CrossRef]
18. Peersman, G.; Laskin, R.; Davis, J.; Peterson, M. Infection in Total Knee Replacement: A Retrospective Review of 6489 Total Knee Replacements. *Clin. Orthop. Relat. Res.* **2001**, *392*, 15–23. [CrossRef]
19. Hardes, J.; Von Eiff, C.; Streitbuerger, A.; Balke, M.; Budny, T.; Henrichs, M.P.; Hauschild, G.; Ahrens, H. Reduction of Periprosthetic Infection with Silver-coated Megaprostheses in Patients with Bone Sarcoma. *J. Surg. Oncol.* **2010**, *101*, 389–395. [CrossRef]
20. McConoughey, S.J.; Howlin, R.; Granger, J.F.; Manring, M.M.; Calhoun, J.H.; Shirtliff, M.; Kathju, S.; Stoodley, P. Biofilms in Periprosthetic Orthopedic Infections. *Futur. Microbiol.* **2014**, *9*, 987–1007. [CrossRef]
21. Cordero, J.; Munuera, L.; Folgueira, M. The Influence of the Chemical Composition and Surface of the Implant on Infection. *INJ* **1996**, *27*, S/C34–S/C37. [CrossRef]
22. Tanaka, K.; Maehara, H.; Kanaya, F. Vascularized Fibular Graft for Bone Defects after Wide Resection of Musculoskeletal Tumors. *J. Orthop. Sci.* **2012**, *17*, 156–162. [CrossRef] [PubMed]
23. Khira, Y.M.; Badawy, H.A. Pedicled Vascularized Fibular Graft with Ilizarov External Fixator for Reconstructing a Large Bone Defect of the Tibia after Tumor Resection. *J. Orthop. Traumatol.* **2013**, *14*, 91–100. [CrossRef] [PubMed]
24. Donati, D.; Di Liddo, M.; Zavatta, M.; Manfrini, M.; Bacci, G.; Picci, P.; Capanna, R.; Mercuri, M. Massive Bone Allograft Reconstruction in High-grade Osteosarcoma. *Clin. Orthop. Relat. Res.* **2000**, *377*, 186–194. [CrossRef] [PubMed]

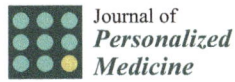

Article

Custom Made Monoflange Acetabular Components for the Treatment of Paprosky Type III Defects

Sebastian Philipp von Hertzberg-Boelch [1,*], Mike Wagenbrenner [1], Jörg Arnholdt [1], Stephan Frenzel [2], Boris Michael Holzapfel [1] and Maximilian Rudert [1]

1. Department of Orthopaedic Surgery, Orthopädische Klinik König-Ludwig-Haus, University of Wuerzburg, 97070 Wuerzburg, Germany; m-wagenbrenner.klh@uni-wuerzburg.de (M.W.); j-arnholdt.klh@uni-wuerzburg.de (J.A.); b-hozapfel.klh@uni-wuerzburg.de (B.M.H.); m-rudert.klh@uni-wuerzburg.de (M.R.)
2. Department of Orthopaedics and Trauma Surgery, Medical University of Vienna, Vienna General Hospital, 1090 Vienna, Austria; stephan.frenzel@meduniwien.ac.at
* Correspondence: s-boelch.klh@uni-wuerzburg.de; Tel.: +49-0941-8030

Abstract: Purpose: Patient-specific, flanged acetabular components are used for the treatment of Paprosky type III defects during revision total hip arthroplasty (THA). This monocentric retrospective cohort study analyzes the outcome of patients treated with custom made monoflanged acetabular components (CMACs) with intra- and extramedullary iliac fixation. Methods: 14 patients were included who underwent revision THA with CMACs for the treatment of Paprosky type III defects. Mechanism of THA failure was infection in 4 and aseptic loosening in 10 patients. Seven patients underwent no previous revision, the other seven patients underwent three or more previous revisions. Results: At a mean follow-up of 35.4 months (14–94), the revision rate of the implant was 28.3%. Additionally, one perioperative dislocation and one superficial wound infection occurred. At one year postoperatively, we found a significant improvement of the Western Ontario and McMaster Universities Arthritis Index (WOMAC) score ($p = 0.015$). Postoperative radiographic analysis revealed good hip joint reconstruction with a mean leg length discrepancy of 3 mm (−8–20), a mean lateralization of the horizontal hip center of rotation of 8 mm (−8–35), and a mean proximalization of the vertical hip center of rotation of 6 mm (13–26). Radiolucency lines were present in 30%. Conclusion: CMACs can be considered an option for the treatment of acetabular bone loss in revision THA. Iliac intra- and extramedullary fixation allows soft tissue-adjusted hip joint reconstruction and improves hip function. However, failure rates are high, with periprosthetic infection being the main threat to successful outcome.

Keywords: patient specific implant; custom made implant; revision hip; Paprosky; pelvic discontinuity

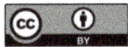

1. Introduction

The revision burden after total hip arthroplasty (THA) will increase [1]. Acetabular bone loss is a major surgical challenge in revision THA (rTHA), particularly in re-revisions or after implant migration. Successful acetabular reconstruction with long-term component fixation requires sufficient primary stability for secondary osteointegration. A broad range of surgical strategies are available, of which the most popular are antiprotrusion cages [2], hemispherical or asymmetrical cups with intra- or extramedullary fixation [3–5] and modular, highly porous acetabular revision systems with and without metal wedges, buttress augments, and cage options [6,7]. However, it has not yet been defined which strategy should be considered as the benchmark [8].

Although custom made implants consume great organizational and financial resources, they are a further treatment option for large osseous defects that otherwise cannot be managed with standard implants. Based on computed tomography (CT), custom made acetabular components offer the surgeon the option to add metal sockets to the implant volume according to the defect of the hemipelvis, to adjust flanges for fixation devices to the remaining bone stock, and to plan the reconstruction of the hip center of rotation (COR) [9].

Most custom made acetabular components are designed as triflanges. These custom made triflange acetabular components (CTACs) are intended to "span the gap" by bridging the periacetabular defect and provide fixation options at the Os ilium, the Os pubis, and the Os ischium. However, these components were initially designed for the posterior approach, and the approach has to be relatively extensile to position all three flanges correctly. Consequently, results for these acetabular implants are highly variable [10].

At the study institution, high-grade acetabular bone defects are treated with different types of "off the shelf" acetabular reconstruction systems via the anterior but mainly the lateral or anterolateral approach. One of these systems relies on the combination of extra- and intramedullary iliac fixation using an iliac flange and an optional intramedullary press-fit stem and has proven good results in various studies [4,5]. However, there are defect situations in which "off the shelf implants" do not seem to be appropriate, for instance, in cases with significant loss of supportive bone from the anterior or posterior acetabular rim maybe with additional resorption of the dome. For these patients, a custom made monoflanged acetabular component (CMAC) seems warranted. The iliac flange is fixed to the gluteal surface of the ilium and can be positioned via the standard anterior or lateral approaches. The implant can be armed with an intramedullary press-fit stem for additional fixation.

In the following, we report on the patients who have been treated with this implant for reconstruction of the acetabulum after complicated rTHA.

2. Methods

2.1. Patient Selection

Approval for this retrospective study was given by the institution's review board (Reference number 2016072801). We retrospectively identified 18 cases that underwent acetabular reconstruction with CMACs between January 2010 and December 2019 at our department. Three cases were excluded since the indication for CMAC was malignancy, and one patient died during CMAC implantation.

2.2. Implant

The CMAC is designed using data obtained via high-resolution CT imaging of the pelvis with an implant-specific algorithm (WinCad, Fa. AQ Solutions). Scans can be performed with or without a prosthesis or spacer in place. Figure 1 illustrates crucial templating steps that can be modified by the surgeon. After design approval by the surgeon, the implant is produced by laser melting of a titanium alloy (TiAl6V4) in a monoblock fashion with a 3D comb surface structure and with optional HA or CAP layering. The variability in form is reflected by Figures 1, 3 and 4. Manufacturing and delivering takes about 6 to 8 weeks.

2.3. Parameters Assessed

All presented data were extracted from the electronic patient charts. Preoperative acetabular defect situation was classified according to the modified Paprosky classification system based on preoperative radiographs and CT scans as described previously [11]. Post-operative radiographs were evaluated for reconstruction of the hip joint's COR according to Rannawat [12]. Leg length discrepancy (LLD) was assessed by comparing the position of the trochanter minores to the connection line between Kohler's teardrops.

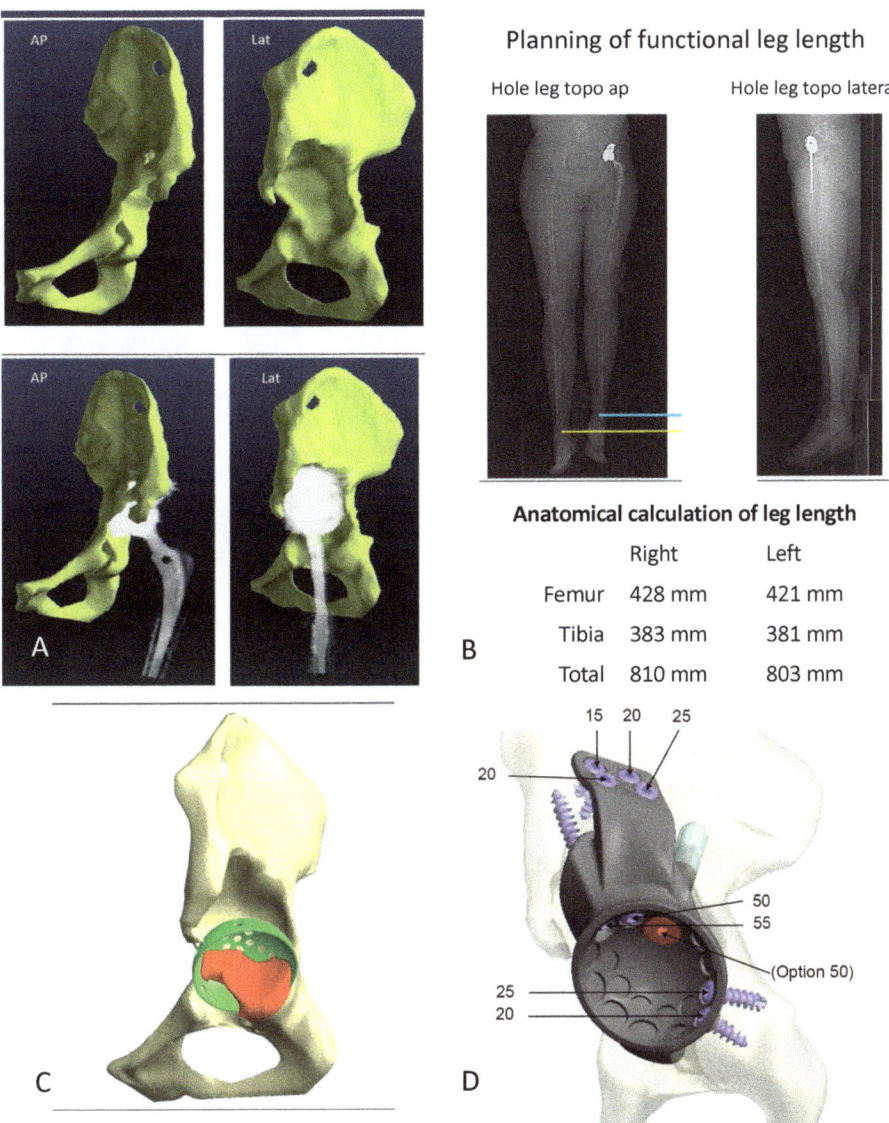

Figure 1. Selected templating steps for a custom made monoflanged acetabular component (CMAC) with optional stem for intra- and extramedullary iliac fixation for a Paprosky IIIA defect: (**A**) Assessment and 3D visualization of the defect situation with and without subtraction of the implant. (**B**) CT-based estimation of leg length discrepancy (LLD) respecting pelvic tilt and joint contractures. (**C**) Virtual reconstruction of the hip center of rotation (COR) by positioning a standard acetabular component of a specific size at the anatomical COR. Bone that has to be reamed to position the original implant is colored in red. (**D**) Design features of the CMAC: The large segmental iliac defect is filled by the implant's metallic monoblock assembled socket. Screws are positioned in areas of the pelvis that are characterized by intact host bone with a recommendation for their length in millimeters. For further primary stability, the surgeon can implant an additional intramedullary press-fit stem (entrance point colored in red). Planning and defect classification have previously been described in detail by our group (11).

Perioperative complications were defined as complication within 3 months after CMAC implantation and were tabulated as documented in the electronic patient chart. Implant revision after CMAC implantation was considered a failure. Failures were excluded from functional follow-up. Functional outcome was assessed using the Western Ontario and McMaster Universities Arthritis Index (WOMAC) Score that was recorded prospectively before and one year after CMAC implantation. Latest ap pelvic radiographs were examined for signs of implant loosening. Therefore, radiolucency lines thicker than 2 mm with sclerotic demarcation were considered significant [13]. Since the Charnley and DeLee zones are not applicable, 4 zones around the implant were defined: the cup, the metal socket, the iliac stem, and the iliac flange.

2.4. Patients

The cohort consisted of 14 patients, 5 men and 9 women. The operations were performed by hip and knee arthroplasty surgeons with additional specialization in revision cases. The operating surgeon indicated treatment with CMAC. Major decision criterion was bone loss at the ilium that did not enable adequate hip COR reconstruction with "off the shelf" cup and cage constructs or asymmetrical cups with intra- or extramedullary fixation. The mean age was 69.5 years (55–83), and the mean body mass index (BMI) was 28.0 kg/m^2 (24.5–30.9), respectively. A total of 11 patients were classified as ASA III, and 3 patients as ASA II. Seven patients had no previous rTHA, the other 7 patients underwent 3 or more previous revisions. Indications for CMACs were spacer implantation after infection in 4 and aseptic loosening in 10 patients.

2.5. Statistics

Parameters are shown as mean and range. A Kaplan–Meier analysis for revision-free survival was performed. The Wilcoxon test was used to test paired samples for significance. A p-value <0.05 was assumed significant. Statistics were conducted with SPSS.

3. Results

Characterization of treated acetabular defects and treatment strategy is shown in Table 1. No additional osteosynthesis at the pelvis was performed during CMAC implantation.

Table 1. Classification of acetabular defects with treatment strategy and failures (number = N; pelvic discontinuity = PD).

Paprosky Classification with and without PD	N	Iliac Stem N	Failure N (Mode)
IIIa	2	0	1 (infection)
IIIa with PD	5	5	1 (aseptic)
IIIB	5	5	0
IIIB with PD	2	2	2 (one each)
total	14	12	4

3.1. Intraoperative Parameters

All patients were operated in supine position. A transgluteal Bauer approach was used in all but two patients, for which an anterolateral approach was more suitable. A semiconstrained liner was cemented into the acetabular construct in all but two patients who received a standard liner. Five patients underwent complete THA removal and spacer implantation before proceeding to CMAC implantation. The mean operation time for the seven patients with additional femoral stem exchange was 181 min (107–249). The mean operation time for the seven patients with only acetabular component exchange was 175 min (93–243). Postoperative weight bearing was restricted for 6 weeks in 11 patients and for 12 weeks in the remaining 3.

3.2. Perioperative Complications

One patient suffered from postoperative dislocation, which was managed with closed reduction. Another patient had a superficial wound infection that was managed with debridement. We did not observe perioperative fracture, nerve injury, or deep vein thrombosis.

3.3. Failures

The mean follow-up was 35.4 months (14–94). We observed two acute septic failures (14.3%) at 10 and 35 months after CMAC implantation, which were treated with debridement, antibiotic therapy, irrigation, and implant retention. However, moving parts were exchanged in these two cases. Further, we observed two aseptic CMAC loosenings (14.3%). One patient was converted to a jumbo head after 14 months, and the other revised and the acetabular component replaced with a modular revision system 20 months after CMAC implantation. Figure 2 depicts the cumulative revision-free survival.

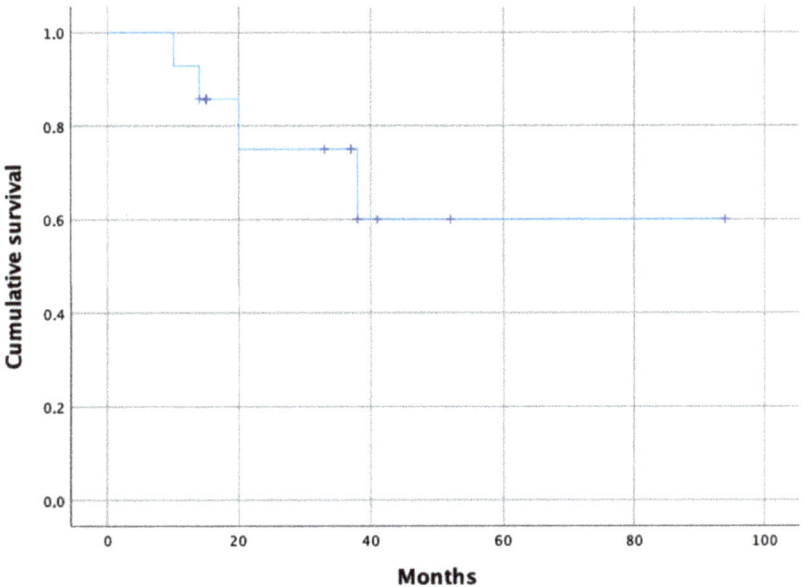

Figure 2. Kaplan–Meyer estimate of revision free-survival.

3.4. Function

Table 2 shows significant improvement of the WOMAC score and its subgroups pain and physical function in patients without failure one year after CMAC implantation. One patient did not complete the WOMAC questionnaires completely.

Table 2. Patient-reported function assessment with the Western Ontario and McMaster Universities Arthritis Index (WOMAC) score (number = N); * only complete pairs were included.

	Preoperative (N)	1 Year Postoperative (N)	p *
pain	51.00 (10–92) (10)	21.27 (10–70) (11)	0.038
stiffness	53.50 (10–100) (10)	28.18 (10–60) (11)	0.068
physical function	72.30 (30–94) (10)	32.36 (1–85) (10)	0.007
all	63.89 (27–82) (10)	29.45 (11–78) (11)	0.015

3.5. Radiographic Evaluation

Results of radiographic evaluation are shown in Table 3. Two patients were planned with intentional extra-anatomic reconstruction of COR as depicted in Figures 3 and 4.

Table 3. Radiographic evaluation.

	Mean (Min to Max)
Leg Length Discrepancy in mm	+3 (−8 to 20)
Lateralization of COR in mm	+8 (−8 to 35)
Proximalization of COR in mm	+6 (−13 to 26)

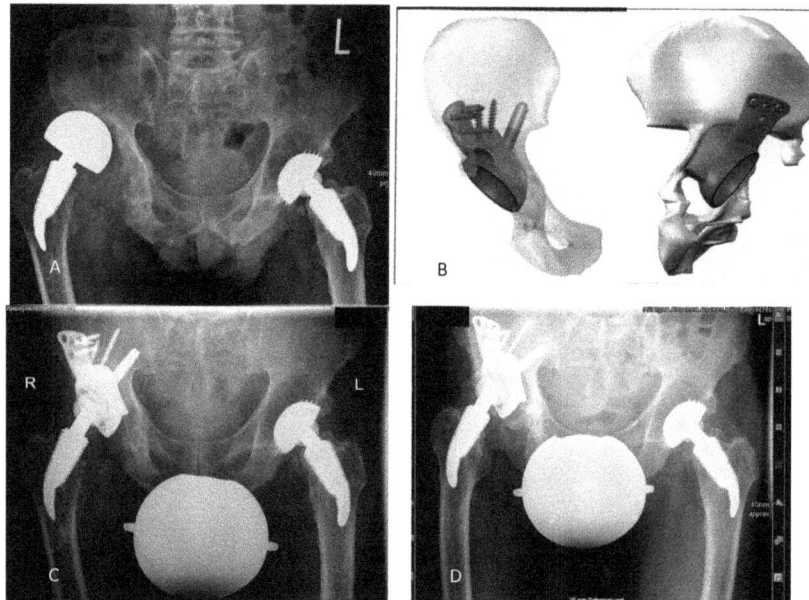

Figure 3. Radiolucency lines without need for revision: (**A**) Preoperative radiographic situation showed the acetabular "up-and-out" defect after implantation of a large head because of acetabular bone loss. (**B**) Anterior to posterior (left) and posterior to anterior (right) views show the intended proximalization of the COR in the virtual 3D reconstruction. The cup is not placed at the level of the Kohler's tear drop. (**C**) Radiograph after revision and CMAC implantation showed restoration of leg length with a high COR. (**D**) Significant radiolucency lines developed around the whole implant at 3 years of follow-up. Although implant migration cannot be excluded, the patient was not revised because he reported daily walks of up to 10 km supported by a cane. Thus, this case was not considered a failure.

For the 10 patients without failure, significant radiolucency lines were found around the socket for one patient, around the acetabular construct for another patient, and around the whole CMAC for the last (Figure 3):

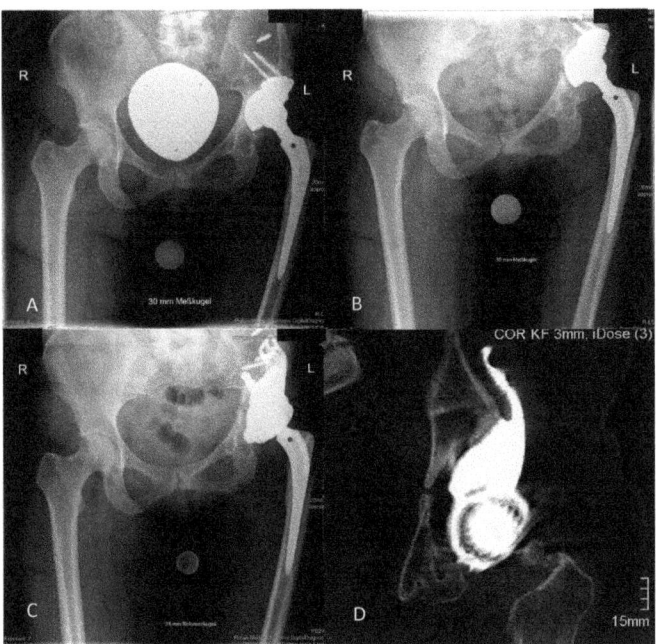

Figure 4. Osteointegration of the socket at follow-up. (**A**) Preoperative situation demonstrated an "up and out" defect that was filled by the loosened cup and augment construct. (**B**) The radiographic control after 2 years displayed PD with complete disruption of the ilio-ischial line and medial protrusion of the cup. (**C**) Radiographic situation 2 years after revision showed no sign of loosening. (**D**) In the CT, spot welds, as sign of osteointegration at the HA-coated socket, were seen.

4. Discussion

Acetabular bone loss remains a major surgical challenge in complicated rTHA. With the presented CMAC we found acceptable results with significant improvement of function one year after implantation and an implant revision rate of 28.6% at a mean follow-up of 35.4 months.

The reported outcome is certainly influenced by patient-related presuppositions for acetabular reconstruction, which are anteceding or even subliminal infection and massive bone loss. In the current study, all patients had at least a Paprosky type III acetabular defect and 42.86% of patients even displayed PD. The optimal surgical strategy for those patients has not yet been defined. A stable pelvic ring is discussed as the "conditio sine qua non" for prevention of mechanical failure of acetabular constructs [7]. Antiprotrusion cages and CTACS as well as cup cage constructs aim to fulfill this strategy [14]. In contrast, the presented implant design abandons this strategy and relies on a combination of intra- and extramedullary iliac fixation for primary stability. However, positioning of the stem can be challenging. In two cases with a IIIa defect but with sufficient medial abutment by the remaining bone, the stems were dispensed. Implant loosening was not observed in these cases. However, whenever possible the iliac stem should by applied for optimal fixation. A rigid fixation of the CMAC to the Os ilium allows osteointegration as depicted in postoperative CT scans (Figure 4).

Irrespectively of the fixation strategy, component fixation seems to be rather successful while other complications are frequent. This statement is underlined by the literature and the data presented data here with high complication rates but acceptable acetabular component survival: In the review of CTACs by Chiarlone et al., the acetabular component survival rate ranged from 86.5% to 100%, but the reoperation rate was 24.5% [15]. In the review by De Martino et al., aseptic loosening of CTACs occurred in only 1.7%. However, the complication rate was 29% [10]. CTACs are designed to span the periacetabular gap by fixation to the iliac, the ischial, and the pubic bone. In contrast, Burastero et al. described a modular press-fit implant design with an antiprotrusion collar for patient-specific acetabular reconstruction and observed osteointegration of all implants at follow-up [8]. The acetabular component survival rate in the current study was 85.72%. However, overall complications occurred in 42.86%. This extremely high rate is comparable to the rate reported in the literature. De Martino et al. and Chiarlone et al. reported reoperation and complication rates ranging from 0 to 66.7% [10,15].

To the best of our knowledge, there is only one other study analyzing the outcome of CMACs. Walter et al. investigated and compared the outcomes of different designs of CTACs. With a mean follow-up of 79.8 months for the CTAC group and 43.0 months in the CMAG group, they found no significant difference regarding the implant survival rate, which was 28.6% and 21.6%, respectively [16].

In comparison to the three-point fixation for CTACs, the iliac fixation is advantageous because it requires less preparation at the ischium. Additionally, it can routinely be implanted in supine position, which facilitates leg length evaluation.

There are limitations to this study. Acetabular defects were assessed based on the preoperative templating CTs, instead of radiographs as initially described by Paprosky. This is warranted for the following reasons: First, radiographic evaluation is not feasible if the volume of the indwelling prosthesis covers bony landmarks. Second, PD does not always match the Paprosky classification [7] and finally, radiographic evaluation has demonstrated high inter- and intraobserver variability and tends to underestimate the acetabular defect situation [11,17]. However, it remains the most popular classification system for acetabular bone loss.

The mean follow-up reflects only the short-term outcome, and the number of patients is limited. Because this study focused on CMACs as revision implants, three patients were excluded due to malignancy. Although the revision burden is increasing, patients that do not meet the criteria for the treatment with an "off the shelf" acetabular revision system are still rare. This limitation is reflected by the overall small number of only 579 and 627 patients in the aforementioned reviews [10,15]. To the best of our knowledge, the current study reports the largest cohort study of patients treated for acetabular bone loss after rTHA failure with one special CMAC design.

Due to the retrospective design of this study, we cannot directly compare the results to those of CTACs. In our hands, the advantages of monoflange fixation are so convincing that we prefer it over the use of CTACs. However, we do observe a trend to highly porous cup-cage constructs with optional wedges and buttress augments. This is mainly based on the instant availability and intraoperative flexibility. However, the surgical strategy used and its success is still highly dependent on the surgeon's skills and his/her experience with a particular implant. CMACs should be considered in cases with a high-grade acetabular defect situation, in which particularly cranial or caudal acetabular bone loss endangers successful reconstruction.

5. Conclusions

CMACs can be considered an option for the treatment of acetabular bone loss in rTHA. Preoperative CT-based 3D planning yields reproducible results for leg length and hip COR. The limited available data show that iliac intra- and extramedullary fixation allows soft tissue-adjusted hip joint reconstruction and improves hip function. However, failure rates are high with periprosthetic infection being the main threat to successful outcome.

Author Contributions: All authors contributed to the study conception and design. Material preparation, data collection, and analysis were performed by M.W., S.P.v.H.-B. and J.A. The first draft of the manuscript was written by S.P.v.H.-B. and all authors commented on previous versions of the manuscript. All authors have read and agreed to the published version of the manuscript.

Funding: This publication was supported by the Open Access Publication Fund of the University of Wuerzburg.

Institutional Review Board Statement: Approval for this retrospective study was given by the institution's review board (Reference number 2016072801).

Informed Consent Statement: Not applicable.

Data Availability Statement: The datasets used and/or analyzed during the current study are available from the corresponding author on reasonable request.

Conflicts of Interest: The authors declare that they have no known competing financial interest or personal relationships that could have appeared to influence the work reported in this paper.

References

1. Bozic, K.J.; Kamath, A.F.; Ong, K.; Lau, E.; Kurtz, S.; Chan, V.; Vail, T.P.; Rubash, H.; Berry, D.J. Comparative Epidemiology of Revision Arthroplasty: Failed THA Poses Greater Clinical and Economic Burdens Than Failed TKA. *Clin. Orthop. Relat. Res.* **2015**, *473*, 2131–2138. [CrossRef] [PubMed]
2. Makita, H.; Kerboull, M.; Inaba, Y.; Tezuka, T.; Saito, T.; Kerboull, L. Revision Total Hip Arthroplasty Using the Kerboull Acetabular Reinforcement Device and Structural Allograft for Severe Defects of the Acetabulum. *J. Arthroplast.* **2017**, *32*, 3502–3509. [CrossRef]
3. Hoberg, M.; Holzapfel, B.M.; Steinert, A.F.; Kratzer, F.; Walcher, M.; Rudert, M. Treatment of acetabular bone defects in revision hip arthroplasty using the Revisio-System. *Orthopade* **2017**, *46*, 126–132. [CrossRef]
4. Prodinger, P.M.; Lazic, I.; Horas, K.; Burgkart, R.; von Eisenhart-Rothe, R.; Weissenberger, M.; Rudert, M.; Holzapfel, B.M. Revision Arthroplasty Through the Direct Anterior Approach Using an Asymmetric Acetabular Component. *J. Clin. Med.* **2020**, *9*, 3031. [CrossRef] [PubMed]
5. Rudert, M.; Holzapfel, B.M.; Kratzer, F.; Gradinger, R. Standardized reconstruction of acetabular bone defects using the cranial socket system. *Oper. Orthop. Traumatol.* **2010**, *22*, 241–255. [CrossRef]
6. Wassilew, G.I.; Janz, V.; Perka, C.; Muller, M. Treatment of acetabular defects with the trabecular metal revision system. *Orthopade* **2017**, *46*, 148–157. [CrossRef]
7. Frenzel, S.; Horas, K.; Rak, D.; Boelch, S.P.; Rudert, M.; Holzapfel, B.M. Acetabular Revision With Intramedullary and Extramedullary Iliac Fixation for Pelvic Discontinuity. *J. Arthroplast.* **2020**. [CrossRef]
8. Burastero, G.; Cavagnaro, L.; Chiarlone, F.; Zanirato, A.; Mosconi, L.; Felli, L.; de Lorenzo, F.D.R. Clinical study of outcomes after revision surgery using porous titanium custom-made implants for severe acetabular septic bone defects. *Int. Orthop.* **2020**, *44*, 1957–1964. [CrossRef]
9. Von Lewinski, G. Custom-made acetabular implants in revision total hip arthroplasty. *Orthopade* **2020**, *49*, 417–423. [CrossRef] [PubMed]
10. De Martino, I.; Strigelli, V.; Cacciola, G.; Gu, A.; Bostrom, M.P.; Sculco, P.K. Survivorship and Clinical Outcomes of Custom Triflange Acetabular Components in Revision Total Hip Arthroplasty: A Systematic Review. *J. Arthroplast.* **2019**, *34*, 2511–2518. [CrossRef]
11. Horas, K.; Arnholdt, J.; Steinert, A.F.; Hoberg, M.; Rudert, M.; Holzapfel, B.M. Acetabular defect classification in times of 3D imaging and patient-specific treatment protocols. *Orthopade* **2017**, *46*, 168–178. [CrossRef]
12. Schofer, M.D.; Pressel, T.; Heyse, T.J.; Schmitt, J.; Boudriot, U. Radiological determination of the anatomic hip centre from pelvic landmarks. *Acta Orthop. Belg.* **2010**, *76*, 479–485. [PubMed]
13. Abrahams, J.M.; Kim, Y.S.; Callary, S.A.; De Ieso, C.; Costi, K.; Howie, D.W.; Solomon, L.B. The diagnostic performance of radiographic criteria to detect aseptic acetabular component loosening after revision total hip arthroplasty. *Bone Jt. J.* **2017**, *99*, 458–464. [CrossRef] [PubMed]
14. Martin, J.R.; Barrett, I.; Sierra, R.J.; Lewallen, D.G.; Berry, D.J. Construct Rigidity: Keystone for Treating Pelvic Discontinuity. *J. Bone Jt. Surg. Am.* **2017**, *99*, e43. [CrossRef] [PubMed]
15. Chiarlone, F.; Zanirato, A.; Cavagnaro, L.; Alessio-Mazzola, M.; Felli, L.; Burastero, G. Acetabular custom-made implants for severe acetabular bone defect in revision total hip arthroplasty: A systematic review of the literature. *Arch. Orthop. Trauma Surg.* **2020**, *140*, 415–424. [CrossRef] [PubMed]
16. Walter, S.G.; Randau, T.M.; Gravius, N.; Gravius, S.; Froschen, F.S. Monoflanged Custom-Made Acetabular Components Promote Biomechanical Restoration of Severe Acetabular Bone Defects by Metallic Defect Reconstruction. *J. Arthroplast.* **2020**, *35*, 831–835. [CrossRef] [PubMed]
17. Telleria, J.J.; Gee, A.O. Classifications in brief: Paprosky classification of acetabular bone loss. *Clin. Orthop. Relat. Res.* **2013**, *471*, 3725–3730. [CrossRef] [PubMed]

MDPI
St. Alban-Anlage 66
4052 Basel
Switzerland
Tel. +41 61 683 77 34
Fax +41 61 302 89 18
www.mdpi.com

Journal of Personalized Medicine Editorial Office
E-mail: jpm@mdpi.com
www.mdpi.com/journal/jpm

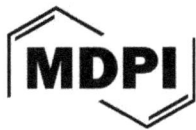

www.ingramcontent.com/pod-product-compliance
Lightning Source LLC
LaVergne TN
LVHW070458100526
838202LV00014B/1746